Functional Anatomy

of the Pelvis *and the* Sacroiliac Joint

A Practical Guide

John Gibbons

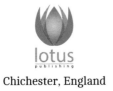
lotus
publishing

Chichester, England

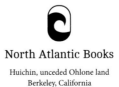
North Atlantic Books

Huichin, unceded Ohlone land
Berkeley, California

First published in 2017 and redesigned in 2021 by
Lotus Publishing
Apple Tree Cottage, Inlands Road, Nutbourne, Chichester, PO18 8RJ, and
North Atlantic Books
Huichin, unceded Ohlone land
Berkeley, California

Drawings Amanda Williams
Photographs Ian Taylor
Cover Design Wendy Craig
Text Design Medlar Publishing Solutions Pvt Ltd., India
Printed and Bound Kultur Sanat Printing House, Turkey

Functional Anatomy of the Pelvis and the Sacroiliac Joint: A Practical Guide is sponsored and published by North Atlantic Books, an educational non-profit based on the unceded Ohlone land Huichin (Berkeley, CA), that collaborates with partners to develop cross-cultural perspectives, nurture holistic views of art, science, the humanities, and healing, and seed personal and global transformation by publishing work on the relationship of body, spirit, and nature.

North Atlantic Books' publications are distributed to the US trade and internationally by Penguin Random House Publishers Services. For further information, visit our website at www.northatlanticbooks.com.

Medical Disclaimer
The following information is intended for general information purposes only. Individuals should always consult their health care provider before administering any suggestions made in this book. Any application of the material set forth in the following pages is at the reader's discretion and is his or her sole responsibility.

British Library Cataloging-in-Publication Data
A CIP record for this book is available from the British Library
ISBN 978 1 905367 66 5 (Lotus Publishing)
ISBN 978 1 62317 102 5 (North Atlantic Books)

Library of Congress Cataloging-in-Publication Data
Names: Gibbons, John, 1968- author.
Title: Functional anatomy of the pelvis and the sacroiliac joint : a
    practical guide / John Gibbons.
Description: Berkeley, California : North Atlantic Books ; Nutbourne,
    Chichester : Lotus Publishing, 2017. | Includes bibliographical references
    and index. | Description based on print version record and CIP data
    provided by publisher; resource not viewed.
Identifiers: LCCN 2016020570 (print) | LCCN 2016019896 (ebook) |
ISBN 9781623171032 (ebook) | ISBN 9781623171025 (pbk.)
Subjects: | MESH: Pelvis—anatomy & histology | Sacroiliac Joint—anatomy & histology |
    Movement—physiology
Classification: LCC QM115 (print) | LCC QM115 (ebook) | NLM WE 760 | DDC
611/.96—dc23
LC record available at https://lccn.loc.gov/2016020570

Contents

Preface

I first realized that there were many areas of the body that still needed more attention when I was trying to consolidate the text for the last chapter of my first book, on muscle energy techniques (METs), which focused specifically on potential muscle weaknesses mainly caused by shortened and tight antagonistic muscles. In particular, I wrote about the effects (possible weakness/inhibition) of the shortened antagonistic muscles of the hip flexors on the gluteal musculature. This last chapter of the MET book inspired me so much to pursue this avenue that I decided to write an entire text on the glutes. Then, while I was writing the book on the glutes, I found that the region of the pelvic girdle and sacroiliac joint (SIJ) kept on cropping up in one way or another in most of the chapters, and so I thought it would be a marvelous idea (at the time of course!) to devote a whole book to the pelvis and SIJ.

So, after many months of contemplation and internal debate, I started writing this book in July 2014, as the initial thought of writing my fourth book had taken me a while to get my head around. Because my book on the glutes had demanded such a vast amount of my time and effort, I wasn't sure if I actually wanted to carry on writing. However, that particular week in July

when *Vital Glutes* went to the printers was a huge stepping stone for me. I could finally focus all my attention on writing a new book, this time on what I felt was one of the most neglected areas of the body—the pelvic girdle and in particular the SIJ.

Having taught courses on the specific areas of the pelvic girdle and lower back for many years, I have always wanted to write a book on the SIJ. The course notes each year seem to get thicker and thicker, because of the increasing amount of material. I thought to myself: now is the perfect time in my life to continue writing, and it would also make perfect sense to put pen to paper and write an entire book about this specialized and fascinating area of the body. I would love to think that, in time, this particular book will be used as a core textbook by physical therapy students and potentially serve as their main reference guide.

Another reason for writing this book was because of what I remember a good friend of mine once saying to me, while he was at university studying for a physiotherapy degree. He told me that on one occasion during the first semester, as he was being taught all the different aspects of the specific area relating to the hip joint, the tutor of the course announced that in the following semester the focus would be on the lumbar spine. My friend casually said to the tutor: "What about the bit in the *middle*?" (He was referring to the pelvis and the SIJ.) The tutor replied: "That bit in the middle doesn't move, so don't worry about it"!

I am pleased to say that things have moved on over the last few years, and we now know that the fascinating joints that make up the pelvic girdle do actually have some movement.

People who have come to know me over the last few years, either through attending my courses or as patients or athletes attending the clinic, will know that I am a qualified osteopath. I can honestly say with hand on heart that these individuals naturally presume that all osteopaths spend many years studying the pelvic girdle and SIJ as well as the lumbar spine, and so on. Many patients who present to the osteopathic and chiropractic clinic typically have lower back, neck, or pelvic pain. I have taught a multitude of osteopaths and chiropractors over the years, and all of them seem to have encountered different training methodologies, especially when it comes to their core knowledge base and understanding of the pelvic girdle, and this appears to reflect the specific institute of training they attended.

The reason I refer to osteopaths in particular, and the way they are perceived in terms of their knowledge, is because I want to mention something that shocked and disappointed me. I can recall a time where I was lecturing a four-day intensive course at my venue at the University of Oxford; the course in question was the Advanced Therapy Master-Class. This particular course is designed to deal specifically with the areas of the pelvis and SIJ. As well as many sports therapists and physiotherapists, there were four recently qualified osteopaths attending the course. As the course gradually progressed over the four days they all mentioned to me (individually) that the specific assessment and treatment techniques I was showing them for the area of the pelvis, SIJ, and hip, and even the lumbar spine, were new to them and that they had not been taught those specific assessment and treatment techniques during their own five-year intensive training courses. These four osteopaths were from two different training establishments; I could have understood it if they had been from a single training center, but to have all of them not being taught what I would call basic palpatory, assessment, and treatment techniques not only surprised me but actually disappointed me as well. I am pleased to say that by the end of the course those osteopaths, as well as the other therapists attending the course, had a far better understanding of how to assess and treat athletes and patients presenting with specific lower back and pelvic pain at their own clinics.

Hopefully, this text will answer some (though maybe not all) of the questions you have been asking yourself with regard to your own athletes and patients, or it might even help you gain a better understanding during your own studies of the pelvis and SIJ. You may be reading this text not as a physical therapist, but as someone who actually has pain in the area of the lower back or pelvis, and you may be trying to better understand why that might be and, more importantly, what you can do about it. Whichever of these applies to you, I sincerely hope that you find what you need in this book.

Acknowledgments

The first person I would like to thank is Jon Hutchings of Lotus Publishing. Once again I sincerely thank you for having the confidence in me to continue with the dream of writing, as without you all of my books, including this one, would not have been written and subsequently published. Thanks again, Jon, for having the faith in me to come up with the goods (so to speak). My thanks also to Ian Taylor, who spent a vast amount of time and effort taking and editing the photographs for this book, and to the copy-editor, Steve Brierley, without whose patience and input this book would definitely not read as well as it does!

I would like to include here my recognition of the outstanding work of four particular pioneers in this field of manual therapy—Andry Vleeming, Diane Lee, Philip Greenman, and Wolf Schamberger. Without the dedication and participation of these individual role models this book would not have been written, and for that I truly thank you all.

I am especially grateful to the musculoskeletal physiotherapist Gordon Bosworth, the person who guided me through my initial osteopathy training. Although I acknowledged him in my previous book, I have to include him here too, because the actual fine-tuning with regard to my assessment and treatment skills in the area of the pelvic girdle and SIJ is all down to Gordon. He made my learning and understanding of this fascinating but complex area a pleasure, and for that I thank him with all my heart. I do consider him to be one of the best physical therapists—if not *the* best—I have ever met. He was (and still is) an inspiration to me in becoming the person I am today—so thanks a million, Gordon, for all that effort. I hope mentoring me was as rewarding for you as it was for me!

For their inspiration and moral support during the creation of this book, I must thank my sister, Amanda Williams, her husband, Philip Williams, and their children, James and Victoria; and my mother, Margaret Gibbons. It gives me great pleasure to include this brief tribute to these much-loved people in my book. My only regret is that my father, John Andrew Gibbons, is not here to see or read my books. I am sure, however, that he is looking down on us all with a smile on his face.

Since the passing of my son, I have begun to realize my purpose in life, and that is to educate as many therapists throughout the world as I can, to try to help them achieve great things in their lives. I hope to do that through my lectures and books. I therefore personally want to thank you, the readers, as without your continual support I definitely would not be able to do what I do.

I always seem to acknowledge a person who has been in my life the longest (apart from family) at the end of this section. Maybe that's just the way it is—you mention one of the most important people in your life at the end. That person is Denise Thomas; we have been together many years at the time of writing of this book and I must say I have had the most amazing time with her. Thanks for being the model in the photographs, and thanks a million for all your support.

John Gibbons

Dedication

*To my amazing son Thomas Rhys Gibbons, who sadly left my world
at 10.51 pm on the 28 February 2017, at the age of 17 years and 17 days.
Rest in peace my little Tom-Tom – you will be truly missed.
We will meet again and that's for sure, but not yet as I have too much
to achieve with my life first and sadly you have made me realize that!*

Abbreviations

AAJ	atlantoaxial joint		**Gmax**	gluteus maximus
AHC	anterior horn cell		**Gmed**	gluteus medius
AIIS	anterior inferior iliac spine		**Gmin**	gluteus minimus
ASIS	anterior superior iliac spine		**GTO**	golgi tendon organ
ASLR	active straight leg raise		**HVT**	high-velocity thrust
COG	center of gravity		**ILA**	inferior lateral angle
CT	computerized tomography		**ITB**	iliotibial band
DDD	degenerative disc disease		**LLD**	leg length discrepancy
DLS	deep longitudinal sling		**L-on-L**	left-on-left
ERS	extension, rotation, side bending		**L-on-R**	left-on-right
FABER	flexion, abduction, external rotation		**MET**	muscle energy technique
FAI	femoroacetabular impingement		**MR**	magnetic resonance
FAIR	flexion, adduction, internal rotation		**MRI**	magnetic resonance imaging
FRS	flexion, rotation, side bending		**MTA**	middle transverse axis

NR	neutral, rotation	**R-on-L**	right-on-left
OAJ	occipitoatlantal joint	**R-on-R**	right-on-right
PGP	pelvic girdle pain	**SCM**	sternocleidomastoid
PHC	posterior horn cell	**SIJ**	sacroiliac joint
PIIS	posterior inferior iliac spine	**SPD**	symphysis pubis dysfunction
PIR	post-isometric relaxation	**SPJ**	symphysis pubis joint
PLS	posterior longitudinal sling	**STJ**	subtalar joint
PSIS	posterior superior iliac spine	**TFL**	tensor fasciae latae
QL	quadratus lumborum	**TMJ**	temporomandibular joint
RI	reciprocal inhibition	**TP**	transverse process
ROM	range of motion	**TVA**	transversus abdominis

Anatomy of the Pelvis and the Sacroiliac Joint

The pelvic girdle is composed of the sacrum, the coccyx, and the three so-called "hipbones"—the ilium, ischium, and pubis. The bones of the adult pelvis join together to form four joints: the left and right sacroiliac joints (SIJs), the sacrococcygeal joint, and the symphysis pubis joint (SPJ), as shown in Figure 1.1.

At birth the ilium, ischium, and pubis bones are separated by hyaline cartilage; by the end of puberty these bones will have naturally conjoined (fused together), with complete ossification normally occurring by the time a person has reached the age of approximately 20–25. The three bones, once fusion has taken place, are collectively called the *innominate bone*, or simply the *innominate*. On the lateral side of the innominate bone is the acetabulum; this area forms the articulation with the head of the femur to create the iliofemoral (hip) joint (see Figure 1.2).

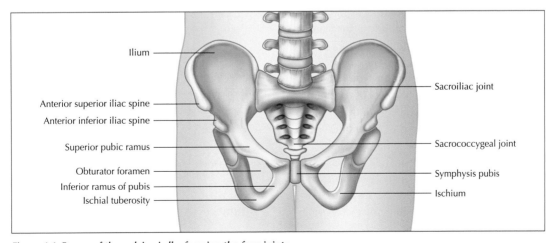

Figure 1.1. Bones of the pelvic girdle, forming the four joints.

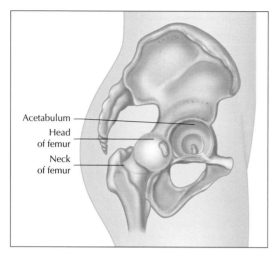

Figure 1.2. Iliofemoral (hip) joint.

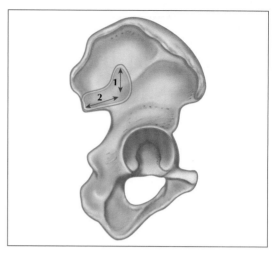

Figure 1.3. L shape of the short (vertical [1]) and long (horizontal [2]) arms of the ilium.

Innominate Bones

Ilium

The ilium is fan shaped and is the most superior as well as the largest of the three hipbones; it makes up approximately two-fifths of the deep, cuplike socket of the hip joint, called the *acetabulum*. The body of the ilium together with the sacrum forms the SIJ. This L-shaped articulation is located on the posterior superior aspect of the ilium and has a vertically (vertical plane) orientated "short arm" and a more horizontally (anteroposterior plane) positioned "long arm" (Figure 1.3).

If you place one hand on your hip, you can feel the curved ridge of the superior aspect of the ilium: this is known as the *iliac crest*. From this crest, if you lightly move your fingers down inferior to the anterior aspect of the ilium, you should feel a bony projection known as the *anterior superior iliac spine (ASIS)*; this area allows the attachment of soft tissues (e.g. the sartorius muscle). If you continue slightly inferior to the ASIS, you will come to another bony landmark called the *anterior inferior iliac spine (AIIS)*; this is where one part of the rectus femoris muscle attaches. Palpating the posterior aspect of the ilium as it curves inferiorly, you will feel the

bony prominence of the *posterior superior iliac spine (PSIS)*; again this is an attachment for soft tissues. These two bony projections (ASIS and PSIS) are commonly used as palpatory landmarks when one is assessing the position of the pelvic girdle (Figure 1.4).

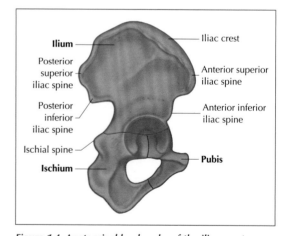

Figure 1.4. Anatomical landmarks of the iliac crest.

Ischium

The ischium is narrower than the ilium bone and is located inferior to the ilium and behind the pubis. The ischium has an easily palpable landmark called the *ischial tuberosity* (Figure 1.5); it is commonly

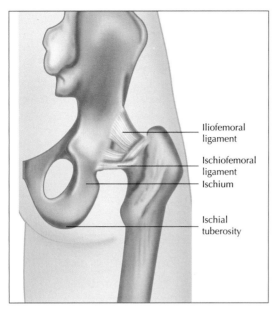

Figure 1.5. Ischium and ischial tuberosity.

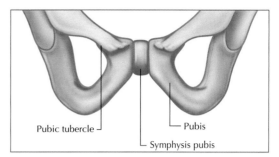

Figure 1.6. Pubis, pubic tubercle and SPJ.

called the *sit bone* and provides the necessary landmark for the attachment of the hamstrings. It is this part of the ischium (tuberosity), along with the coccyx, on which you rest your body weight while adopting a sitting position. The ischium is the strongest of the three bones and forms approximately two-fifths of the acetabulum (hip socket).

Pubis

The pubis, or pubic bone, is the most anterior as well as the smallest of all the three hipbones and makes up approximately one-fifth of the acetabulum. The body of the pubis is wide, strong, and flat, and together with the opposite pubic bone makes up the SPJ. This joint is classified as an *amphiarthrosis*, as it is connected centrally by a broad piece of fibrocartilage (Figure 1.6). On the superior aspect of the pubis there is a bony projection called the *pubic tubercle*; this structure allows the attachment of the inguinal ligament and is also used as a palpatory landmark when one is assessing the position of the pelvic girdle.

Sacrum

The sacrum (sacred bone) is a large triangular bone located at the base of the lumbar spine and forms the back part of the pelvic cavity. The sacrum starts out from birth as five individual bones before starting to fuse between the ages of 16 and 18; the sacrum is considered to have fully fused into a single bone by the time you have reached 34 years of age.

Considerable differences in the shape of the sacrum between individuals, as well as structural differences between the left and right sides, are well documented. The connection of the sacrum to the ilium forms the SIJ.

The superior aspect of the sacrum is called the *sacral base* and is primarily made up of the 1st sacral segment; the base is angled in a forward direction to form a concavity. The opposite end of the sacrum is called the *sacral apex* and this is made up of the fifth sacral segment (see Figure 1.7). The natural position of the sacrum is called the *sacral angle* and is generally thought to be in the range 40–44 degrees (see Figure 1.8), although, as discussed by some authors, the angle can be anywhere from 30 to 50 degrees. Moreover, a specific type of motion called *nutation* (a nodding motion, which will be discussed later) can be responsible for an increase in this angle by anywhere between 6 and 8 degrees on standing up (from a sitting position). The sacral angle increases because of the change in the

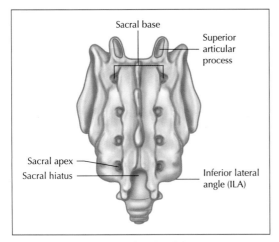

Figure 1.7. Anatomical landmarks of the sacrum (posterior view).

curvature of the lumbar spine, from an initial flexion curvature when sitting, to an extension curvature (lumbar lordosis) when standing, as one performs the motion from a sitting to a standing posture. This sacral movement allows the whole of the spinal column to adopt an upright position.

On the lateral sides of the sacrum located between the levels of the first three sacral vertebrae (S1–S3) are the *alae* (wings): these auricular (earlike) L-shaped areas of the sacrum make up the articulation with the ilium—i.e. the SIJ. In an earlier paragraph regarding the ilium I mentioned that there is a short vertical arm and a long anteroposterior (horizontal) arm (Figure 1.8),

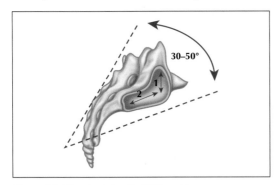

Figure 1.8. The short (vertical [1]) and long (horizontal [2]) arm of the sacrum, and the sacral angle (lateral view).

which will naturally dovetail with each other, like pieces of a jigsaw puzzle.

Another way of looking at the sacrum is as a continuation of the lumbar spine, while the SIJs on either side are mimicking what I generally call *atypical facet joints*. You can think of the sacrum as a single vertebra, and the left and right SIJs as the articulating facet joints, with the superior articular facet being the ilia component and the inferior articular facet being the sacral component (see Figure 1.11).

Coccyx

The coccyx is the continuation and endpoint of the vertebral column and is commonly referred to as the *tailbone*. It has between three and five (normally four) vertebral segments called the *coccygeal vertebrae*, and most textbooks state that these are actually fused; some authors, however, maintain that the coccygeal vertebrae are indeed separate and individual entities (Figure 1.9).

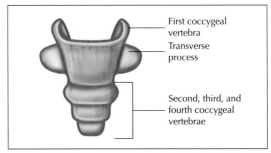

Figure 1.9. Coccyx bone and the individual segments.

There are many muscles with attachments directly on the coccyx: for example, the pelvic floor muscles attach to the anterior surface of the coccyx, and the gluteus maximus (Gmax) muscle and ligaments attach to the posterior surface. Likewise, some ligaments attach directly to the coccyx, such as the sacrococcygeal ligament and some of the fibers of the sacrospinous and sacrotuberous ligaments. The coccyx also plays a role in weight bearing (while sitting), as it forms part of the *tripod* structure, working in conjunction with the left and right ischial tuberosities (sit bones).

Symphysis Pubis Joint

The symphysis pubis joint (SPJ) is classified as a *non-synovial fibrocartilaginous amphiar-throsis*, connecting the left and right pubic bones.

In adults only 0.08" (2mm) of movement (shift) and one degree of rotation are considered to be possible in this joint; however, these values will increase in women during pregnancy and childbirth. The available movement of the SPJ is also influenced by the natural shape of the joint, and by muscular activation from the adductor and abdominal muscles.

The ends of each pubic bone are covered by hyaline cartilage that connects to the piece of fibrocartilage located in the center of the SPJ. The joint has strong superior and inferior ligaments and a thinner posterior ligament (Figure 1.10).

One can think of the design of the symphysis pubis as being similar to the intervertebral discs of the spine, with a central disc of fibrocartilage that cushions against compressive loads, as well as providing shock absorption and contributing to

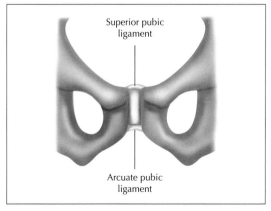

Superior pubic ligament

Arcuate pubic ligament

Figure 1.10. Symphysis pubis joint and associated ligaments.

passive stabilization. Because of this similarity, the articular disc of the SPJ is also vulnerable to both degeneration and trauma, particularly when the joint is subjected to traumatic or repetitive shear forces (e.g. osteitis pubis).

Functionally, the SPJ helps to resist tension, shearing, and compression forces, and remarkably is able to widen during pregnancy. The anatomist Andreas Vesalius, who challenged the Hippocratic belief that the pubic bones separated during childbirth, was the first to recognize this joint in 1543.

Sacroiliac Joint

Lower back pain and the link with the sacroiliac joint (SIJ, or SI joint) date back to the era of Hippocrates (c.460–377 BC); the medical practitioners (obstetricians) at the time felt that under normal conditions the SIJs were immobile. I am very pleased to say that things have progressed enormously over the last few decades with all the information now readily available in respect of the general consensus of the role and function of the pelvic girdle, and in particular of the SIJ. I can guarantee, though, that over time some things will nevertheless change, so this book may well need to be updated in the future.

I have been lecturing courses on the pelvic girdle, and on the SIJ in particular, for many years at my venue based at the University of Oxford, which means I have come into contact with thousands of physical therapists, ranging from osteopaths and physiotherapists to chiropractors and lots of sports therapists, to mention but a few. If I am honest with myself, I personally consider that the area of the pelvis is a relatively difficult subject to try to get across to my students (mainly therapists); this is because I consider the SIJ to be something of a "mystery" to many therapists, and it becomes especially difficult when I am trying to explain the subject matter to my athletes and patients.

The majority of physical therapists attending the course on the pelvic girdle tell me at some point that they see patients and athletes on a daily basis with what they consider to be a presentation of *sacroiliac joint dysfunction*. In the past, patients with presenting SIJ issues have even been referred directly to them by the local GP or a colleague.

Vleeming et al. (2007) say that mobility of the pelvic joints is difficult to measure objectively, especially in the weight bearing position, and that feeling motion at the sacroiliac joint during active and passive motion is difficult to prove.

Bearing in mind the above quote, you can imagine that teaching a specific course on this fascinating

but undoubtedly complex area of the body is not as straightforward as one might think.

Anatomy

The SIJ (Figure 1.11), is located between the sacrum and the ilium and is classified as a *true synovial arthrodial joint*, as it contains a joint capsule, synovial fluid, articular cartilage, and a synovial membrane.

The SIJ is unique: on the ilia side, the cartilage is made up mainly of fibrocartilage, whereas on the sacral side, the cartilage consists of hyaline, or articular, cartilage. The articular (hyaline) cartilage is thicker (0.04–0.12", or 1–3mm) on

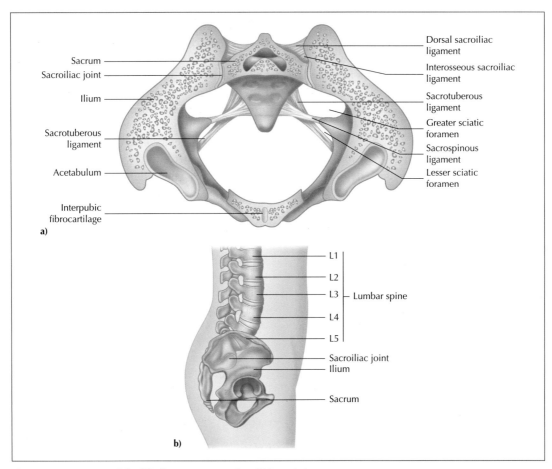

Figure 1.11. Anatomy of the SIJ; a) transverse section; b) lateral view.

the sacral side than on the ilia side. Kampen and Tillman (1998) found that in adults the cartilage on the sacral surface of the joint can reach 0.16" (4mm) in thickness, but does not exceed 0.04–0.08" (1–2mm) on the iliac surface. The lack of thickness of the cartilage on the ilia side might be one of the factors responsible for hardening (sclerosis).

The SIJs have an auricular L-shaped appearance, similar to a kidney, with a short (vertical) upper arm and a longer (horizontal) lower arm (as already mentioned earlier).

Regarding the shape of the SIJ, different characteristics between individuals have been clinically proven; moreover, there can be significant structural differences between the left and right sides of the joint surfaces within the SIJs of the same individual. There is also clear evidence of the fact that the paired SIJs, and even the PSISs, are generally asymmetric in appearance, which can also be the case in patients and athletes who present with no symptoms of pain or dysfunction (i.e. are asymptomatic).

In terms of motion, the pelvis is capable of moving in all three planes of the body: flexion and extension in the sagittal plane (forward and backward bending); lateral flexion (side bending) in the frontal plane; and rotation of the trunk in the transverse plane. It has been debated that the SIJ can move anywhere between 2 and 18 degrees, but more recent evidence provided by many clinicians demonstrates that there are roughly 2–4 degrees of rotation and 0.04–0.08" (1–2mm) of translation. Studies have shown us that movement is possible, but only in very small amounts; this was demonstrated by Egund et al. (1978) and Sturesson et al. (1989, 2000a, 2000b), who found the motion of the SIJ to be at best approximately 2–4 degrees in rotation and 0.08" (2mm) in translation.

We know that when we are developing through the natural aging process, the SIJ characteristics change. In early life the SIJ surfaces are in general initially flat, but as we start to walk and progress through puberty, these surfaces develop distinct ridges and grooves and lose their naturally flattened appearance. These ridges and grooves actually fit into one another to some extent; this will potentially aid the overall stability of the SIJ, while still allowing some degree of movement.

The text *Greenman's Principles of Manual Medicine* (DeStefano 2011) mentions that "during the aging process, there is an increase in the grooves on the opposing surfaces of the sacrum and ilium that appears to reduce available motion and enhance stability." The author also says that "it is of interest to note that the age at which the incidence of disabling back pain is highest (range: 25 to 45 years) is the same age when the greatest amount of motion is available in the sacroiliac joints."

Because of the relationship of the three main pelvic joints (the two sacroiliac and the symphysis pubis), as well as their relationship to the iliofemoral joint (hip joint), a dysfunction existing in any one of these joints can have a direct impact on the other two/three joints.

Ligaments of the SIJ

The SIJ has very strong ligaments, which increase the joint's stability and make potential dislocations very rare.

Stability of the SIJ is provided partly through ligamentous attachments. These specific ligaments will provide joint integrity as well as resistance to shearing-type forces. The ligaments that bind the sacrum directly to the innominate are (see Figure 1.12):

- Sacrotuberous
- Sacrospinous
- Interosseous
- Long dorsal (posterior sacroiliac)

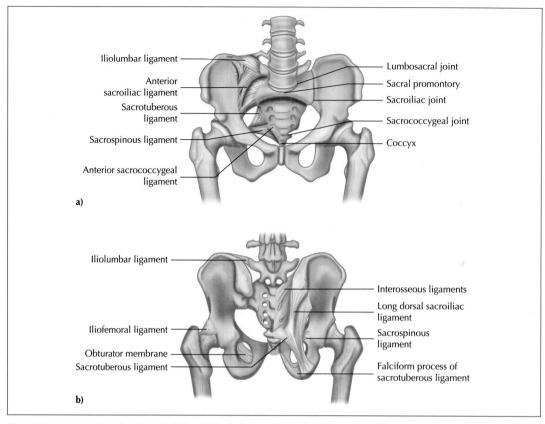

Figure 1.12. Ligaments relating to stability of the SIJ; a) anterior view, b) posterior view.

The iliolumbar ligament will also have a stabilizing influence on the SIJ as well as on the lumbar spine.

Sacrotuberous Ligament

The sacrotuberous ligament attaches from the PSIS and also has an attachment to the posterior sacroiliac ligaments. The ligament then continues and attaches onto the ischial tuberosity and splits into three individual bands: the outer (lateral) side attaches from the PSIS to the ischial tuberosity; the inner (medial) band attaches from the coccyx to the ischial tuberosity; and the superior band connects the PSIS to the coccyx.

Four muscles have an attachment directly to the sacrotuberous ligament and will contribute to the overall stability of the SIJ:

- Biceps femoris
- Gluteus maximus (Gmax)
- Multifidus
- Piriformis

Vleeming et al. (1989a) found that in approximately 50% of subjects the lower border of the sacrotuberous ligament was directly continuous with the tendon of the origin of the long head of biceps femoris; this muscle could therefore act to stabilize the SIJ via the sacrotuberous ligament.

Part of the role of the sacrotuberous ligament is to resist the anterior nodding type of motion of the sacrum known as *nutation*. This ligament will also prevent posterior rotation of the innominate bone with respect to the sacrum. If for some reason there is laxity in the sacrotuberous ligament (along with the sacrospinous ligament), the decreased tension can result in a posterior rotation of the innominate bone, and also lead to increased nutation of the sacrum.

Sacrospinous Ligament

The sacrospinous ligament has an attachment from the lateral aspect of the sacrum and coccyx and attaches to the spine of the ischium, appropriately named the *ischial spine*. The ligament has the appearance of a thin triangle and, together with the sacrotuberous ligament, it modifies the greater sciatic notch in the greater sciatic foramen. In one respect, the function of the sacrospinous ligament is similar to that of the sacrotuberous ligament: it prevents posterior rotation of the innominate bone relative to the sacrum, and also limits nutation (forward motion) of the sacrum relative to the innominate bone.

Interosseous Ligament

The interosseous ligament consists of a dense, short, thick collection of strong collagenous fibers that run in a horizontal plane and connect the sacral tuberosities of the sacrum to the ilium. This ligament lies deep in the narrow recess between the sacrum and the ilium, and has deep and superficial components to it. The main function of the interosseous ligament is to prevent a separation or abduction of the SIJ by strongly binding the sacrum to the ilium, as this will help secure the SIJ interlocking mechanism.

Long Dorsal Ligament (Posterior Sacroiliac Ligament)

The long dorsal ligament attaches from the medial and lateral crests of the sacrum and to the PSIS. There is also a connection of this ligament to the thoracolumbar fascia, as well as to the multifidus and erector spinae muscles.

The long dorsal ligament mainly resists counter-nutation of the sacrum (posterior nutation) as well as anterior rotation of the innominate bone. Consequently, this ligament will naturally slacken when the sacrum is in a state of nutation and/or if there is posterior rotation of the innominate bone.

If sacral torsion is present (discussed in later chapters) and the sacral base is found to be "posterior," this ligament will be under constant tension and may be tender when palpated.

Lee (2004, p. 22) mentions that the skin overlying the long dorsal sacroiliac ligament is a frequent area of pain in patients with lumbosacral and pelvic girdle dysfunction, and that tenderness on palpation of the ligament does not necessarily incriminate this tissue, given the nature of pain referral from both the lumbar spine and the SIJ.

Iliolumbar Ligament

The iliolumbar ligament is a very strong ligamentous structure; it attaches from the transverse processes (TPs) of L4/5 and travels to the inner border of the ilium.

This ligament, which has five individual bands, is one of three vertebrae–pelvis ligaments responsible for stabilizing the lumbosacral spine in the pelvis, along with the two mentioned already, namely the sacrospinous and sacrotuberous. The main function of the iliolumbar ligament is essentially to limit the motion of the lumbosacral junction by stabilizing the connection between the pelvis and the lower lumbar vertebrae (L4 and L5).

Function of the SIJs

The SIJs' primary responsibility is to transfer the weight of the upper body to the lower extremities. The body weight is transferred through the vertebral column to the lumbar spine (L5), to the sacrum and across the SIJs to the ischial tuberosities, and then out to the acetabula of the hip joints. This mechanism of bony attachments demonstrates the SIJs' role as weight-bearing joints (Figure 1.13). The SIJs are also able to transfer

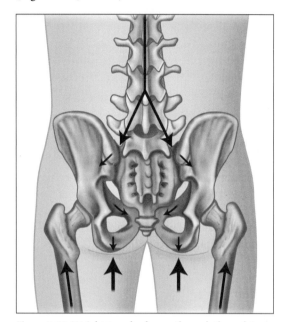

Figure 1.13. Weight transfer forces through the pelvis and the SIJs.

the forces in the opposite direction when one is walking, standing, or sitting: the pressure is directed through the legs to the innominates and the sacrum, and then dissipated upward through the lumbosacral junction.

In their secondary role, the SIJs can be thought of as shock absorbers (mainly at the point of heel contact), as they help cushion the increased stress that is forced upon the lumbar spine and in particular upon the lower lumbar intervertebral discs. Authors in the past have suggested that the incidence of lower lumbar disc disease/degeneration increases when the SIJs present with pathological changes.

Lee and Vleeming (2007) discussed the analysis of gait mechanics and demonstrated that the SIJs provide sufficient flexibility for the intra-pelvic forces to be transferred effectively to and from the lumbar spine and lower extremities.

Motion of the Pelvis and the Sacroiliac Joint

Previous authors have suggested that there are approximately 14 individual types of dysfunction possible within the pelvic girdle complex. This in itself suggests to me that, because there are so many types of potential dysfunction which can be present within the pelvic girdle, there logically have to be just as many types of natural motion available as well.

Pelvis Motion

Put in a relatively simple way, there are three main types of motion available within the pelvic girdle:

- Sacroiliac motion, which comprises the motion of the sacrum on the innominate bone.
- Iliosacral motion, which comprises the motion of the innominate bone on the sacrum.
- Symphysis pubis motion, which typically relates to the motion of the pubic bone on one side with respect to the bone on the other side.

Sacroiliac Motion

Sacroiliac motion is the movement of the sacrum within the innominate bone, and there are two main types: (1) anterior/forward motion, or

nutation (think of this as sacral flexion); and (2) posterior/backward motion, or counter-nutation (think of this as sacral extension). Bilateral movement of the sacrum occurs with forward and backward bending of the trunk; on the other hand, unilateral movement of the sacrum occurs with flexion and extension of the hip joint and lower limbs, such as when we initiate the walking/gait cycle.

Nutation

The word *nutation* actually means "nodding", and this motion of the sacral base (top part of the sacrum) is directed anteriorly and inferiorly, while the sacral apex (bottom part of the sacrum)/coccyx moves posteriorly and superiorly relative to the innominate bone (see Figure 2.1(a)).

During nutation (which is also known as *anterior nutation*), the sacrum is considered to glide inferiorly down the short (vertical) arm and posteriorly along the long (horizontal) arm of the L-shaped articular surface (see Figure 2.2).

The natural wedge shape of the sacrum, as well as the ridges and grooves of the articular surfaces,

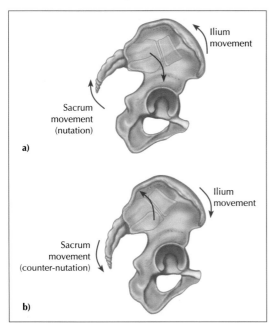

Figure 2.1. (a) Sacral nutation. (b) Sacral counter-nutation.

limits nutation. In addition, the interosseous, sacrotuberous, and sacrospinous ligaments will limit how much nutation is possible, as they become taught in this position; this is considered to be the most stable position.

Vrahas et al. (1995) mention that nutation represents a movement that tightens most of the SIJ ligaments, among which are the vast

interosseous and dorsal sacroiliac ligaments (with the exception of the long dorsal ligament), thereby preparing the pelvis for increased loading.

Counter-Nutation

In counter-nutation the sacral base moves posteriorly and superiorly, while the sacral apex/coccyx moves anteriorly and inferiorly relative to the innominate bone (Figure 2.1(b)). During this type of motion (which is also known as *posterior nutation*), the sacrum is considered to glide anteriorly along the long arm and superiorly up the short arm of the L-shaped articular surface (Figure 2.3).

The long dorsal ligament limits this specific motion of counter-nutation. Because of the laxity of the interosseous and sacrotuberous ligaments, this sacral position of counter-nutation is considered to be the least stable.

Iliosacral Motion

Iliosacral motion is the movement permitted by the innominate bone on the sacrum. Bilateral movement (anterior and posterior rotation) of

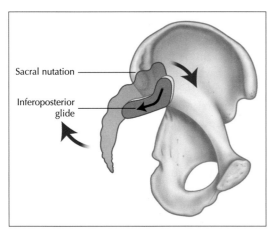

Figure 2.2. Sacral nutation: the sacrum glides inferiorly down the short arm and posteriorly along the long arm.

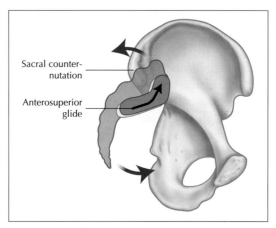

Figure 2.3. Sacral counter-nutation: the sacrum glides anteriorly along the long arm and superiorly up the short arm.

the innominate bones occurs with forward and backward bending of the trunk; on the other hand, unilateral movement (anterior and posterior rotation) of the innominate bone occurs with flexion and extension of the hip joint and lower limbs, for example during the gait cycle (similar to unilateral sacral motion).

Anterior Innominate Motion

When the hip and lower limb are extended, the innominate rotates anteriorly as the L-shaped articular surface glides inferiorly down the short arm and posteriorly along the long arm (Figure 2.4). This anterior motion of the innominate is reminiscent of counter-nutation of the sacrum.

Posterior Innominate Motion

When the hip and lower limb are flexed, the innominate rotates posteriorly as the L-shaped articular surface glides anteriorly along the long arm and superiorly up the short arm (Figure 2.5). This posterior motion of the innominate is reminiscent of nutation of the sacrum.

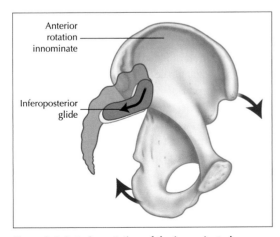

Figure 2.4. Anterior rotation of the innominate bone: the L-shaped articular surface glides inferiorly down the short arm and posteriorly along the long arm.

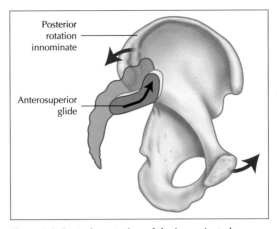

Figure 2.5. Posterior rotation of the innominate bone: the L-shaped articular surface glides anteriorly along the long arm and superiorly up the short arm.

Symphysis Pubis Motion

Anteriorly, the two hipbones are joined together to form a connection known as the *symphysis pubis joint*. During normal walking, the symphysis pubis joint acts as a type of pivot point for the motion of the two hipbones.

Although movement is possible at the symphysis pubis joint, it is normally restricted because of the attachments of the strong superior and inferior ligaments. The limited motion that is available mainly occurs during the walking cycle; however, movement is also possible at this joint when one adopts a stabilized standing position while balancing on one leg.

Symphysis pubis dysfunction (SPD) is generally classified according to the position in which the joint is fixed—either a *superior symphysis pubis* or an *inferior symphysis pubis* (see Figure 2.6).

Studies have shown that if you were to maintain a one-legged standing position for a few minutes, a superior motion (shear) of the symphysis pubis would be seen. If the one-legged motion is maintained over an extended period of time, recurrent SPD can result.

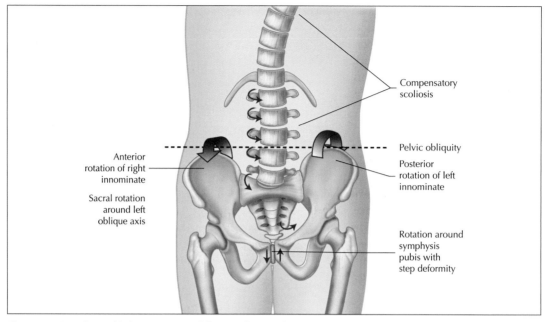

Figure 2.6. Superior and inferior motion of the symphysis pubis joint.

SPD is commonly associated with pregnancy and childbirth; it is thought to affect to varying degrees around one in five women who are pregnant, with around 5–7% of them continuing to experience ongoing painful symptoms after childbirth. During pregnancy, and especially during childbirth, the symphysis pubis ligaments become more lax in order to allow a natural separation of this joint, since this increased movement is needed to widen the internal diameter of the pelvic bowl.

Combined Sacroiliac and Iliosacral Motion

We have looked at the individual motion of the sacrum during nutation and counter-nutation within the innominate bones (sacroiliac) and how the innominate bone rotates around the sacrum (iliosacral). Next, we will combine the motion of the sacroiliac, iliosacral, lumbar, and hip joints during forward and backward bending of the trunk.

When the pelvic girdle, i.e. the two innominate bones and the sacrum, rotate as a unit through

the hip joint, this motion is known as an *anterior pelvic tilt* or a *posterior pelvic tilt*.

Bilateral Motion—Forward Bending

Bilateral (both sides) nutation and counter-nutation are the natural movements that the sacrum performs when we forward and backward bend our trunk while in a stable position on two legs.

On the initiation of forward bending of the trunk, the pelvic girdle will shift posteriorly to control the center of gravity in order to maintain the balance. The sacrum will be in a position of nutation and will stay there throughout the full range of motion (ROM). The left and right innominates rotate symmetrically on the femur in an anterior direction (anterior pelvic tilt), and the PSIS will move symmetrically in a cephalic direction (superior) as the lumbar spine (L5) flexes on the sacrum. As trunk flexion continues, there will come a natural point when tension is increased within the sacrotuberous ligament, biceps femoris, and thoracolumbar fascia, and

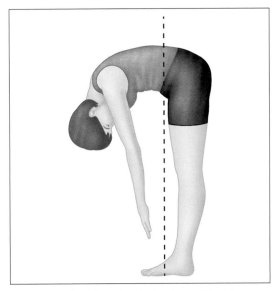

Figure 2.7. Bilateral motion during forward bending.

a position where sacral nutation ceases. At this point the innominate bones continue rotating anteriorly; however, because of the increased tension in the soft tissues (explained earlier), especially the hamstrings, the final position of trunk flexion is that in which the sacrum is considered to be in a position of *relative* counter-nutation, even though the sacrum will appear to be in a position of nutation (Figure 2.7).

On the return to a standing position, the sacrum remains in a position of nutation until the erect posture is achieved; at this crucial point, the sacrum slightly counter-nutates to maintain a suspension between the two innominate bones. (Note that, even though I have mentioned counter-nutation, the sacrum still maintains an overall position of nutation.)

Bilateral Motion—Backward Bending

This time, on the initiation of backward bending, the pelvic girdle will shift anteriorly, while the innominate bones symmetrically rotate posteriorly on the femur (posterior pelvic tilt); the PSIS can be seen and felt to rotate in a caudal direction (inferiorly), while the thoracolumbar

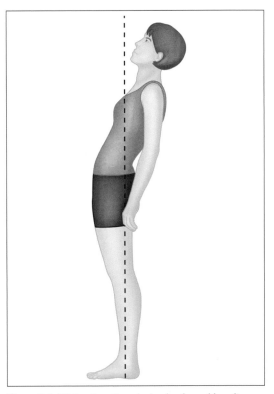

Figure 2.8. Bilateral motion during backward bending.

spine continues extension until L5 extends on the sacrum (Figure 2.8). The sacrum remains in a position of nutation throughout backward bending; this position is considered to be the most stable because of the compression of the SIJs.

Unilateral (One Side) Motion of the Sacrum

During the walking/gait cycle, the sacrum is required to perform its natural motion in a way that is completely opposite to that during forward and backward bending movements. This time we need a specific type of unilateral (one-sided) motion of the sacrum, not a bilateral motion. What I mean by this is the following: as we walk from point A to point B, we need one side of the sacrum (e.g. the left side) to move forward into *nutation*, while at the same time the opposite side (right side in this case) is moving backward into *counter-nutation* (or posterior nutation). This movement gets a little bit more complex, as the nutation/counter-nutation will naturally induce a movement of *sacral rotation*. The problem we encounter now is that when you have a rotation of the sacrum (or in fact any vertebrae), a coupled (combined) motion with side bending also occurs; the general rule (according to the current research) is that the side bending motion will be coupled to the opposite side of the sacral rotation. This follows what is typically known as a *Type I* or *neutral mechanic* (see Chapter 6), in which the rotation and side bending are coupled to the opposite side; for instance, the sacrum can perform a side bending motion to the left side, but it will rotate to the opposite side (to the right side in this case).

Consider the following example to illustrate what I am trying to say. If the *left* side of the sacrum goes forward into anterior nutation, it will rotate to the *right* side (the sacral base will palpate deeper on the left side) and will also side bend to the *left* (Figure 2.9). However, the *right* side of the sacrum will also rotate to the *right* side, but this time the sacral base will be in a posterior nutation position (counter-nutation, as the sacral base will now palpate shallow on the right side).

The movement discussed above, in which you have a rotation to one side and a side bending motion to the other, is also known as a *sacral torsion*; this

specific type of sacral movement is considered to occur around an oblique axis (Figure 2.10).

Sacral Axis

There are approximately six types of sacral axis (Figure 2.10):

- Superior transverse axis
- Middle transverse axis
- Inferior transverse axis
- Left oblique axis
- Right oblique axis
- Vertical axis

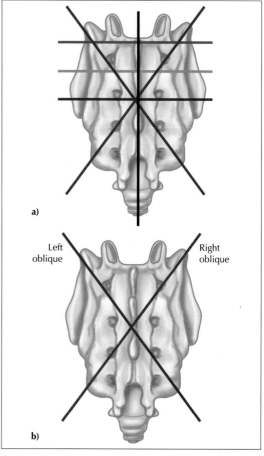

Left oblique

Right oblique

a)

b)

Figure 2.10. (a) Sacral axis, (b) Left oblique axis and right oblique axis.

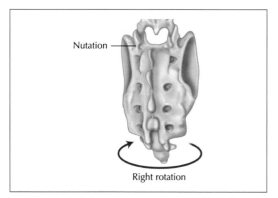

Nutation

Right rotation

Figure 2.9. Example of a unilateral motion of the sacrum.

It is not within the scope of this book to cover all the different sacral axis variations. For this text, however, the one of particular relevance is the middle transverse axis (MTA), because sacral dysfunctions are palpated and treated about this horizontal axis, according to Mitchell terminology. Moreover, this axis is considered to undergo a transformation during the gait cycle into the *oblique axis*, which is the specific axis that will be focused on in this text.

Oblique Axis

It has been suggested by some authors that there is a left oblique axis and a right oblique axis (Figure 2.10(b)). The *left oblique axis* runs through the left sacral base and continues through the right inferior lateral angle (ILA); the *right oblique axis* runs through the right sacral base and continues through the left ILA.

In Chapter 3 I will take you through exactly how the oblique axis is utilized in combination with the movements of the kinetic chain as we perform sacral motion during the walking/gait cycle. For now, however, we will focus on the two natural physiological motions that the sacrum is capable of: "left rotation on the left oblique axis," which is typically called a *left-on-left* (L-on-L) sacral torsion, and a "right rotation on the right oblique axis," commonly known as a *right-on-right* (R-on-R) sacral torsion.

There are, however, also two non-physiological motions of the sacrum: "left rotation on the right oblique axis," which is typically called a *left-on-right* (L-on-R) sacral torsion, and a "right rotation on the left oblique axis," commonly known as a *right-on-left* (R-on-L) sacral torsion.

When authors mention the word "sacral torsion," they can mean one of two things: a naturally occurring motion of the sacrum that is performed, for example, during the gait cycle (Chapter 3 will explain this); or a dysfunction of the sacrum,

in that it becomes fixed in this specific type of position or torsion.

Physiological Motions (Anterior Motion Fixation/Nutation)

Before we look at sacral torsions, let's just remind ourselves of the *neutral* position of the sacrum (Figure 2.11(a) & (b)).

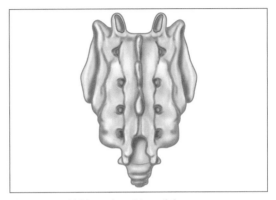

Figure 2.11. (a) Neutral position of the sacrum.

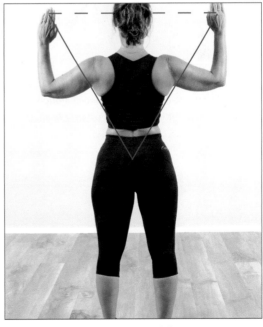

Figure 2.11. (b) Neutral position of the sacrum, *as indicated by the model.*

Left-on-Left (L-on-L)

Let's discuss a L-on-L sacral motion/torsion a bit further: it relates to the sacral bone being in a position of left rotation on the left oblique axis. This will be specific to the case where the sacrum has rotated to the left side, so the sacral sulcus (the area that is naturally formed by the junction of the sacral base with the corresponding ilium) will palpate as deep on the right. Moreover, the ILA as well as the sacral sulcus will palpate as posterior (shallow) on the left side, which will indicate that

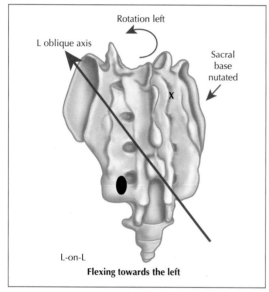

Figure 2.12. (a) Left-on-left (L-on-L) sacral motion/ torsion. X = Anterior or deep. ● = Posterior or shallow.

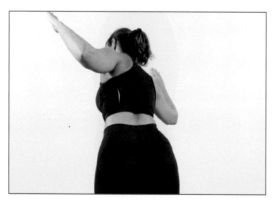

Figure 2.12. (b) L-on-L sacral torsion, as demonstrated by the model—sacral nutation is shown on the right side.

the *right* side of the sacrum has anteriorly nutated to the *left* (Figure 2.12(a)).

The specific motion of a L-on-L sacral torsion is demonstrated in Figure 2.12(b).

Right-on-Right (R-on-R)

A R-on-R sacral torsion relates to a right rotation on the right oblique axis. This will be specific to a sacrum that has rotated to the right side, so the sacral sulcus will palpate as deep on the left side. The ILA and the sacral sulcus will palpate as posterior (shallow) on the right, which will indicate that the *left* side of the sacrum has anteriorly nutated to the *right* (Figure 2.13(a)).

The model in Figure 2.13(b) is demonstrating the specific motion of a R-on-R sacral torsion.

Physiological Summary

As I have already mentioned, L-on-L and R-on-R sacral torsions are naturally occurring motions

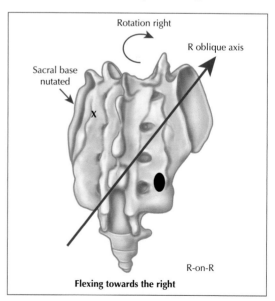

Figure 2.13. (a) Right-on-right (R-on-R) sacral motion/ torsion. X = Anterior or deep. ● = Posterior or shallow.

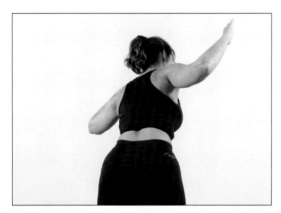

Figure 2.13. (b) R-on-R sacral torsion, as demonstrated by the model—sacral nutation is shown on the left side.

around the sacrum, although these specific motions can be fixed in a position of nutation. For example, if you have a dysfunctional position, say a L-on-L sacral torsion, then the sacrum is capable of performing this movement, as it is already fixed in this position and is potentially capable of rotating back to a "neutral" position. However, it is unable to perform a "R-on-R" sacral torsion due to the fact that the left side of the sacrum is unable to counter-nutate (posterior nutation), as this side (left) is held in a fixed position of anterior nutation.

You will read in Chapter 3 that most of the activity of our musculoskeletal system will involve the walking/gait cycle. As humans, we especially need to be able to maintain ongoing L-on-L and R-on-R sacral (torsion) motions, since these are of paramount importance to enable us to ambulate normally through the gait cycle. If the sacrum cannot perform these naturally occurring sacral torsions (motion), dysfunction occurs as a consequence.

Non-Physiological Motions (Posterior Motion Fixation/Counter-Nutation)

Non-physiological motions of the sacrum are a little bit more complex to grasp, as they are considered to be *unnatural* motions that occur

around an oblique axis of the sacrum. If you do happen to find this type of posterior sacral dysfunction with your patients, it often tends to be caused by the lumbar spine/trunk being placed into a position of increased (forced) flexion with a combined movement of rotation (as in the motion of rotating your body to pick up a heavy weight from the floor).

It may take you a while to think about and understand this next concept but I will try my best to explain this in a relatively simple way, even though many people will still have difficulty understanding what it is I am trying to portray due to the natural complexity of this fascinating area.

Before we start I would like you to think of this motion simply as a backward/posterior torsion, whereas the other two types I mentioned in the earlier paragraphs are forward/anterior torsions.

Left-on-Right (L-on-R)

A *L-on-R sacral torsion* relates to a left rotation on the right oblique axis, and this will be specific to the case where the sacrum has rotated to

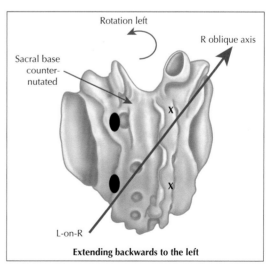

Figure 2.14. (a) Left-on-right (L-on-R) sacral torsion. X = Anterior or deep. ● = Posterior or shallow.

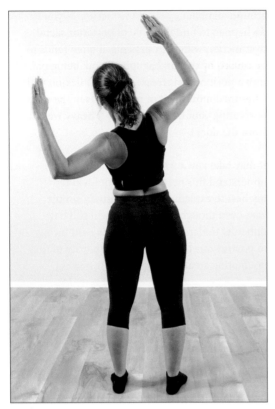

Figure 2.14. (b) L-on-R sacral torsion, as demonstrated by the model—sacral counter-nutation is shown on the left side.

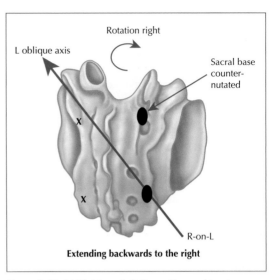

Figure 2.15. (a) Right-on-left (R-on-L) sacral torsion. X = Anterior or deep. ● = Posterior or shallow.

the *left* side. However, because of the posterior motion of the left side of the sacrum, the sacral sulcus will now palpate as shallow on the *left*, and the ILA will palpate as posterior (shallow) on the *left*; this will indicate that the *left* side of the sacrum has counter-nutated or posteriorly nutated (see Figure 2.14(a)).

This specific motion of a L-on-R sacral torsion is demonstrated by the model in Figure 2.14(b).

Right-on-Left (R-on-L)

It follows that a *R-on-L sacral torsion* must be the opposite of a L-on-R sacral torsion; thus, the

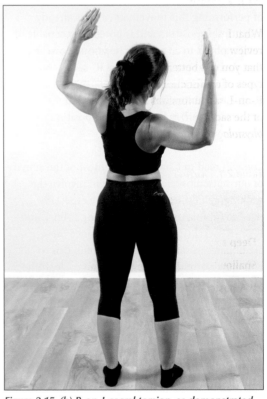

Figure 2.15. (b) R-on-L sacral torsion, as demonstrated by the model—sacral counter-nutation is shown on the right side.

sacral torsion this time relates to a right rotation on the left oblique axis, and this will be specific to the sacrum having rotated to the *right* side. Because of the posterior motion of the right side of the sacrum, however, the sacral sulcus will now palpate as "shallow" on the *right*, and the ILA will palpate as posterior (shallow) on the *right*. This will indicate that the *right* side of the sacrum has counter-nutated, or (if easier to understand) that the sacrum has posteriorly nutated (think of this simply as a backward motion), as shown in Figure 2.15(a).

Figure 2.15(b) illustrates the specific motion of a R-on-L sacral torsion, as demonstrated by the model.

Non-Physiological Summary

What I would like to do now is give a brief review of the main points discussed above, so that you can better understand these specific types of dysfunction. We know that L-on-R and R-on-L sacral torsions are *unnatural* motions of the sacrum, hence their being termed *non-physiological*. These specific motions can be fixed

in a position of counter-nutation or a backward torsion. For example, if you have a dysfunctional position of a L-on-R sacral torsion, the sacrum is capable of performing this backward type of movement, as it is already fixed in that position. The sacrum is, however, unable to perform the normal physiological motion of a L-on-L or a R-on-R sacral torsion, because of the fact that the *left* side of the sacrum is unable to nutate, since it is held in a fixed position. Another way of thinking about this is that the left side of the sacrum cannot perform the motion of anterior nutation, or simply go forward on the left, as it is held backward in a fixed position of counter-nutation or posterior nutation.

Sacral Torsions Summary

Tables 2.1 and 2.2 (overleaf) summarize the physiological and non-physiological motions of the sacrum. You will notice that the tables contain extra components, namely the position of L5, seated flexion test, lumbar spring test, sphinx test, lumbar lordosis curvature, and position of the medial malleolus. All of these will be explained in more detail in later chapters, especially

Table 2.1. Normal physiological motion: anterior/forward sacral torsions.

	L-on-L sacral torsion Forward/nutation	R-on-R sacral torsion Forward/nutation
Deep sacral sulcus (neutral)	Right	Left
Shallow sacral sulcus (neutral)	Left	Right
ILA posterior	Left	Right
L5 rotation	Right—ERS(R)	Left—ERS(L)
Seated flexion test	Right	Left
Lumbar spring	Negative	Negative
Sphinx test	Sacral sulci level	Sacral sulci level
Lumbar lordosis	Increased	Increased
Medial malleolus (leg length)	Short left	Short right

Table 2.2. Non-physiological motion: posterior/backward sacral torsions.

	L-on-R sacral torsion Backward/counter-nutation	R-on-L sacral torsion Backward/counter-nutation
Deep sacral sulcus (neutral)	Right	Left
Shallow sacral sulcus (neutral)	Left	Right
ILA posterior	Left	Right
L5 rotation	Right—FRS(R)	Left—FRS(L)
Seated flexion test	Left	Right
Lumbar spring	Positive	Positive
Sphinx test	Left sacral sulcus shallow (right sacral sulcus deeper)	Right sacral sulcus shallow (left sacral sulcus deeper)
Lumbar lordosis	Decreased	Decreased
Medial malleolus (leg length)	Short left	Short right

Chapter 12, but have been mentioned here because my aim in this chapter is to whet your appetite to continue reading. For now, I just wanted you to be aware of all the different types of physiological and non-physiological motion that the sacrum is capable of before we progress through the rest of the chapters.

Sacroiliac Joint Stability, Muscle Imbalances, and the Myofascial Slings

As the incidence of pelvic and lower back pain continues to increase, we will need to look at and understand the muscular relationships that affect the core and lumbo–pelvic–sacral stability. We will then have to decide how to incorporate this knowledge into an assessment and treatment plan, especially for patients and athletes who present with pain associated with the area of the pelvic girdle and lower back.

There are two main factors that affect the stability of the pelvis (or to be more precise the sacroiliac joint (SIJ)): form closure and force closure. These two mechanisms collectively assist in a process known as the *self-locking mechanism*.

Form closure arises from the anatomical alignment of the bones of the innominate and the sacrum, where the sacrum forms a kind of keystone between the wings of the pelvis. The SIJ transfers large loads and its shape is adapted to this task. The articular surfaces are relatively flat, which helps to transfer compression forces and bending movements. However, a relatively flat joint is vulnerable to shear forces. The SIJ is protected from these forces in three ways. First, the sacrum is wedge (triangular) shaped and thus is stabilized

between the innominate bones, similarly to a keystone in a Roman arch, and is kept in a state of "suspension" by the ligaments acting upon it. Second, in contrast to other synovial joints, the articular cartilage is not smooth but rather irregular (think back to Chapter 1). Third, a frontal dissection through the SIJ reveals cartilage-covered bone extensions protruding into the joint—the so-called "ridges" and "grooves." They seem rather irregular, but are in fact complementary to each other, and this unusual irregularity is very relevant as it serves to stabilize the SIJ when compression is applied.

According to Vleeming et al. (1990a), after puberty most individuals develop a crescent-shaped ridge running the entire length of the iliac surface with a corresponding depression on the sacral side; this complementary ridge and groove are now believed to lock the surfaces together and increase stability of the SIJ.

If the articular surfaces of the sacrum and the innominate bones fitted together with perfect form closure, mobility would be practically impossible. However, form closure of the SIJ is not perfect and mobility—albeit small—is possible, and therefore stabilization during loading is required. This is

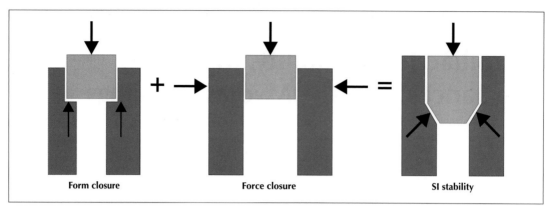

Figure 3.1. The relationship between form/force closure and sacroiliac stability.

achieved by increasing compression across the joint at the moment of loading; the anatomical structures responsible for this compression are the ligaments, muscles, and fasciae. The mechanism of compression of the SIJ by these additional forces is what is commonly called *force closure*. When the SIJ is compressed, friction of the joint increases and consequently reinforces form closure (Figure 3.1). According to Willard et al. (2012), force closure reduces the joint's "neutral zone," thereby facilitating stabilization of the SIJ.

Force closure is accomplished as follows. The first method is by nutation of the sacrum, which is achieved either by anterior motion of the sacral base or by posterior rotation of the innominate bone. These two types of motion result in a tightening of the sacrotuberous, sacrospinous, and interosseous ligaments; this tightening assists in activating the force closure mechanism, thereby increasing the compression of the SIJ. Counter-nutation, on the other hand, decreases the stability of the SIJ because of the reduced tension in the above-mentioned ligaments.

Cohen (2005) states that because the ilium and sacrum only meet at approximately one-third of their surfaces, the associated ligaments provide the rest of the stability between these bones.

In the second method, force closure is assisted by the activation/contraction of the inner and outer

core muscles (local and global muscle systems), as you will read later on in this chapter.

The terms *form closure* and *force closure* delineate the active and passive components of this self-locking mechanism and were first identified by Vleeming et al. (1990a, 1990b). Below is a quote from Vleeming et al. (1995) that I personally believe explains the above text.

"Shear in the sacroiliac joints is prevented by the combination of specific anatomical features (form closure) and the compression generated by muscles and ligaments that can be accommodated to the specific loading situation (force closure). If the sacrum would fit the pelvis with perfect form closure, no lateral forces would be needed. However, such a construction would make mobility practically impossible."

Sacroiliac Stability

Several ligaments, muscles, and fascial systems contribute to force closure of the pelvis: these are collectively referred to as the *osteo-articular-ligamentous system*. Recall that when the body is working efficiently, the shear forces between the innominate bones and the sacrum are adequately controlled, and loads can then be transferred between the trunk, pelvis, and legs.

Vleeming and Stoeckart (2007) mention that various muscles are involved in force closure of the SIJ, and that even muscles such as the rectus femoris, sartorius, iliacus, Gmax, and hamstrings have adequate lever arms to influence movement in the SIJ. The effect of these muscles is dependent on open or closed kinematic movements, and whether the pelvis is sufficiently braced.

As you will read shortly, and also in later chapters, there is one muscle in particular that plays a highly significant role in stabilizing the SIJs—this muscle is the Gmax. Some of the Gmax fibers merge and attach onto the sacrotuberous ligament as well as onto a connective tissue structure known as the *thoracolumbar fascia*. Vleeming et al. (1989a) demonstrated this fact on 12 cadaver dissections; they found that the Gmax muscle was directly attached to the sacrotuberous ligament in all cases.

The Gmax connects, via the thoracolumbar fascia, to the contralateral latissimus dorsi to form what is known as the *posterior oblique myofascial sling* (see section "The Outer Core Unit: The Integrated Myofascial Sling System (Global System)" later in this chapter). It has been shown that weakness, or possibly a misfiring sequence, of the Gmax will predispose the SIJ to injury by decreasing the function of this (posterior oblique) myofascial sling. A weakness or misfiring of the Gmax is a potential cause of a compensatory overactivation of the contralateral latissimus dorsi; walking and running (gait cycle, explained in Chapter 4) impose high loads on the SIJ, so this weight-bearing joint will need to be self-stabilizing in order to reduce the effect of the altered compensatory mechanism.

Research has shown that sacral nutation (a nodding type of movement of the sacrum between the innominate bones) is the best position for the pelvic girdle to be at its most stable. As I have already explained in earlier chapters, nutation occurs when moving (for example) from a sitting position to standing, and full nutation occurs during forward or backward bending of the trunk. This motion of sacral nutation tightens the major ligaments (sacrotuberous, sacrospinous, and interosseous) of the posterior pelvis, and the resulting tension increases the compressive force across the SIJ. The increased tension provides the required stability that is needed by the SIJ during the gait cycle as well as when simply rising from a sitting to a standing position.

Vleeming et al. (1989b) showed how load application to the sacrotuberous ligament, either directly to the ligament or through its continuations with the long head of biceps femoris or the attachments of the Gmax, significantly diminishes forward rotation of the sacral base. They demonstrated that this increases the coefficient of friction, thus decreasing movement of the SIJ by force closure.

Sacral Nutation and Counter-Nutation

I find it very beneficial at certain times, especially for you the reader, to try to discuss alternative ways of explaining a relatively complex motion. I therefore thought I would introduce an opinion by another author, Evan Osar (2012), who states that *nutation* is the anterior inferior motion of the sacral base, while *counter-nutation* is the posterior superior motion of the sacral base. Nutation is necessary for the locking of the SIJ during unilateral stance (see Figure 3.2(a)). The inability to nutate the sacrum is a leading cause of unilateral stance instability and one of the causes of the classic Trendelenburg gait. Counter-nutation, on the other hand, is necessary in order to unlock the SIJ to allow anterior rotation of the innominate and extension of the hip joint (see Figure 3.2(b)). The inability to unlock or counter-nutate the sacrum leads to compensatory increases in lumbopelvic flexion, which in turn lead to and perpetuate lumbar instability.

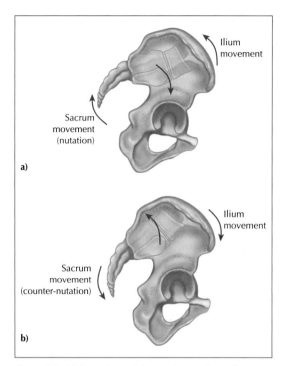

Figure 3.2. (a) Posterior pelvic rotation and sacral nutation. (b) Anterior pelvic rotation and sacral counter-nutation.

Force Closure Ligaments

The main ligamentous structures that influence force closure (Figure 3.3) are: (1) the sacrotuberous ligament, which connects the sacrum to the ischium and has been termed the *key* or *lead* ligament; and (2) the long dorsal sacroiliac ligament, which connects the third and fourth sacral segments to the PSIS and is also known as the *posterior sacroiliac ligament.*

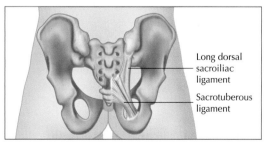

Figure 3.3. Sacrotuberous ligament (key) and the long dorsal sacroiliac ligament.

Ligaments can increase articular compression when they are tensed or lengthened by the movement of the bones to which they attach, or when they are tensed by the contraction of muscles that insert onto the bones.

Tension in the sacrotuberous ligament can be increased in one of three ways:

1. Posterior rotation of the innominate bone relative to the sacrum.
2. Nutation of the sacrum relative to the innominate bone.
3. Muscular contraction of any one of the four muscles that have a direct attachment to the sacrotuberous ligament, namely biceps femoris, piriformis, Gmax, and multifidus.

The main ligamentous tissue to restrain counter-nutation of the sacrum, or anterior rotation of the innominate, is the long dorsal sacroiliac ligament (posterior sacroiliac ligament). This is a less stable position (compared with the position of nutation) for the pelvis to resist horizontal and/or vertical loading, since the SIJ is under less compression and is not self-locked. The long dorsal ligament is commonly a source of pain and can be palpated just below (inferior to) the level of the PSIS.

By themselves, ligaments cannot maintain a stable pelvis—they rely on several muscle systems to assist them. There are two important groups of muscles that contribute to stability of the lower back and pelvis: collectively they are called the *inner unit* (core) and the *outer unit* (myofascial sling systems). The inner unit consists of the transversus abdominis (TVA), multifidus, diaphragm, and muscles of the pelvic floor—also collectively known as the *core*, or *local stabilizers*. The outer unit consists of several "slings," or systems of muscles (global stabilizers and mobilizers that are anatomically connected and functionally related). The inner and outer units will be discussed later on in this chapter.

Force Couple

Definition: A *force couple* is a situation where two forces of equal magnitude, but acting in opposite directions, are applied to an object and pure rotation results, as mentioned by Abernethy et al. (2004).

Any altered positioning of the pelvis caused by potential muscle imbalances will subsequently affect the rest of the kinetic chain. There are several force couples responsible for maintaining proper positioning and alignment of the pelvis. The force couples responsible for controlling the position of the pelvis in the sagittal and frontal planes are shown schematically in Figures 3.4(a–f) and 3.5 (overleaf).

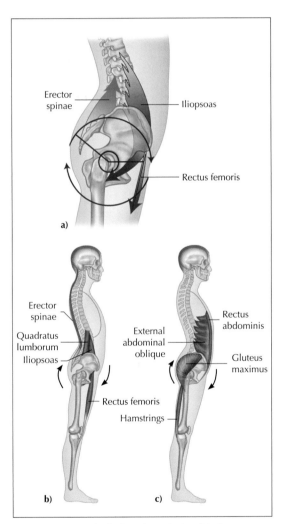

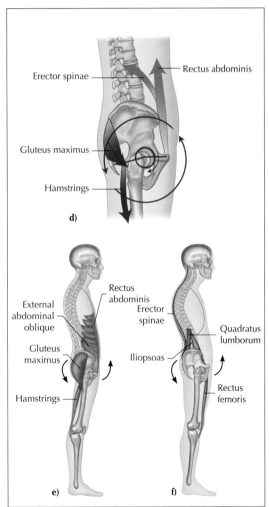

Figure 3.4. (a) Sagittal plane (anterior) pelvic force couple. (b) Anterior tilt: muscles held in a shortened position. (c) Anterior tilt: muscles held in a lengthened position.

Figure 3.4. (d) Sagittal plane (posterior) pelvic force couple. (e) Posterior tilt: muscles held in a shortened position. (f) Posterior tilt: muscles held in a lengthened position.

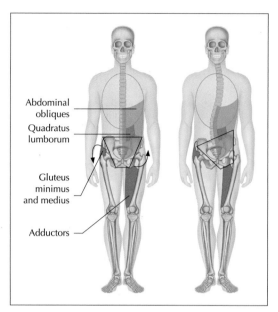

Abdominal
obliques
Quadratus
lumborum

Gluteus
minimus
and medius

Adductors

Figure 3.5. Frontal plane (lateral) pelvic force couples.

Posture

Definition: *Posture* is the attitude or position of the body, as discussed by Thomas (1997).

According to Martin (2002), posture should fulfill three functions:

1. Maintain the alignment of the body's segments in any position: supine, prone, sitting, all fours, and standing.
2. Anticipate change to allow engagement in voluntary, goal-directed movements, such as reaching and stepping.
3. React to unexpected perturbations or disturbances in balance.

From the above, it can be seen that posture is an active as well as a static state, and that it is synonymous with balance. Optimal posture must be maintained at all times, not only when holding static positions (e.g. sitting and standing) but also during movement.

If optimal posture and postural control are to be encouraged during exercise performance, the principles of good static posture must be fully appreciated. Once these are understood, poor posture can be identified and corrective strategies adopted.

- *Good posture* is the state of muscular and skeletal balance that protects the supporting structures of the body against injury or progressive deformity, irrespective of the attitude (e.g. erect, lying, squatting, or stooping) in which these structures are working or resting.
- *Poor posture* is a faulty relationship of the various parts of the body, producing increased strain on the supporting structures, and resulting in less efficient balance of the body over its base of support.

Poor Posture

Poor posture may be a result of many different contributing factors. It may be caused by trauma suffered by the body, some form of deformity within the musculoskeletal system, or even faulty loading. Because sitting has become a position maintained by our bodies for long periods of time (possibly 8+ hours), most people in today's society are losing the fight against gravity and altering their center of gravity (COG). With correct posture, your postural muscles are fairly inactive and energy efficient, only responding to disruptions in balance in order to maintain an upright position. As you move away from an ideal alignment, postural muscle activity therefore increases, thus leading to higher energy expenditure.

Pain Spasm Cycle

Ischemia will be a primary source of pain in the initial stages of poor posture. The blood flow through a muscle is inversely proportional to the level of contraction or activity, reaching almost zero at 50–60% of contraction. Some

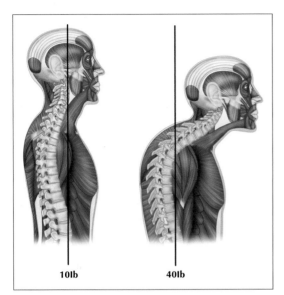

Figure 3.6. (a) The result of a forward head posture.

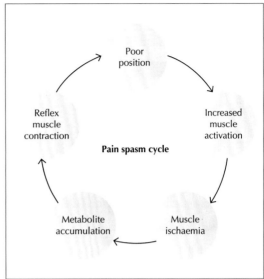

Figure 3.6. (b) Pain spasm model.

studies have indicated that the body is not able to maintain homeostasis with a sustained isometric contraction of over 10%.

Consider the following example: the weight of the head is approximately 7% of total body weight (shoulders and arms are around 14%). This means that for a person weighing 176lbs (80kg), the head will weigh around 11–13lbs (5 to 6kg). If the head and shoulders move forward, out of ideal alignment, the activation of the neck extensors will increase dramatically, resulting in restricted blood flow. Previous authors have stated that for every inch of forward head posture, the weight of the head on the spine can increase by approximately 10lb (4.5kg). For example, if the weight of the head is normally 10lb (4.5kg), it will now potentially weigh 20lb (9kg) for just a 1" (2.5cm) increase in forward head posture, 30lb (13.5kg) for a 2" (5cm) increase, and an unbelievable 40lb (18kg) if the head translates 3" (7.5cm), as shown in Figure 3.6(a).

This prolonged isometric contraction will force the muscles into anaerobic metabolism and increase lactic acid and other irritating metabolite

accumulation. If adequate rest is not given, a reflex contraction of the already ischemic muscles may be initiated. This person will have now entered the pain spasm cycle (Figure 3.6(b)).

The neuromuscular system, as we know, is made up of *slow-twitch* and *fast-twitch* muscle fibers, each having a different role in the body's function. Slow-twitch fibers (Type I) are active in sustained low-level activity, such as maintaining correct posture, whereas fast-twitch fibers (Type II) are used for powerful, gross movements. Muscles can also be broken down into two further categories—*tonic* (or *postural*) and *phasic*.

Tonic (Postural) and Phasic Muscles

Janda (1987) identified two groups of muscles on the basis of their evolution and development. Functionally, muscles can be classified as *tonic* or *phasic*. The tonic system consists of the flexors, which develop later on to become the dominant structure. Umphred et al. (2001) identified that the tonic muscles are involved in repetitive or rhythmic activity and are activated in flexor synergies, whereas the phasic system consists of the extensors and emerges shortly after birth. The phasic muscles work eccentrically against the force of gravity and are involved in extensor synergies. The division of muscles into predominantly phasic and predominantly postural is given in Table 3.1.

Previous authors have suggested that muscles which have a stabilizing function (postural) have a natural tendency to shorten when stressed, and that other muscles which play a more active/moving role (phasic) have a tendency to lengthen and can subsequently become inhibited (Table 3.2). The muscles that tend to shorten have a primary

Table 3.1. Phasic and postural muscles of the body.

Predominantly postural muscles	Predominantly phasic muscles
Shoulder girdle	
Pectoralis major/minor	Rhomboids
Levator scapulae	Lower trapezius
Upper trapezius	Mid trapezius
Biceps brachii	Serratus anterior
Neck extensors: Scalenes/Cervical erectors/Sternocleidomastoid	Triceps brachii
	Neck flexors: Supra- and infrahyoid/Longus colli
Forearm	
Wrist flexors	Wrist extensors
Trunk	
Lumbar and cervical erectors	Thoracic erectors
Quadratus lumborum	Abdominals
Pelvis and thigh	
Hamstrings	Vastus medialis
Iliopsoas	Vastus lateralis
ITB	Gluteus maximus
Rectus femoris	Gluteus minimus and medius
Adductors	
Piriformis/Tensor fasciae latae	
Lower leg	
Gastrocnemius/Soleus	Tibialis anterior/Fibularii

postural role and are related to the potential inhibition weakness of the gluteal muscles (which you will read about later).

Table 3.2. Lengthening and shortening of muscles.

	Postural	**Phasic**
Function	Posture	Movement
Muscle type	Type I	Type II
Fatigue	Late	Early
Reaction	Shortening	Lengthening

There are some exceptions to the rule which states that certain muscles follow the pattern of becoming shortened while others become lengthened—some muscles are capable of modifying their structure. For example, some authors suggest that the scalene muscles are postural in nature, while others suggest that they are phasic. We know from specific testing, depending on what dysfunction is present within the muscle framework, that the scalenes can be found to be held in a shortened position and tight, but at other times they can be observed to be lengthened and weakened.

There is a distinction between postural and phasic muscles; however, many muscles can display characteristics of both and contain a mixture of Type I and Type II fibers. The hamstring muscles, for example, have a postural stabilizing function, yet are polyarticular (cross more than one joint) and are notoriously prone to shortening.

Postural Muscles

Also known as *tonic muscles*, the postural muscles have an antigravity role and are therefore heavily involved in the maintenance of posture (Figure 3.7). Slow-twitch fibers are more suited to maintaining posture: they are capable of sustained contraction but generally become shortened and subsequently tight.

Postural muscles are slow-twitch dominant because of their resistance to fatigue, and are innervated by a smaller motor neuron. They therefore have a lower excitability threshold, which means the nerve impulse will reach the postural muscle before the phasic muscle. With this sequence of innervation, the postural muscle will inhibit the phasic (antagonist) muscle, thus reducing its contractile potential and activation.

Phasic Muscles

Movement is the main function of phasic muscles. These muscles, which are often more superficial than postural muscles and tend to be polyarticular, are composed of predominantly Type II fibers and are under voluntary reflex control (Figure 3.7).

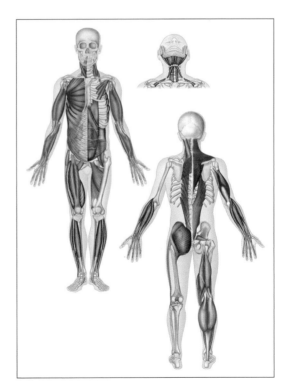

Figure 3.7. Postural and phasic muscles: (a) anterior view; (b) posterior view. The blue muscles are predominantly postural, and the red muscles predominantly phasic.

A shortened, tight postural muscle often results in inhibition of the associated phasic muscle, whose function becomes weakened as a result. The relationship between a tightness-prone muscle and an associated weakness-prone muscle is one way. As the tightness-prone muscle becomes tighter and subsequently stronger, this causes an inhibition of the weakness-prone muscle, resulting in its lengthening and consequent weakening: think about how this might affect the relationship, for example, between the iliopsoas and the gluteal muscles, or between the pectoralis major/minor and the rhomboids.

Muscle Activity Before and After Stretching

Let's take a look at some electromyography (EMG) studies of trunk muscle activity before and after stretching hypertonic muscles, in this case the erector spinae. In Table 3.3 the hypertonic erector spinae are indicated as being active during trunk flexion. After stretching, these muscles are suppressed both in trunk flexion (which allows greater activation of the rectus abdominis) and in trunk extension (dorsal raise).

Effects of Muscle Imbalance

The research results of Janda (1983) indicate that tight or overactive muscles not only hinder the agonist through Sherrington's law of reciprocal inhibition as stated by Sherrington (1907), but also become active in movements that they are not normally associated with. This is the reason why, when trying to correct a musculoskeletal imbalance, you would encourage *lengthening* of an overactive muscle by using a muscle energy technique (MET), prior to attempting to *strengthen* a weak elongated muscle (METs will be explained in Chapter 7).

Think about the following words before you continue reading:

"A *tight* muscle will pull the joint into a dysfunctional position and the *weak* muscle will allow this to happen."

One possible way to address this, therefore, is to simply apply the following rule: "lengthen before you strengthen."

If muscle imbalances are not addressed, the body will be forced into a compensatory position, which increases the stress placed on the musculoskeletal system, eventually leading to tissue breakdown,

Table 3.3. EMG recordings of muscle activity. (Source: Hammer 1999)

Muscle	First recording			Second recording		
Rectus abdominis	⫽⫽⫽	⫽⫽⫽	∿	⫽⫽⫽	⫽⫽⫽	∿
Erector spinae	⫽⫽	⫽⫽	⫽⫽⫽	∿	∿	⫽⫽⫽

irritation, and injury. You are now in a vicious circle of musculoskeletal deterioration as the tonic muscles shorten and the phasic muscles lengthen (Table 3.4).

Muscle imbalances are ultimately reflected in posture. As mentioned earlier, postural muscles are innervated by a smaller motor neuron and therefore have a lower excitability threshold. Since the nerve impulse reaches the postural muscle before the phasic muscle, the postural muscle will inhibit the phasic (antagonist) muscle, thus reducing the contractile potential and activation.

When muscles are subject to faulty or repetitive loading, the postural muscles shorten and the phasic muscles weaken, thus altering their length–tension relationship. Consequently, posture is directly affected because the surrounding muscles displace the soft tissues and the skeleton.

Table 3.4. The vicious circle of musculoskeletal deterioration.

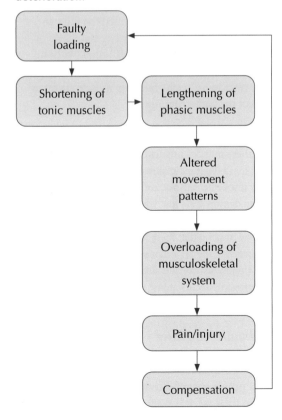

Core Muscle Relationships

Inner Core Unit (Local System)

> **Definition:** *Static stability* is the ability to remain in one position for a long time without losing good structural alignment, as mentioned by Chek (1999).

Static stability is also often referred to as *postural stability*, although this might be somewhat misleading, since as Martin (2002) states: "… posture is more than just maintaining a position of the body such as standing. Posture is active, whether it is in sustaining an existing posture or moving from one posture to another."

The inner core unit (Figure 3.8) consists of:

* Transversus abdominis (TVA)
* Multifidus
* Diaphragm
* Muscles of the pelvic floor

Only the TVA and multifidus will be covered in this book, as these muscles are specifically related to postural and phasic imbalances and are easily palpated by the physical therapist.

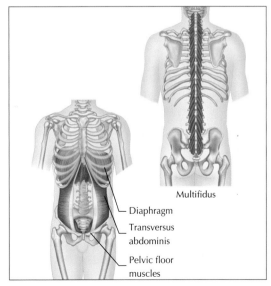

Multifidus

Diaphragm

Transversus abdominis

Pelvic floor muscles

Figure 3.8. The inner core unit.

Since the diaphragm and muscles of the pelvic floor are difficult to palpate, they will not be discussed here.

Transversus Abdominis

The transversus abdominis (TVA) is the deepest of the abdominal muscles. It originates at the iliac crest, inguinal ligament, lumbar fascia, and associated cartilage of the inferior six ribs, and attaches to the xiphoid process, linea alba, and pubis.

The main action of the TVA is to compress the abdomen via a "drawing-in" of the abdominal wall. This drawing-in is observable as a movement of the umbilicus (belly button) toward the spine. The muscle neither flexes nor extends the spine. Kendall et al. (2010) also state that "this muscle has no action in lateral flexion except that it acts to … stabilize the linea alba, thereby permitting better action by anterolateral trunk muscles [internal and external obliques]."

The TVA appears to be the key muscle of the inner unit. Richardson et al. (1999) found that in people without back pain, the TVA fired 30 milliseconds prior to shoulder movements and 110 milliseconds before leg movements. This corroborates the key role of the TVA in providing the stability necessary to perform movements of the appendicular skeleton. As the TVA contracts during inspiration it pulls the central tendon inferiorly and flattens, thereby increasing the vertical length of the thoracic cavity and compressing the lumbar multifidus.

Multifidus

The multifidus is the most medial of the lumbar back muscles, and its fibers converge near the lumbar spinous processes to an attachment known as the *mammillary process*. The fibers radiate inferiorly, passing to the TPs of the vertebrae that lie two, three, four, and five levels below. As well as some fibers uniting distally with the sacrotuberous

ligament, those fibers that extend below the level of L5 anchor to the ilium and the sacrum.

The multifidus is considered to be a series of smaller muscles, which are further divided into *superficial* and *deep* components. There is more muscle mass of the multifidus near the base of the sacrum than at the apex, especially filling the space between the PSISs rather than the ILAs.

The role of the multifidus in producing an extension force is essential to the stability of the lumbar spine, as well as functioning to resist forward flexion of the lumbar spine and the shear forces that are placed upon it. The multifidus muscle also functions to take pressure off the intervertebral discs, so that the body weight is evenly distributed throughout the whole vertebral column. The superficial muscle component acts to keep the vertebral column relatively straight, while the fibers of the deep muscle component contribute to the overall stability of the spine.

Richardson et al. (1999) identified the lumbar multifidus and the TVA as the key stabilizers of the lumbar spine. Both muscles link in with the thoracolumbar fascia to provide what Richardson et al. refer to as "a natural, deep muscle corset to protect the back from injury."

More recently, Richardson et al. (2002) investigated how these muscles impact the SIJ using the Echo Doppler (a diagnostic ultrasound device, which can show if specific muscles are contracting). They were able to demonstrate that when the TVA and multifidus co-contract, the stiffness of the SIJ increases, thereby proving that these muscles are essential to compressing the SIJ and stabilizing the joint under load (force closure) and also that it is critical that this compression occurs at just the right time.

Hydraulic Amplifier

Described by Osar (2012), the hydraulic amplifier effect occurs with the contraction of muscles within their fascial envelopes. All muscles are invested inside fascia and, as they contract, push out into the fascia, thus creating a stiffening effect around the joint. In the spine, contraction of the lumbar erector spinae and multifidus within the thoracolumbar fascia creates an extension force, assisting extension of the spine. Osar says that when the lumbosacral multifidus contracts, it broadens posteriorly into the lumbodorsal fascia (Figures 3.9 & 3.10).

This effect is aided by contraction of the TVA, which pulls the thoracolumbar fascia tight around the contracting erector spinae and multifidus, thereby creating a stable column (Figure 3.11).

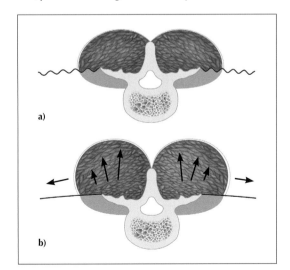

Figure 3.9. As the multifidus contracts, it pushes into the thoracolumbar fascia and, along with contraction of the TVA, provides intersegmental stability.

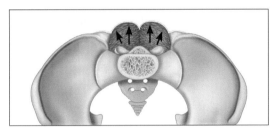

Figure 3.10. (a) The relaxed multifidus muscle in transverse section. (b) Co-contraction of the TVA and multifidus creates a stiffening tension on the thoracolumbar fascia, thereby providing intersegmental stability.

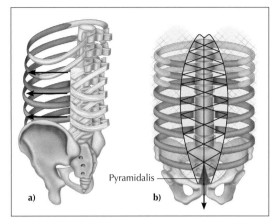

Figure 3.11. (a) As the TVA contracts, it tenses the thoracolumbar fascia, which allows the multifidus and lumbar erector spinae to contract against it and aid spinal elongation and stiffness. (b) Contraction of the pyramidalis tenses the linea alba (central tendon), creating a stable base for contraction of the TVA.

Outer Core Unit (Global System)

The force closure muscles of the outer core unit consist of four integrated myofascial sling systems (Figures 3.12–3.15):

- Posterior (deep) longitudinal sling
- Lateral sling
- Anterior oblique sling
- Posterior oblique sling

These myofascial slings provide force closure and subsequent stability for the pelvic girdle; failure or even weakness of any of these slings to secure pelvic stability can lead to lumbopelvic pain and dysfunctions. Although the muscles of the outer core unit can be trained individually, effective force closure requires specific coactivation and release of these myofascial slings for optimal function and performance.

The integrated myofascial sling system represents many forces and is composed of several muscles. A muscle may participate in more than one sling,

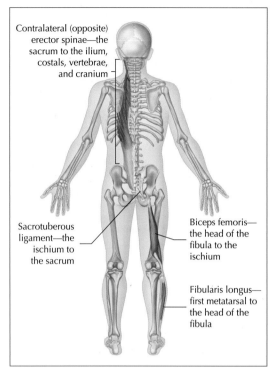

Contralateral (opposite) erector spinae—the sacrum to the ilium, costals, vertebrae, and cranium

Sacrotuberous ligament—the ischium to the sacrum

Biceps femoris—the head of the fibula to the ischium

Fibularis longus—first metatarsal to the head of the fibula

Figure 3.12. Posterior (deep) longitudinal sling.

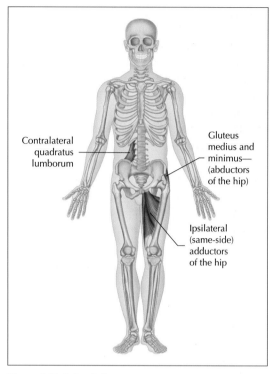

Contralateral quadratus lumborum

Gluteus medius and minimus—(abductors of the hip)

Ipsilateral (same-side) adductors of the hip

Figure 3.13. Lateral sling.

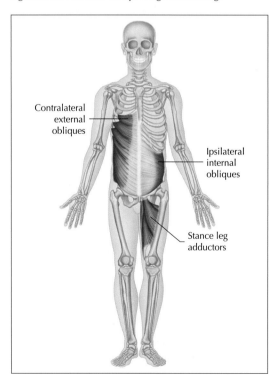

Contralateral external obliques

Ipsilateral internal obliques

Stance leg adductors

Figure 3.14. Anterior oblique sling.

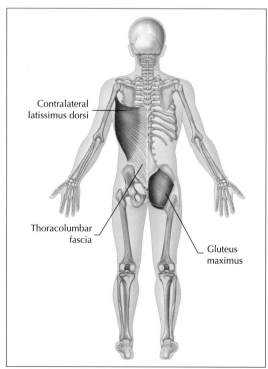

Contralateral latissimus dorsi

Thoracolumbar fascia

Gluteus maximus

Figure 3.15. Posterior oblique sling.

and the slings may overlap and interconnect, depending on the task in hand. There are several slings of myofascial systems in the outer unit, including (but probably not limited to) a *coronal* sling (having medial and lateral components), a *sagittal* sling (having anterior and posterior components), and an *oblique spiral* sling. The hypothesis is that the slings have no beginning or end, but rather connect as necessary to assist in the transference of forces. It is possible that the slings are all part of one interconnected myofascial system, and a sling that is identified during any particular motion could merely be a result of the activation of selective parts of the whole sling (Lee 2004).

The identification and treatment of a specific muscle dysfunction (such as weakness, inappropriate recruitment, or tightness) is important when restoring force closure (second component of stability) and for understanding why parts of a sling may be restricted in motion or lacking in support. Note the following points:

- The four systems of the *outer core unit* are dependent upon the *inner core unit* for the joint stiffness and stability necessary for creating an effective force generation platform.
- Failure of the inner unit to work in the presence of outer unit demand often results in muscle imbalance, joint injury, and poor performance.
- The outer unit cannot be effectively conditioned by the use of modern resistance machines, as the specific training provided by these types of machine generally does not relate to day-to-day functional movements.
- Effective conditioning of the outer unit should include exercises that require integrated function of the inner and outer units, using movement patterns common to any given client's work or sport environment (Chek 1999).

In Chapter 4 I will discuss the walking cycle (gait cycle); if you have a good understanding of the information regarding the myofascial sling systems, then, hopefully, it should make perfect sense how these slings are now incorporated into this cycle. I truly hope that as you read that particular chapter, the pieces of the jigsaw puzzle will slowly begin to form a recognizable picture. My goal is for you to come back to each specific chapter time and time again, to try to understand and digest what I have written. More importantly, however, I want you to be able to use this information in your own clinical setting to assess and treat your own athletes and patients.

Exercising the Outer Core

I personally believe that when most people go to the gym to exercise, they generally perform routines that are typically frontal-plane or sagittal-plane types of exercise: they either lift a weight to the sides (frontal plane) of their body or to the front (sagittal plane). If one were to ask these individuals to demonstrate an exercise to train their *core*, and also to perform that specific exercise in the transverse plane, I am sure that after some thought they would probably lie on their back and perform an abdominal crunch type of motion with a rotation; in other words, their elbow would be directed toward their opposite knee while performing the crunch movement (Figure 3.16(a)).

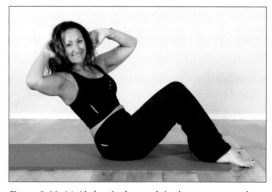

Figure 3.16. (a) Abdominal crunch in the transverse plane.

Let's be a little realistic here. Apart from when we get out of bed in the morning, when do we ever perform that type of motion on a daily basis? When do we lie on our back and rotate the elbow toward the opposite knee? I would call this exercise *non-functional*, even though the majority of gym users routinely perform this exercise for their core muscles every day in their personal exercise routines.

If you think about it, most sporting movements, or simply walking come to that, normally involve some type of action in the *transverse plane* (movement across the body) of motion. Does it not make perfect sense, therefore, to train specifically within the parameters of the transverse plane, in combination with training in the sagittal (coronal) and frontal planes?

Movement-Based Exercise

The inner core unit musculature is generally made up of postural (tonic) muscle types that function mainly as stabilizers. These inner core muscles effectively stabilize the spine and SIJ at low levels of muscular contraction, with a low susceptibility to fatigue. Coordination of the inner core is critical for proper stabilization, which then allows a coordinated recruitment of the muscles of the outer core unit. The ability of the inner core unit muscles to contract prior to force production by the phasic muscles (biased toward movements) is actually considered more important than their inherent strength.

The outer core unit is mainly a phasic system, with large muscles that have the ability, because of the fact that they are very well orientated, to produce enough force to subsequently propel the body forward. The outer core, consisting of the four myofascial slings, also plays a very important role in stabilization of the pelvis, as all of the four individual slings mentioned earlier cross this area and naturally assist in force closure of the SIJ.

With regard to functional types of exercise, movement patterns must be identified and resistance applied to those patterns in a specific way. This is what resistance training is all about … resisting movements!

If specific movements performed by athletes and patients on a daily basis can be identified, these can be replicated by using some form of resistance training, thereby creating a stability protocol. This stability protocol will be further enhanced if these movements can be performed at a speed of contraction that mimics their daily functions. This will not only improve levels of overall fitness but also promote force closure of the pelvis, and subsequently promote a stable foundation. Each exercise will now have a direct purpose and function, instead of just increasing the size of the cross-sectional area of a particular muscle.

Before embarking on a training program for the outer and inner core, it is important to understand the meanings of the words "rep" and "set."

Repetitions and Sets

Definition: A *repetition* (or *rep*) is one complete motion of an exercise. A *set* is a group of consecutive repetitions.

You may have heard someone comment that they performed, for example, three sets of 12 reps on the bench press machine. This means that they did 12 consecutive bench presses, had a break (rest), and then repeated the process a further two times.

There is no simple answer to the question of how many repetitions and sets should be performed, as the number of repetitions required depends on many factors, including where the patient/athlete is in their current training and what their individual goals are. Remember, the purpose of this book/chapter is to improve the optimum functionality of the pelvis through activation of the outer core unit so that your patient/athlete can perform the activities needed for everyday life, as well as participate in any sports-related activities. I suggest we aim for between 10 and 12 reps and between one and two sets of each exercise, at least to start with.

Please also remember that, as with any training program, the workouts will need to be progressive. For example, let's say the patient/athlete starts with two or three exercises that I have chosen from the above primary movement patterns, and they perform two sets of 10 reps for each exercise; when the patient gets to the stage where they find these exercises to be relatively easy, it is then time to progress. This might happen after one week or it might take longer, perhaps three or four weeks. The exercise can be made more difficult by simply changing the number of repetitions, reducing the rest period between sets, adding in another exercise, or changing the resistance of the band (another color), as shown in Figure 3.16(b). For example, the green band is level 1 (easy), the blue band is level 2 (moderate), and the black band is level 3 (hard).

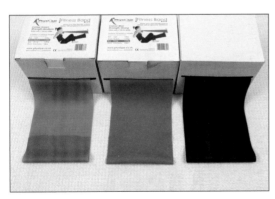

Figure 3.16. (b) Color of band indicates the level of resistance.

To progress in the program, you could, for example, ask the patient to either increase the number of repetitions, i.e. perform two sets of 12 reps (instead of 10 reps), or rest for only 30 seconds (instead of 45 seconds) between the sets. I highly recommend that everything be written down, as it is very easy to forget what was done in the previous training session—trust me on this! I can guarantee that within a few weeks the patient/athlete will easily be doing three sets of 12–15 reps for six or seven different types of outer core exercise.

The following exercises do not specify the number of repetitions and sets next to the exercise diagram, as I want to demonstrate how to perform the individual exercises correctly. Refer to Appendix 2 at the end of the book for an "Exercise Stabilization Sheet" for the outer core muscles; it has been designed specifically for you to photocopy and give out to your athletes and patients (or even for your own personal use). The blank boxes allow you to record the number of repetitions and sets for your patient's rehabilitation program for the pelvis.

Unfortunately, there are a multitude (indeed, an almost infinite number) of movements that are performed in everyday life, making it near impossible to ensure that they are all included in every gym-based training program. However, I have selected the following six exercises, which can be incorporated into any strength and stability training regime, as they will specifically target the global muscles of the outer core sling system.

Primary Movement Patterns

The following exercises are what I consider to be the primary movement patterns, and one or more of these demonstrated exercises can be included in any functional, strength, or stability training program. The therapist/trainer should nevertheless be able to modify and adapt these primary movement exercise patterns accordingly (I will explain later in this chapter). This adaptability protocol will make the exercises far more functional, as well as being more interesting and specific to the needs and demands of your athletes and patients.

Some of the exercises I mention will activate one particular sling more than another; remember, however, that there is a natural cross-over on each exercise, so it is difficult to exercise and target only one specific sling at a time. This is because all of the four slings I have mentioned have to be involved in one way or another, depending on the particular movement one is performing. For example, the anterior and posterior oblique sling will be classified as agonist and antagonist (opposite to each other); however, I consider them to be also synergists (helpers to each other), because when you walk or run in a forward direction, the right arm moves in a forward motion, subsequently activating the anterior oblique sling, but at the same time the left arm moves in a backward type of motion, activating the posterior oblique sling. Hence the opposite and synergistic theory!

I believe the theory above is explained very well by the following:

"When walking or running, every forward motion of the right limb elicits an automatic backward motion of the left limb, and vice versa. You cannot have one movement without the other."

The six primary movement pattern exercises are:

1. Push
2. Pull
3. Squat—Bend to Extend
4. Bend to Extend with Rotation
5. Single-Leg Stance
6. Rotation

Each of these movement patterns can be reproduced in a gym environment using specific exercise machines (e.g. cable machine) or resistance bands; they can, however, also be performed practically anywhere, as the majority of the exercises that I demonstrate in this chapter simply involve using a single piece of resistance exercise band, a core ball, and some dumbbells. Example movement/exercises for incorporating sling patterns are presented in the following sections.

1. Push

The first exercise I propose is very effective at utilizing the *anterior oblique* sling. If you look at the start position in Figure 3.17(a), you will notice that the exercise band (alternatively a cable machine can be used) is held with the athlete's right hand at shoulder height, and their left arm and left leg are placed in a forward position. The exercise motion is shown in Figure 3.17(b): the athlete pushes the band forward across their body, using their stance leg adductors, internal oblique, and contralateral external oblique. At the same time, the left arm comes backward, as this induces a rotation of the trunk to the left side, subsequently working the anterior oblique sling in the transverse plane of motion.

All day-to-day movements will work this muscle sling, but particularly good examples are the actions of walking, running, and throwing.

> **Note:** It is very important that the athlete control the motion in both phases, i.e. the concentric (shortening) phase and the

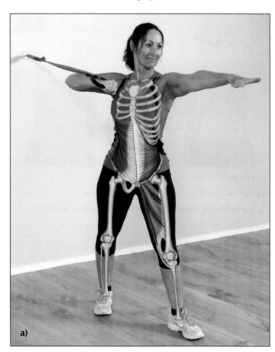

Figure 3.17. Anterior Oblique Sling: (a) start position.

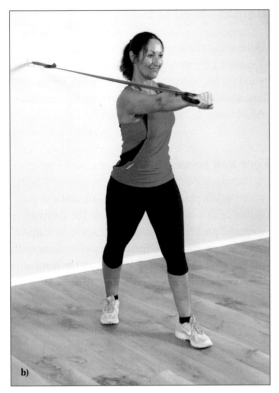

Figure 3.17. Anterior Oblique Sling: (b) finish position.

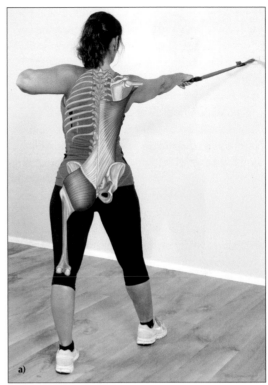

Figure 3.18. Posterior Oblique Sling: (a) start position.

eccentric (lengthening) phase, and not let the band control the movement. Moreover, one has to be very aware of the activation of the inner core musculature in order to provide the necessary stability to perform all of these exercises I describe. If you are unsure about performing these exercises, please seek professional advice before you begin any type of resistance training.

I always say the following to my athletes and patients during the demonstrations, as I consider it to be relevant to all of the sling exercises:

"You control the movement—don't let the movement control you."

2. Pull

This particular exercise is one of my personal favorites, as it is very effective in utilizing the

posterior oblique sling. If you look at the start position in Figure 3.18(a), you will see that the exercise band/cable is held with the athlete's right hand at shoulder height, and their left leg and left arm are placed in a backward position. The exercise motion is shown in Figure 3.18(b): using the latissimus dorsi, thoracolumbar fascia, and contralateral Gmax, the athlete pulls the band backward across their body with their right arm. At the same time, the left arm comes forward, as this induces a rotation of the trunk to the right side, subsequently working the posterior oblique sling in the transverse plane of motion.

I often say the following when teaching a class, or even to my athletes and patients, as I personally believe it reinforces perfectly the motion in the two exercises outlined above:

"Every pull is a push and every push is a pull—you cannot have one without the other."

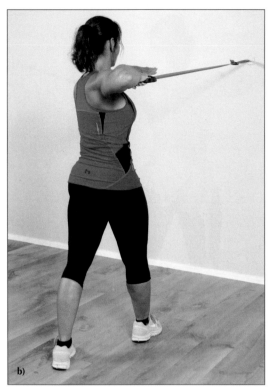

Figure 3.18. Posterior Oblique Sling: (b) finish position.

3. Squat—Bend to Extend

Any exercise or motion that incorporates a bend-to-extend type of motion, such as a typical squat or a dead lift, will incorporate the *posterior (deep) longitudinal sling* as well as involving the *posterior oblique sling*.

Core Ball Squat

A core ball is placed against the wall, and the patient positions themselves so that the core ball is located near their lower back (Figure 3.19(a)). From this position, the patient steps forward slightly, with their knees shoulder-width apart. The patient is then asked to activate the inner core and slowly squat (eccentric phase) until they reach a position of approximately 90 degrees (Figure 3.19(b)). The therapist makes sure that the tracking of the patella is toward the patient's second toe and that the patella does not pass beyond the level of the toes, as indicated by the arrows in Figure 3.19(b). The patient is then

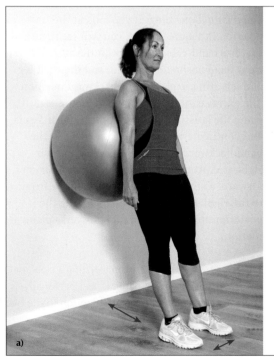
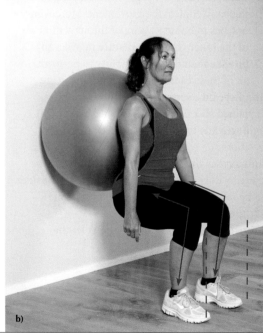

Figure 3.19. Core Ball Squat: (a) start position; (b) full-squat position.

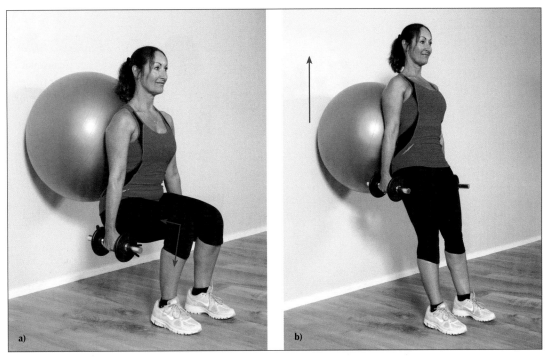

Figure 3.20. Core Ball Squat with Weight: (a) start position; (b) concentric phase.

instructed to stand up on the return (concentric phase) for a count of two; they are also instructed to squeeze their glutes just before the end phase of the squat.

Progression 1: With Weight

The Core Ball Squat exercise is performed as explained above, except the patient now holds a light weight in each hand, as shown in the start position in Figure 3.20(a). The concentric phase of the squat is shown in Figure 3.20(b).

Progression 2: With Weight and Without a Core Ball

The start position of this progression is shown in Figure 3.21(a): the athlete holds a dumbbell in each hand, with their knees shoulder-width apart. The squat is then performed to reach a knee-bend of approximately 90 degrees (Figure 3.21(b)) overleaf.

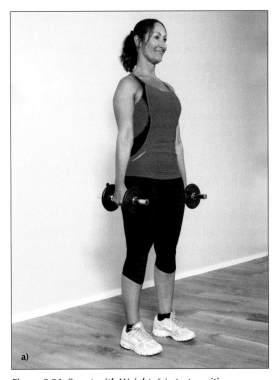

Figure 3.21. Squat with Weight: (a) start position.

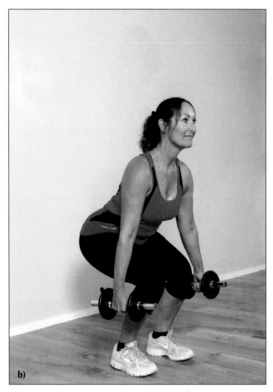

Figure 3.21. Squat with Weight: (b) finish position.

Please remember that the patella follows an imaginary line to the second toe and does not pass the level of the toes. From the 90-degree position, the athlete then rises to return to the start position. (This exercise can be performed with or without dumbbells.)

4. Bend to Extend with Rotation

A bend-to-extend type of movement with a rotation is an excellent way of incorporating the *posterior (deep) longitudinal sling* as well as the *posterior oblique sling*, all at the same time. In the start position (Figure 3.22(a)), the athlete's right hand holds the exercise band/cable at shoulder height in a forward position, and their left arm is placed in a backward position. Notice that the athlete has adopted a type of squat position, which can vary in terms of depth; the athlete here has adopted an angle of 45 degrees, but one can choose

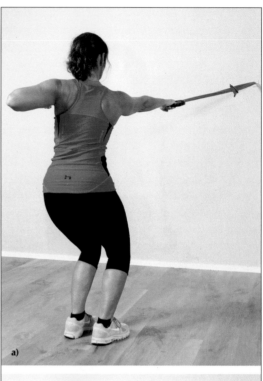

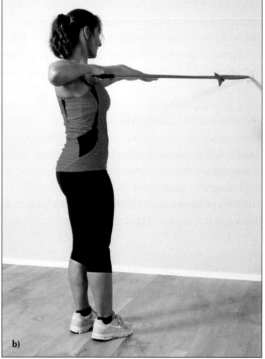

Figure 3.22. Posterior (deep) Longitudinal and Posterior Oblique Sling: (a) start position; (b) finish position.

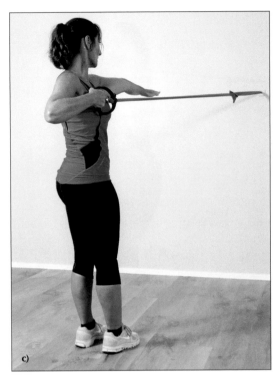

Figure 3.22. Posterior (deep) Longitudinal and Posterior Oblique Sling: (c) alternative position for the arm at the end of motion.

to start at a smaller or greater angle, depending on requirements.

The exercise motion is shown in Figure 3.22(b): the athlete pulls the band backward across their body, using both of their posterior slings. At the same time, the left arm comes forward as the athlete returns to the erect position. Figure 3.22(c) shows an alternative end position for the right arm, as some patients find this movement easier. What I sometimes suggest is that my athletes vary or alternate the two movements described above.

5. Single-Leg Stance

The *lateral sling* system helps to stabilize the body in the frontal plane. During any type of single-leg stance the hip abductors—gluteus medius (Gmed) and gluteus minimus (Gmin)—and the adductors of the supporting leg work in conjunction with the contralateral (opposite) quadratus lumborum (QL) to stabilize the pelvis. The internal and external oblique abdominal musculature also works synergistically to secure a stable spine and pelvis. Dysfunction of the lateral sling system is a common source of injury to the back, the SIJ, and also the supporting leg. If you think about it, most sports are single-leg dominant in nature. During walking, but especially running and sprinting, the body is propelled forward through powerful single-leg actions, so the need for a strong and functional lateral sling system is of paramount importance. This specific sling system will help improve overall athletic performance and conserve energy expenditure, as well as reducing the possibility of sustaining musculoskeletal types of injury.

Any exercises which incorporate a movement that relies on being in a single-leg stance position will activate the muscles of the lateral sling. The last chapter of *The Vital Glutes: Connecting the Gait Cycle to Pain and Dysfunction* (Gibbons 2014) specifically targets exercises that are biased toward a single-leg stance position in order to activate the Gmed muscle in particular of the lateral sling system. For this text I will therefore include an exercise that is demonstrated on one leg; however, I am also going to simultaneously target the anterior and oblique slings while performing a push and a pull motion as described earlier.

Note: If you have difficulty standing on one leg, possibly because of weakness of the lateral sling, I recommend that you read *The Vital Glutes: Connecting the Gait Cycle to Pain and Dysfunction* (Gibbons 2014) first, so that you will have a better understanding of why and how to initiate the strengthening of the Gmed/lateral sling system before embarking on trying to perform the following exercise.

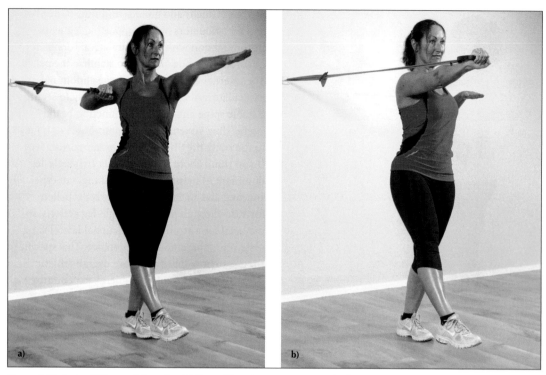

Figure 3.23. Lateral Sling and Anterior Oblique Sling: (a) start position; (b) finish position.

Lateral Sling and Anterior Oblique Sling

Figure 3.23(a) shows the athlete in a single-leg stance position (lateral sling), while at the same time holding the exercise band with their right hand, with the arm raised to 90 degrees; the left arm is held in a forward position and the body is rotated to the right. The athlete then pushes the right arm forward while the left arm moves backward; this will induce a rotation of the trunk to the left side (Figure 3.23(b)), subsequently activating the anterior oblique system and at the same time utilizing the lateral sling musculature.

Lateral Sling and Posterior Oblique Sling

Figure 3.24(a) shows the athlete standing on one leg (lateral sling), while at the same time holding the exercise band with their right hand, with the arm raised to 90 degrees; the left arm is held in a backward position and the body is rotated

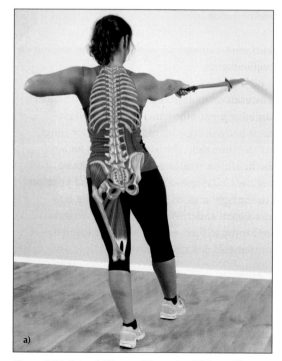

Figure 3.24. Lateral Sling and Posterior Oblique Sling: (a) start position.

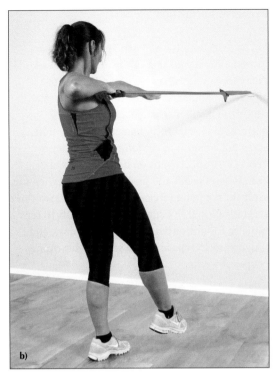

Figure 3.24. Lateral Sling and Posterior Oblique Sling: (b) finish position.

to the left. The athlete then pulls the right arm backward while the left arm moves forward; this will induce a rotation of the trunk to the right side (Figure 3.24(b)), causing an activation of the posterior oblique system and at the same time utilizing the lateral sling muscles.

6. Rotation

The last motion of the primary movement patterns is *rotation*, which will utilize mainly the internal and external obliques as well as the gluteal muscles.

Anterior Rotation

Figure 3.25(a) shows the athlete standing with their legs shoulder-width apart, holding the exercise band with their right hand, and

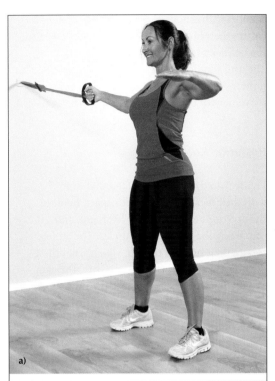

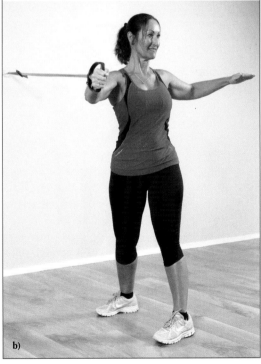

Figure 3.25. Oblique Sling—Anterior Rotation: (a) start position; (b) finish position.

stabilizing the inner core muscles. The athlete rotates their body to the left, which will utilize the oblique muscles (see Figure 3.25(b)). The arm should be relatively fixed, since the motion is from the trunk and not from the movement of the arm.

Posterior Rotation

Figure 3.26(a) shows the athlete standing with their legs shoulder-width apart, holding the exercise band with their left hand, and stabilizing the inner core muscles. The athlete rotates their body to the left, which will utilize the oblique muscles (Figure 3.26(b)). The arm should be relatively fixed, since the motion is from the trunk and not from the movement of the arm.

Exercise Variations

I have demonstrated and explained six primary movement patterns that can be included in an outer core stabilization program. When I see athletes and patients for the first time I normally suggest that only two initial exercises are performed to start with, namely a *pull* motion and a *push* motion. I recommend that they do between 10 and 12 reps on both sides (push exercise on the left and push on the right, then the same for the pull exercise) and repeat for two/three sets (10–12 × 2/3). I suggest starting with 10 reps initially, for one or two sets (once per day), and progress to 15 reps for three sets per day over a couple of weeks.

When patients visit me for their second and third sessions, I will personally check their

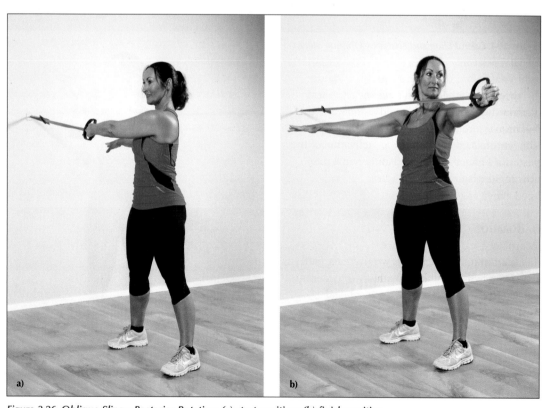

Figure 3.26. Oblique Sling—Posterior Rotation: (a) start position; (b) finish position.

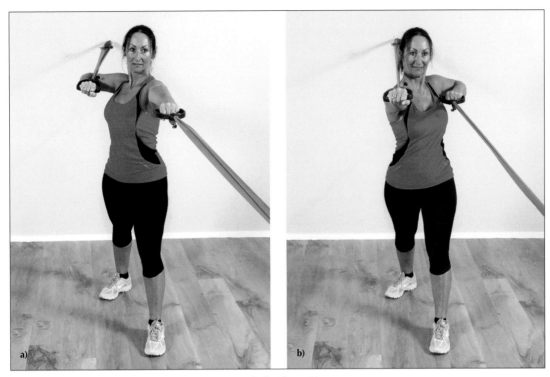

Figure 3.27. Combined Push–Pull: (a) start position; (b) finish position.

technique before I give them another exercise; this way I can make sure that what I showed them initially is being reiterated in their demonstration back to me. When I am happy with what they have shown me, then, and only then, will I give them another one (or possibly two) of the primary movement exercises listed above.

Once all of the six exercises have been incorporated into their exercise regime, we can then start to add a bit of variety and adapt the exercises accordingly to make them more specific and tailored to the athlete, depending on their individual sporting requirements. Although the following exercises are explained and demonstrated for only one side of the body, they would of course be incorporated in a program for both sides (an exercise performed on the right is repeated on the left, and so on).

Combined Push–Pull

The athlete in Figure 3.27(a) holds a piece of exercise band with their left hand and another piece of exercise band with their right hand. They are asked to combine the motion of a push from the right arm and a pull from the left arm (Figure 3.27(b)). It is recommended that the inner core muscles are activated, to make sure that they are stable while performing this motion.

Combined Push–Pull on One Leg

This is the same exercise as above, but this time the athlete adopts a single-leg stance position while grasping the exercise bands (see Figure 3.28(a)). The motion is a combination of a push from the right arm and a pull from the left arm while standing on one leg (see Figure 3.28(b)).

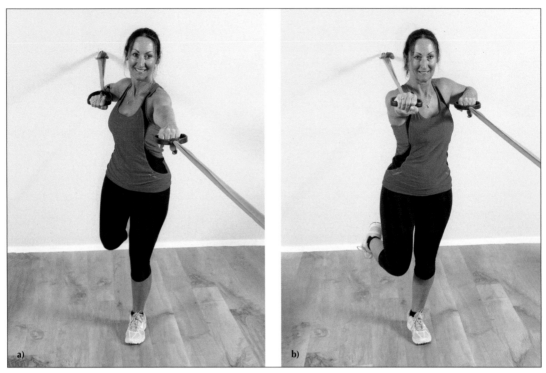

Figure 3.28. Combined Push–Pull on One Leg: (a) start position; (b) finish position.

Push with Lunge

In the start position shown in Figure 3.29(a), the athlete is holding the exercise band with the right hand at shoulder height, and the left arm and left leg are placed in a forward position. The exercise motion is shown in Figure 3.29(b): the athlete pushes the band forward across their body, while at the same time the left arm moves backward as the left knee bends to perform a lunge type of motion. (Note: the left knee does not past the level of the toes, and the patella follows the second toe.)

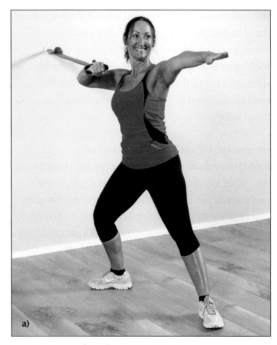

Figure 3.29. Push with Lunge: (a) start position.

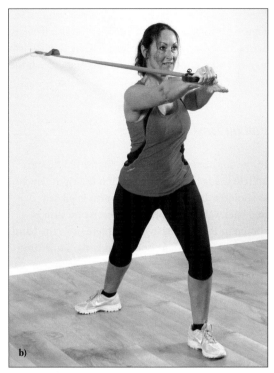

Figure 3.29. Push with Lunge: (b) finish position.

Pull with Lunge

In the start position (Figure 3.30(a)) you will notice that this time the athlete is holding the exercise band with their right hand placed in a forward position at shoulder height; the left arm is held in a backward position, with the left leg forward. The exercise motion is shown in Figure 3.30(b): the athlete pulls the band backward across their body, while at the same time the left arm moves forward as the right knee bends to perform a lunge type of motion. (Note: the right knee does not pass the level of the toes, and the patella follows the second toe.)

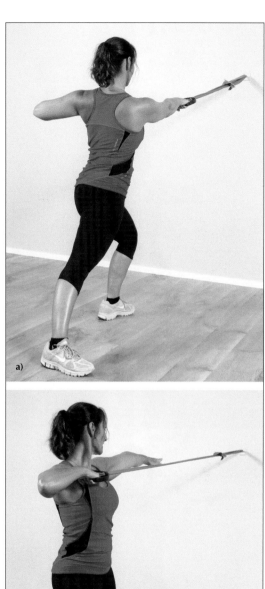

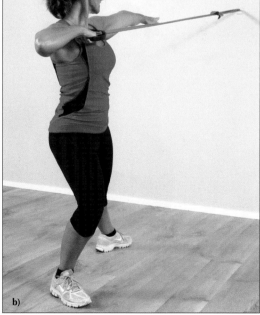

Figure 3.30. Pull with Lunge: (a) start position; (b) finish position.

Push on Unstable Base

In the start position shown in Figure 3.31(a), the exercise band is held in the right hand at shoulder height, and the left arm is placed in a forward position. The exercise motion is shown in Figure 3.31(b): the athlete pushes the band forward across their body, and at the same time the left arm moves backward while maintaining stability on the unstable base.

Pull on Unstable Base

In the start position shown in Figure 3.32(a), the athlete holds the exercise band in the right hand at shoulder height, and the left arm is placed in a backward position. The exercise motion is shown in Figure 3.32(b): the athlete pulls the band backward across their body, and at the same time the left arm moves forward while maintaining stability on the unstable base.

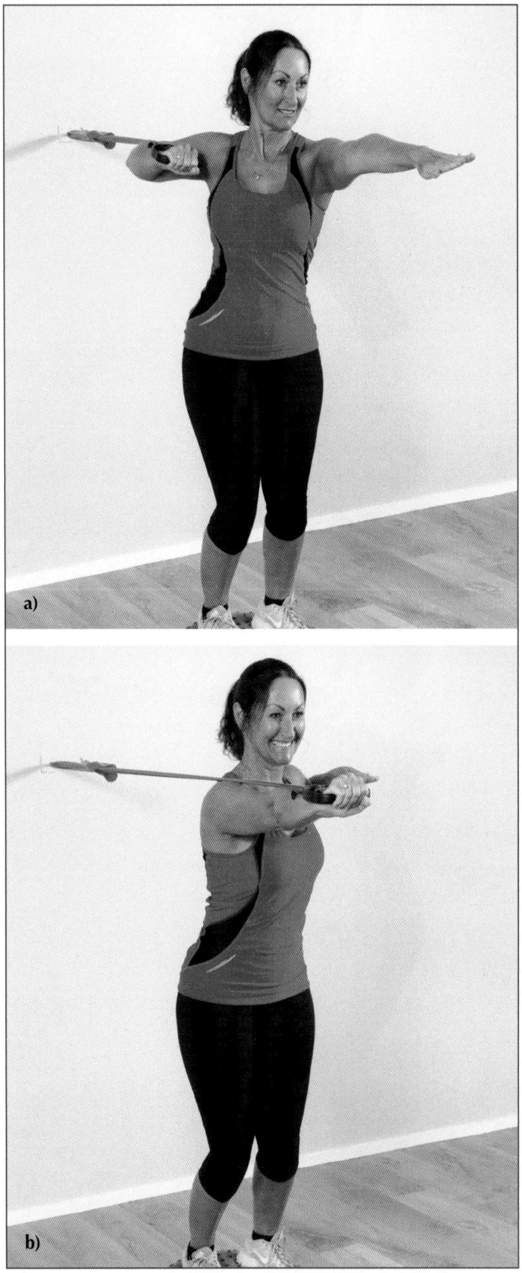

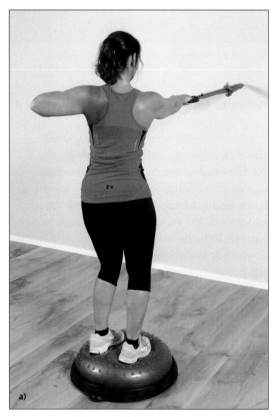

Figure 3.31. Push on Unstable Base: (a) start position; (b) finish position.

Figure 3.32. Pull on Unstable Base: (a) start position.

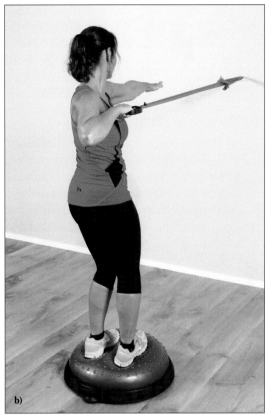

Figure 3.32. Pull on Unstable Base: (b) finish position.

Bend to Extend with Rotation on Unstable Base

In the start position shown in Figure 3.33(a), the athlete holds the exercise band with their right hand at shoulder height and places their left arm in a backward position, while adopting a squat position on the unstable base. The exercise motion is shown in Figure 3.33(b): the athlete pulls the band backward across their body, and at the same time the left arm moves forward as they return to the erect position while maintaining stability on the unstable base.

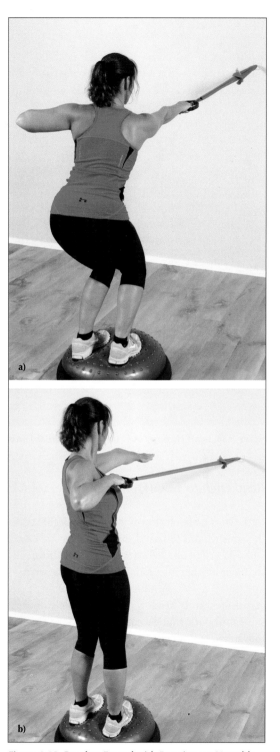

Figure 3.33. Bend to Extend with Rotation on Unstable Base: (a) start position; (b) finish position.

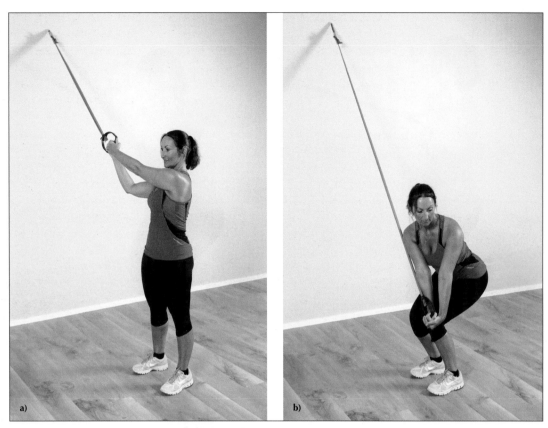

Figure 3.34. Bend High to Low: (a) start position; (b) finish position.

Bend High to Low (Wood Chop)

In the start position shown in Figure 3.34(a), the athlete holds the band simultaneously with their right and left hands at a point above shoulder height. The exercise motion is shown in Figure 3.34(b): the athlete pulls the band across their body to a low position, while at the same time performing a squatting motion. This movement is similar to chopping wood.

Bend Low to High (Reverse Wood Chop)

In the start position shown in Figure 3.35(a), the athlete squats down and holds the band simultaneously in the right and left hands at a point below shoulder height. The exercise motion

is shown in Figure 3.35(b): the athlete pulls the band across their body to a high position, while at the same time rising from the squat to an erect position.

Bend Low to High (Single Arm)

A combination of a bend-low-to-high type of movement with a rotation and a squat is an excellent way of incorporating the posterior longitudinal sling as well as the posterior oblique sling, both at the same time. In the start position (Figure 3.36(a)), you will see that the athlete is holding the exercise band/cable at a lower level with their right hand in a forward position, and the left arm is placed in a backward position; the trunk adopts a position of left rotation.

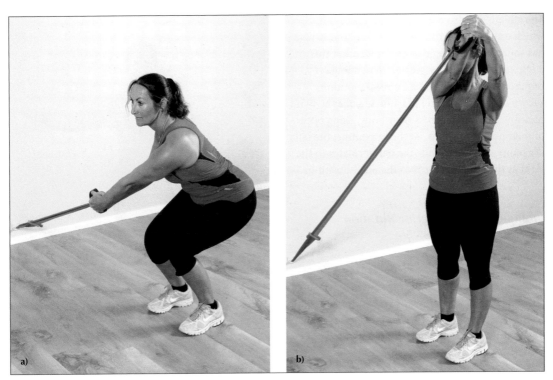

Figure 3.35. Bend Low to High: (a) start position; (b) finish position.

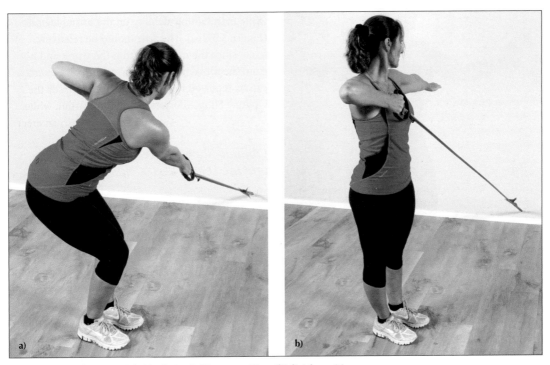

Figure 3.36. Bend Low to High (Single Arm): (a) start position; (b) finish position.

The athlete has also adopted a squat position, which can vary in terms of depth: here the athlete has squatted to an angle of 45 degrees, but this angle can be smaller or greater, depending on requirements. Overleaf the exercise motion is shown in Figure 3.36(b): the athlete pulls the band backward and high across their body, using both of their posterior slings. At the same time, the left arm comes forward while the trunk rotates to the right as the athlete returns to the erect position.

Oblique Sling—Anterior Rotation on Unstable Base

In this demonstration shown in Figure 3.37(a), the athlete starts with their legs shoulder-width apart, and holds the exercise band with their right hand while stabilizing their inner core muscles. The athlete then rotates their body to the left,

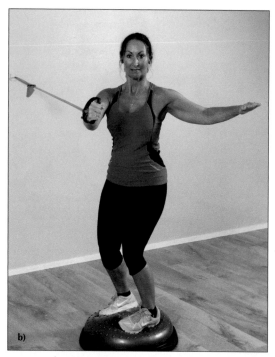

Figure 3.37. Oblique Sling—Anterior Rotation on Unstable Base: (b) finish position.

while maintaining stability on the unstable base (Figure 3.37(b)). The arm should be relatively fixed, since the motion is from the trunk and not from the movement of the arm (the same exercise can be repeated for a posterior rotation; see Oblique Sling—Posterior Rotation).

Oblique Sling—Anterior Rotation on One Leg

Figure 3.38(a) shows the athlete standing with their legs shoulder-width apart and holding the exercise band with their right hand, while stabilizing the inner core muscles. The athlete then rotates their body to the left while performing the exercise in a single-leg stance position (Figure 3.38(b)). The arm should be relatively fixed, since the motion is from the trunk and not from the movement of the arm (the same exercise

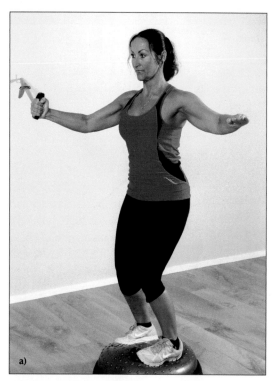

Figure 3.37. Oblique Sling—Anterior Rotation on Unstable Base: (a) start position.

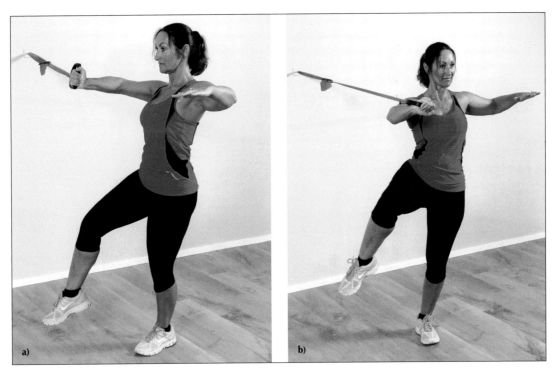

Figure 3.38. Oblique Sling—Anterior Rotation on One Leg: (a) start position; (b) finish position.

can be repeated for a posterior rotation; see Oblique Sling—Posterior Rotation).

Rotation While Kneeling

For an anterior rotation, the athlete in Figure 3.39(a) kneels on an exercise mat, with their knees shoulder-width apart, and holds the exercise band with their left hand while stabilizing the inner core muscles. The athlete then rotates their body to the right while performing the exercise in a kneeling position (see Figure 3.39(b)). The arm should be relatively fixed, since the motion is from the trunk and not from the movement of the arm.

The same exercise can be repeated for a posterior rotation (see Figure 3.40a & b).

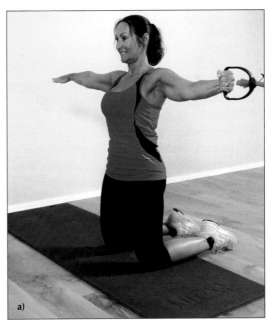

Figure 3.39. Oblique Sling—Anterior Rotation While Kneeling: (a) start position.

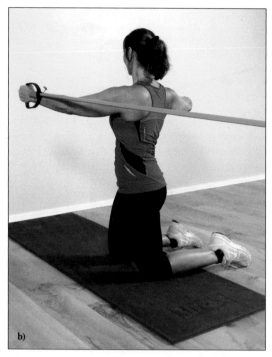

Figure 3.39. Oblique Sling—Anterior Rotation While Kneeling: (b) finish position.

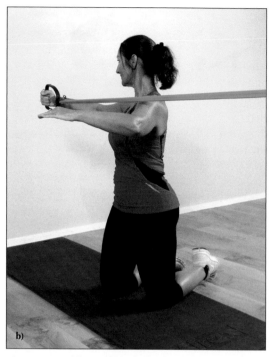

Figure 3.40. Oblique Sling—Posterior Rotation While Kneeling: (a) start position; (b) finish position.

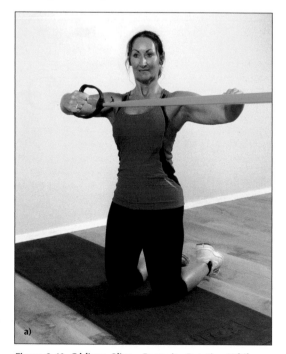

Figure 3.40. Oblique Sling—Posterior Rotation While Kneeling: (a) start position.

Conclusion

We need the inner and outer core units to function synergistically to: (1) stabilize the body; and (2) create powerful and economic movement. Without efficient functioning of the inner unit there is no stability of the spine and SIJs. Moreover, the core will not be able to provide a stable base of contraction for the phasic muscles (outer core) to contract, which can result in a loss of limb power and a reduced economy of movement patterns, as well as an increased susceptibility to musculoskeletal injuries.

A well-conditioned inner core unit is very dependent on strong outer core unit systems, and vice versa, in order to protect the smaller inner unit muscles, the spinal ligaments, and the associated joints of the spine and pelvis.

Let me try to explain this concept with the following example. I have been fortunate to work with the Oxford University Boat Team for many years. When they have been rowing on very flat and calm lakes and rivers, I have mentioned to them many times (mainly during training sessions) that the outer core unit (i.e. the phasic muscles) is doing most of the work to propel the boat through the water, and the inner core unit is relatively relaxed (by comparison), especially on calm water.

I am currently the sports osteopath for the team, so when they finish rowing I always ask them how they feel (in terms of their lower back and pelvis, etc.); I can honestly say that most of the time there are no reports of musculoskeletal issues. However, when the team row on the "tideway" (the River Thames in London) in preparation for the annual Boat Race, it is a completely different story; this river can be very unpredictable—one minute the river is particularly choppy and the next it is calm. The River Thames is tidal fed from the sea, which alters the tone of the water; in addition, passing motorboats produce waves that can also affect the flow and manner of the water. Because of these variable circumstances, if the river appears rougher than usual, then I consider the inner core unit to be working a lot harder than normal, because it has to stabilize each of the individual rowers in their seats. Moreover, the inner core unit is trying to stabilize the rowing boat to prevent it from tilting from side to side, while at the same time the outer core unit is still being utilized to propel the boat forward. At the end of the training session, I ask the rowers the same question (relating to any issues with the lower back); in this case, probably around half of them say that they need to see me for treatment to help reduce the symptoms that they are experiencing.

In order to have a strong outer core unit, it is paramount that the inner core unit be stabilized first, as the most susceptible area in a rower's musculoskeletal system is the lower lumbar spine—usually disc injuries occur to L4/5 or to L5/S1.

Most of the rowers know a bit about core stability training, and some have done one or two exercises before, mainly abdominal trunk curls and planks (two exercises that I typically classify as *non-functional* and definitely not effective for the inner core—hence not recommended). During the times I have been involved in their training, I have tried to make the inner core training fun, as these exercises are generally not appealing to a bunch of fit young rowers who are used to doing only bench presses, squats, and lunges.

For example, I would get all the team (eight in this case, or nine including the cox) to sit on gym balls in a straight line, one behind the other, facing the same way—except for the cox at the end, who would sit facing them. While sitting on the ball, they would then place their feet on the ball in front and try to maintain stability by using their inner core muscles, which is especially challenging, as the feet are now lifted off the floor.

The idea of this exercise was to mimic sitting in a boat on water. From this position, each team member had to keep the line of eight rowers (nine including cox) stable by activating their inner core muscles. Once this had been achieved, we would then try to mimic the motion of rowing while still sitting on the gym balls. Apart from being fun, this is a great way of activating the inner core muscles without having to think about the processes involved.

This exercise is just one example that emphasizes to the team *why* training the inner core unit is every bit as important as training the outer core unit. The mentality of many athletes who I have come into contact with is to train only the muscles they can see and not the ones that they cannot.

Note: I haven't included many inner core exercise explanations/demonstrations, as I feel it is not within the scope of this book. The reason for this is mainly that I wanted to focus my attention on training and stabilizing the outer core muscles in this text, because I feel that this particular area has been neglected in the past. There are numerous books on the shelves that offer specific inner core activation exercises, so may I suggest you consult one of them. I have discussed here only briefly some of the inner core exercises that I incorporate in the rowing training program—my strategy is to train the rowers' inner core muscles, without them actually being aware that they are training them!

The Walking/Gait Cycle and Its Relationship to the Pelvis

4

Most of us, I would say, take walking for granted—it is something that we just do without understanding what exactly is going on … until we suffer pain somewhere in our body, and then the simple action of walking becomes very painful. What I would like to do in this chapter is examine in detail what exactly takes place when we walk (you might want to go through some of the movements yourself as they are described) and the relationship of the gait cycle to both the pelvis and the kinetic chain.

Gait Cycle

Definition: A *gait cycle* is a sequence of events in walking or running, beginning when one foot contacts the ground and ending when the same foot contacts the ground again.

The gait cycle is divided into two main phases: the *stance* phase and the *swing* phase. Each cycle begins at initial contact (also known as *heel-strike*) of the leading leg in a stance phase, proceeds through a swing phase, and ends with the next contact of the ground with that same leg. The stance phase is subdivided into *heel-strike*, *mid-stance*, and *propulsion* phases.

Human gait is a very complicated, coordinated series of movements. An easier way of thinking about the gait cycle is to break it down into phases. The stance phase is the weight-bearing component of each cycle; it is initiated by heel-strike and ends with toe-off from the same foot. The swing

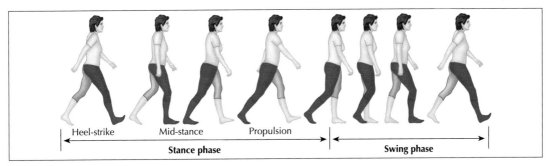

Figure 4.1. Stance and swing phases of the gait cycle.

phase is initiated with toe-off and ends with heel-strike. It has been estimated that the stance phase accounts for approximately 60% of a single gait cycle, and the swing phase for approximately 40% (see Figure 4.1).

Heel-Strike

If you think about the position of your body just before you contact the ground with your right leg during the contact phase of the stance phase, the right hip is in a position of flexion, the knee is extended, the ankle is dorsiflexed, and the foot is in a position of supination (Figure 4.2). The tibialis anterior muscle, with the help of the tibialis posterior, works to maintain the ankle/foot in a position of dorsiflexion and inversion (inversion is one part of the motion referred to as *supination*).

In normal gait, the foot strikes the ground at the beginning of the heel-strike in a supinated position of approximately 2 degrees. A normal foot will then move through 5–6 degrees of pronation at the

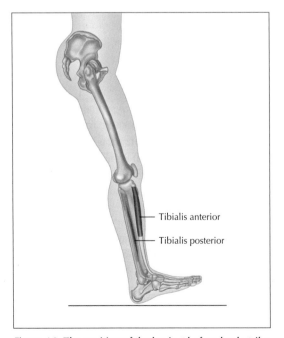

Tibialis anterior

Tibialis posterior

Figure 4.2. The position of the leg just before heel-strike.

subtalar joint (STJ) to a position of approximately 3–4 degrees of pronation, as this will allow the foot to function as a "mobile adaptor."

A Myofascial Link

As a result of the ankle and foot being in a position of dorsiflexion and supination, the tibialis anterior (which is the main muscle responsible for this anatomical position, with an insertion on the medial cuneiform and first metatarsal on the foot) is now part of a link system that we will call a *myofascial sling* (see Chapter 3). This sling, starting from the initial origin of the tibialis anterior, continues as the insertion of the fibularis longus (onto the first metatarsal and medial cuneiform, as in the case of the tibialis anterior) to its muscular origin on the lateral side and head of the fibula. This bony landmark is also where the biceps femoris muscle inserts.

The sling now continues as the biceps femoris muscle toward its origin on the ischial tuberosity, where the muscle attaches to the tuberosity via the sacrotuberous ligament; often the biceps femoris directly attaches to this ligament rather than to the ischial tuberosity, and some authors have mentioned that potentially 30% or more of the biceps femoris attaches directly to the ILA of the sacrum. If you think back to Chapter 1, I mentioned that Vleeming et al. (1989a) found that in 50% of subjects, part of the sacrotuberous ligament was continuous with the tendon of the long head of the biceps femoris.

The sling then carries on as the sacrotuberous ligament, which attaches to the inferior aspect of the sacrum at the ILA and fascially connects to the contralateral (opposite side) multifidi and to the erector spinae, which continue to the base of the occipital bone. This myofascial sling is known as the *posterior longitudinal sling (PLS)* or the *deep longitudinal sling (DLS)*, as shown in Figure 4.3.

Even before you initiate the contact to the ground through heel-strike, dorsiflexion of the ankle

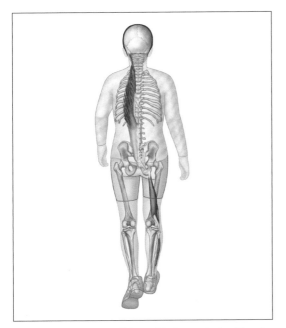

Figure 4.3. A person walking, with the posterior (deep) longitudinal sling muscles highlighted.

(by the contraction of the tibialis anterior) initiates a coactivation of the biceps femoris and fibularis longus just prior to heel-strike. Studies have shown that the biceps femoris communicates with the fibularis longus at the fibular head, transmitting approximately 18% of the contraction force of the biceps femoris through the fascial system into the fibularis longus muscle. This co-contraction therefore serves to "wind up" the thoracolumbar fascia mechanism as a means of stabilizing the lower extremity; this results in the storage of the necessary kinetic energy that will subsequently be released during the propulsive phase of the gait cycle.

The posterior (deep) longitudinal sling as described is being fascially tensioned; the increased tension is focused on the sacrotuberous ligament via the attachment of the biceps femoris (Figure 4.4(b)). This connection will assist the *force closure* mechanism process of the SIJ; in simple terms, this creates a self-locking and stable pelvis for the initiation of the weight-bearing gait cycle. You may also notice that the right ilium (Figure 4.4(a–c)) undergoes posterior rotation

during the swing phase, which will assist the force closure of the SIJ because of the increased tension in the sacrotuberous ligament.

You can also see from Figure 4.4(c), overleaf, that there is now tension developing within the right sacrotuberous ligament because of the contraction of the biceps femoris as well as the posterior rotation of the right innominate; at the same time,

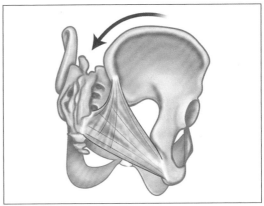

Figure 4.4. (a) Right ilium in posterior rotation— sacrotuberous ligament tensioned.

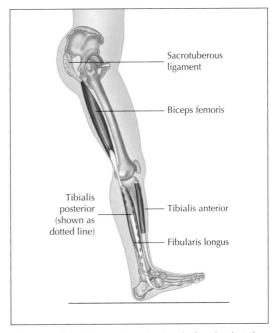

Figure 4.4. (b) Position of the leg just before heel-strike, with the biceps femoris and sacrotuberous ligament tensioned.

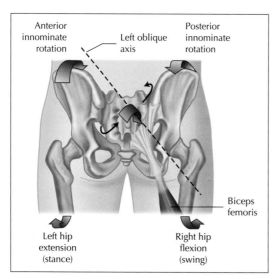

Figure 4.4. (c) Right ilium in posterior rotation—left ilium in anterior rotation and sacrum rotated on the L-on-L axis.

the left innominate is rotating anteriorly and the sacrum has rotated on the left oblique axis (L-on-L). This specific motion of the lumbopelvic hip complex occurs all at the same time as the right heel-strike.

For the next phase, you might want to stand and slowly go through the following movements so that you can get a sense of what happens with your body in the normal walking cycle. As explained above, just before the heel-strike phase your hip will be flexed, your knee extended, and your ankle dorsiflexed with the foot supinated. The tibialis anterior and tibialis posterior maintain this position of the ankle and foot, and as you contact the ground, these two muscles are responsible for controlling the rate of pronation through the STJ by contracting eccentrically.

As your right leg moves from heel-strike to toe-off (stance phase), your body weight begins to move over your right leg, causing your pelvis to shift laterally to the right. As the movement continues toward toe-off, your right pelvic innominate bone begins to rotate anteriorly while your left innominate bone begins to rotate posteriorly.

As you proceed through the gait cycle, you now enter the mid-stance phase of gait. This is where the hamstrings should reduce their tension because of the natural anterior rotation of the pelvis and the slackening of the sacrotuberous ligament. Form closure at this point is gradually lost during the latter part of the stance phase, so that stability at this point is chiefly maintained through force closure. This is the point during the mid-stance phase where the Gmax on the right side should take the role of the continued movement of lower limb extension, as well as working in concert with the contralateral latissimus dorsi (left side). The active contraction of these two muscles increases the tension in the thoracolumbar fascia (posterior oblique sling), thus providing the necessary force closure stability to the right SIJ during the mid-stance phase of gait.

I would like to elaborate a little more on this process. Phasic contraction of the Gmax occurs in the mid-stance phase; the Gmax simultaneously contracts with the contralateral latissimus dorsi—it is this muscle that will extend the arm through what is known as *counter-rotation*, to assist in propulsion. The thoracolumbar fascia, which is a sheet of connective tissue, is located between the Gmax and the contralateral latissimus dorsi; this fascial structure is forced to increase its tension because of the contractions of the Gmax and latissimus dorsi. This increased tension will assist in stabilizing the SIJ of the stance leg through the force closure mechanism.

In Figure 4.5 you can see that just before heel-strike, the Gmax will reach maximum stretch as the latissimus dorsi is being stretched by the forward swing of the opposite arm. Heel-strike signifies a transition to the propulsive phase of gait, at which time the Gmax contraction is superimposed on that of the hamstrings.

As explained in the previous paragraphs, activation of the Gmax occurs in concert with contraction of the contralateral latissimus dorsi, which is now extending the arm in unison with the propelling leg. The synergistic contraction of the Gmax and

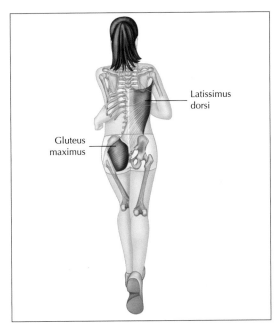

Latissimus dorsi

Gluteus maximus

Figure 4.5. A person running, with the posterior oblique sling muscles highlighted.

the contralateral latissimus dorsi creates a state of tension within the thoracolumbar fascia, which will be released in a surge of energy that will assist the muscles of locomotion. This stored energy within the thoracolumbar fascia helps to reduce the overall energy expenditure of the gait cycle. Janda (1992, 1996) mentions that poor Gmax strength and activation is postulated to decrease the efficiency of gait. The posterior oblique sling also contains a lower component (consisting of the continuations of the Gmax), which acts to increase the tension of the iliotibial band (ITB); this helps to stabilize the knee during the stance phase of gait.

As we progress from the mid-stance phase to heel-lift and propulsion, the foot begins to re-supinate and passes through a neutral position when the propulsive phase begins; the foot continues in supination through toe-off. As a result of the foot supinating during the mid-stance propulsive period, the foot is converted from a "mobile adaptor" (which is what it is during the contact period) to a "rigid lever" as the mid-tarsal joint locks into a supinated position. With

the foot functioning as a rigid lever (as a result of the locked mid-tarsal joint) during the time immediately preceding toe-off, the weight of the body is propelled more efficiently.

Pelvis and SIJ Motion

Next we will take a look at the pelvis and how it functions during the mid-stance phase of the walking cycle. As the right innominate bone starts to rotate anteriorly from an initial posteriorly rotated position, the tension of the right sacrotuberous ligament is reduced, and the sacrum will be forced to move (passively) into a right torsion on the right oblique axis (R-on-R) (recall, the motion of the pelvis and sacroiliac joint in Chapter 2). In other words, the sacrum rotates to the right and side bends to the left, because the left sacral base moves into an anterior nutation position (this is also known as *Type I spinal mechanics*, as the rotation and side bending are coupled to opposite sides—see Chapter 6; the motion is illustrated in Figure 4.6(a) overleaf.

We also need to mention and consider that, as the left side of the sacrum moves forward into nutation, the right side of the sacral base will move backward into counter-nutation *(R-on-R)*; this is mainly because of the slackening of the right sacrotuberous ligament and the continual anterior rotational movement of the right innominate bone during mid-stance.

Owing to the kinematics of the sacrum, the lumbar spine rotates left (opposite to the sacrum) and side bends to the right (Type I mechanics), as shown is Figure 4.6(b) overleaf. The thoracic spine rotates right (same as the sacrum) and side bends to the left, and the cervical spine rotates right and side bends to the right. The cervical spine coupling is opposite to that of the other vertebrae, since its specific spinal motion is classified as *Type II spinal mechanics* (Type II means that rotation and side bending are coupled to the same side—see Chapter 6 for more details).

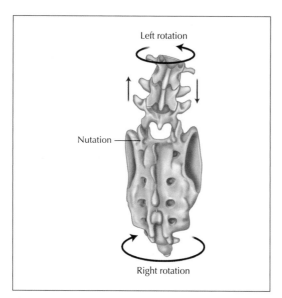

Figure 4.6. (a) Sacral rotation and lumbar counter-rotation.

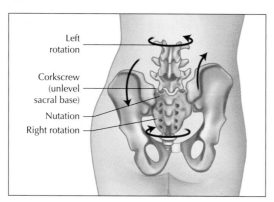

Figure 4.6. (b) Sacral rotation and lumbar counter-rotation superimposed on the pelvic girdle.

As the left leg moves from weight bearing to toe-off, the left innominate, the sacrum, and the lumbar and thoracic vertebrae undergo sacral torsion, rotation, and side bending in a similar manner to that described above, but with movements in the opposite directions.

The anterior oblique also works in conjunction with the stance leg adductors, ipsilateral internal oblique, and contralateral external oblique muscles (Figure 4.7). These integrated muscle contractions help stabilize the body on top of the stance leg and assist in rotating the pelvis forward for optimum propulsion in preparation for the ensuing heel-strike.

The abdominal oblique muscles, as well as the adductor muscle group, serve to provide stability and mobility during the gait cycle.

When looking at the EMG recordings of the oblique abdominals during gait and superimposing them on the cycle of adductor activity in gait, Basmajan and De Luca (1979) found that both sets of muscles (obliques and adductors) contribute to stability at the initiation of the stance phase of the gait cycle, as well as to the rotation of the pelvis and the action of pulling the leg through during the swing phase of gait. (This was also demonstrated by Inman et al. (1981).) As the speed of walking increases to running and sprinting speeds, the activation of the anterior oblique system becomes more prominent as well as a necessity.

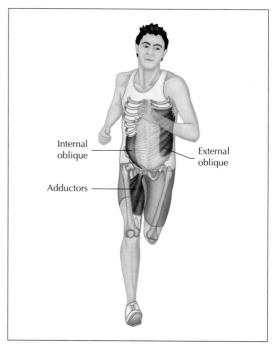

Figure 4.7. A person running, with anterior oblique sling muscles highlighted.

The swing phase of gait utilizes the lateral sling system, as we have now entered the single-leg stance position. This sling connects the Gmed and Gmin of the stance leg, and the ipsilateral (same side) adductors, with the contralateral (opposite) QL. Contraction of the left Gmed and adductors stabilizes the pelvis, and activation of the contralateral QL will assist in elevation of the pelvis; this will allow enough lift of the pelvis to permit the leg to go through the swing phase of gait. The lateral sling plays a critical role, as it assists in stabilizing the spine and hip joints in the frontal plane and is a necessary contributor to the overall stability of the pelvis and trunk.

Not only does the lateral sling system provide stability that protects the working spinal and hip joints, but it is also a necessary contributor to the overall stability of the pelvis and trunk. Should the trunk become unstable, the diminished stability will compromise one's ability to generate the forces necessary for moving the swing leg quickly, as required in many work and sports environments. Attempts to move the swing leg, or to generate force with the stance leg during gait and other functional activities, can easily disrupt the SIJs and symphysis pubis and cause kinetic dysfunction

in joints throughout the entire kinetic chain (Chek 1999).

Maitland (2001) mentions that proper body movement while walking is influenced by the ability of the sacrum to cope with left torsion on the left oblique axis (L-on-L) and right torsion on the right oblique axis (R-on-R). Since most walking is accomplished with the vertebral column relatively upright and vertical, for the purpose of this discussion we will assume that your spine and sacrum are in neutral while you walk.

The way our axial skeletal system alternately undulates in side bending and rotation as we walk is very interesting and extremely important to our overall well-being. It is a movement that is reminiscent of the undulating action of a snake as it slithers through the grass. The big difference between a snake and a human, of course, is that our snakelike spine has ended up being given two legs on which to walk.

Summary of the Sacrum and the Gait Cycle

To summarize the gait cycle and the specific motion of the sacral spine, the sacrum is capable of left rotation on the left oblique axis (L-on-L), from which it then returns to a neutral position. From this neutral position the sacrum then rotates to the right on the right oblique axis (R-on-R) and again returns to neutral. The movement of the sacrum is *anterior* in its nature as it undergoes the earlier-described motion of nutation. The forward nutational movement during walking is anterior on one side, followed by a return to the neutral position; anterior nutation then occurs on the opposite side, before the sacrum again returns to neutral. This process is continually repeated. According to various studies, the motion of posterior nutation (counter-nutation) does not appear to extend past the neutral position during the normal walking/gait cycle.

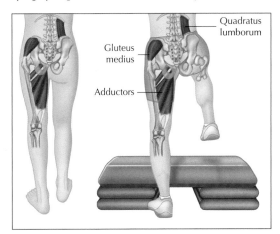

Figure 4.8. An example of the swing phase of gait, with lateral sling muscles highlighted on the single-stance leg.

Quadratus lumborum

Gluteus medius

Adductors

Leg Length Discrepancy and Its Relationship to the Kinetic Chain and the Pelvis

I would personally say that the majority of patients and athletes who visit my clinic in Oxford generally present with pain somewhere in their bodies. Part of my initial screening is to have the patient stand with their back to me; with them in this position, I place both my hands on top of their iliac crest to see if there is any pelvic obliquity; in other words, I look for a low or a high side (Figure 5.1). Very often I do find that there is a discrepancy in the level of the height of the iliac crest between the two sides, which could possibly indicate a leg length discrepancy (LLD), or, as it has been alternatively termed, a *short-leg syndrome* or a *long-leg syndrome.*

LLD is possibly the most significant postural asymmetry that presents itself to the physical therapist. The existence of a considerable difference between the two sides can be very detrimental to how we function on a day-to-day basis, not least during the walking/gait cycle: the discrepancy can significantly affect not just the pelvis and SIJ but also our overall posture.

> **Definition:** *Leg length discrepancy (LLD) is a condition where one leg is shorter than the other.*

One has to decide if there is an "actual" (or "true") anatomical LLD or an "apparent" LLD, as the condition has been implicated in all sorts of deficiencies related to our gait pattern and

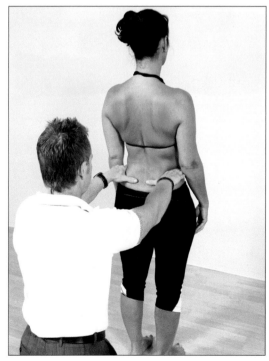

Figure 5.1. Observation of measurement of leg length by palpation of the iliac crest.

running mechanics. LLD has also been linked to postural dysfunctions, as well as to increased incidence of scoliosis, lower back pain, SIJ dysfunction, and osteoarthritis of the spine, hip, and knee. Even stress fractures of the hip, spine, and lower extremity have been related to changes in leg length.

The *actual* (true) leg length measurement is the length that is typically determined by the use of a tape measure from a point on the pelvis—the ASIS—to the medial malleolus (distal part of the tibia), as shown in Figure 5.2; the ASIS is normally used as the landmark, since it is impossible to truly palpate the femur below the iliac crest. Before taking this measurement, it is beneficial to measure

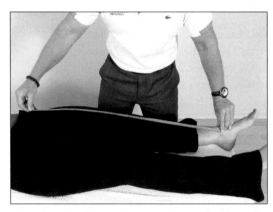

Figure 5.2. True leg length measurement, taken from the ASIS to the medial malleolus.

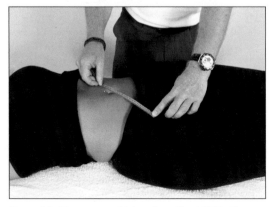

Figure 5.3. Measurement taken from the ASIS to the umbilicus.

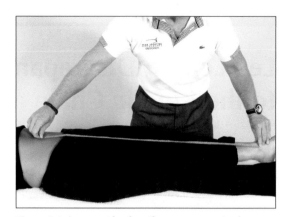

Figure 5.4. Apparent leg length measurement, taken from the umbilicus to the medial malleolus.

the distance from the ASIS on the left and right sides to the umbilicus (Figure 5.3) to ascertain if any pelvic rotation is present. If a difference in the two measurements is found, the pelvic rotations need to be corrected before a reassessment is done (Chapter 13).

If the measurements taken from the ASIS to the medial malleolus on both sides are the same, it can then be assumed that the lengths of the two limbs are effectively equal; on the other hand, if the measurements differ, one can assume that an actual (true) LLD is present.

The *apparent* leg length measurement is taken from the umbilicus to the medial malleolus (Figure 5.4). If the measurements taken on both sides are different, one can assume that a dysfunction exists somewhere, which will require further investigation.

Supine to Long Sitting Test

The supine to long sitting test is commonly used to ascertain the relevance of the SIJ to an apparent or true LLD. With the patient in a supine position, the therapist initially compares the relative positions of the two medial malleoli, to see if a difference exists between these two bony landmarks (Figure 5.5(a) overleaf).

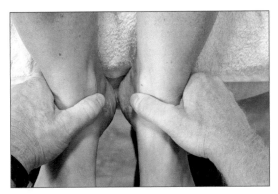

Figure 5.5. (a) Palpation for the positions of the medial malleoli (leg length) in the supine position.

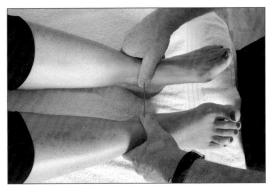

Figure 5.5. (c) Close-up view of the positions of the medial malleoli (leg length) after the supine to long sitting test. The malleoli appear to be level in this case.

Next the patient is asked to sit up, while keeping their legs extended. The positions of the two medial malleoli are compared once again, to see if there is any change (Figure 5.5(b–c)).

If, for example, there is a *posterior* innominate present, the leg that appeared shorter in the supine position will now appear to lengthen with the sitting-up motion. If there is an *anterior* innominate present (very common on the right side), the leg that appeared longer in the supine position will now appear to shorten with the sitting-up motion (Figure 5.5(d)).

If an actual (true) LLD is present, the true long leg will appear to be longer in the supine position as well as in the sitting position, so no obvious

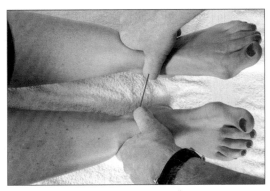

Figure 5.5. (d) Close-up view of the positions of the medial malleoli (leg length) after the supine to long sitting test. The right leg appears shorter, possibly indicating a right anterior innominate rotation.

change will be observed (this, along with further discussion on leg length changes, will be presented in more detail in Chapter 12). For now, it is sufficient to simply note down if there are any changes in the position of the medial malleoli in the supine and long sitting positions.

Note: This test can help in differentiating between a true LLD and a sacroiliac dysfunction. Please be careful when asking your patients to perform this test: the motion of the test (sitting up) can easily exacerbate a patient's symptoms because of the forces needed to perform the action. Assistance by the therapist might sometimes be necessary.

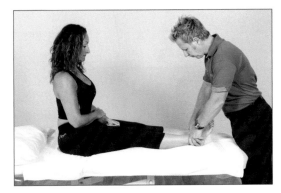

Figure 5.5. (b) Observation of the positions of the medial malleoli (leg length) after the supine to long sitting test.

Types of LLD

LLD can be divided into three main groups:

1. **Structural:** This is an actual (or true) shortening of the skeletal system, typically caused by one of four things:
    *   Congenital defect, e.g. congenital dysplasia of the hip joint
    *   Surgery, e.g. total hip replacement (THR)
    *   Trauma, e.g. fractured femur or tibia
    *   Disease process, e.g. tumor, osteoarthritis, Osgood–Schlatter disease, or Legg–Calvé–Perthes disease

    Fractured bones in children have been known to grow faster for many years after the healing process: this can naturally result in the limb becoming anatomically longer.

2. **Functional:** This can be a development from altered biomechanics of the lower body, such as ankle and foot over-pronation or supination, pelvic obliquity, muscle imbalances (as a result of, for instance, a weak Gmed and abdominals or tight adductors and hip flexors), hip or knee joint dysfunction, and even poor inner core stabilization, to name just a few.

3. **Idiopathic:** If there are obvious findings during the history taking and assessment process, the physical therapist may have an idea as to the cause of the patient's LLD. However, if the therapist cannot ascertain a reason for the change in the presenting leg length, the condition would be classified as *idiopathic*, which means that it arises independently, not as a result of some other condition.

Kiapour et al. (2012) estimate that a LLD of as little as 0.4" (1cm) increases the load across the SIJ fivefold.

Assessment

The therapist has to be very intuitive during the initial assessment. When placing their hands on top of the iliac crest of a patient in a standing position in order to ascertain pelvic obliquity, the therapist needs to be aware of a "pelvic shift" as the patient stands. Let me give you an example: if the patient has a weak Gmed muscle on the left side, the pelvis might appear to drop to the right side and deviate or laterally shift to the left; this will have the effect of the left iliac crest appearing elevated on that side (left), thus giving the natural appearance of a longer left leg (Figure 5.6).

When the patient presents to the clinic, one can assume that the pain has been present for a while; since the pain has persisted for an extended period of time we can safely say that the presenting condition is now in the chronic stage. Because of the natural overcompensatory mechanisms that occur through soft tissue chronicity, the postural muscles are probably held in a shortened and subsequently tight position; one particular lumbar spine muscle that has a natural tendency to shorten as a result of LLD is the QL. A perceived problem can arise when the patient lies on their back (supine position), so that you can observe the positions of the left and right medial malleoli when

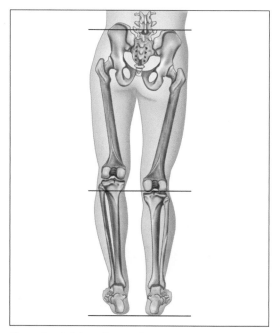

Figure 5.6. Left long-leg syndrome versus right short-leg syndrome.

looking for any LLD. You may notice that the left medial malleolus appears nearer to the patient's head (cephalic) than the one on the right, giving the appearance of a short left leg. This apparent shortness of the leg is possibly a result of a tight left QL muscle. When the patient was standing, however, you may have convinced yourself that the patient's left leg actually looked longer!

This might seem initially confusing, but just think about it for a moment. Could it not simply mean (this is only one example because there are many potential causes of a higher iliac crest) that when the patient adopts a standing position the Gmed on the left side is weak, causing the pelvis to shift to the side of weakness, now giving the appearance of a longer left leg? Conversely, is it not possible that when the patient is in a supine position, the left QL is held in a shortened position, which is responsible for hitching up the pelvis, having the effect of pulling the leg closer to the head and thus making the left leg appear shorter?

The following phrase might help you remember this process:

"When you are standing, the weak muscles show themselves; when you are lying, the short muscles show themselves."

Foot and Ankle Position

One of the most neglected aspects of the body, especially when patients present to the clinic, is the position of the lower limb. Every single day osteopaths, chiropractors, and physical therapists see lots of patients who initially present with lower back, pelvis, and sacroiliac pain. These specialist therapists naturally spend a lot of time observing and assessing the pelvis and lumbar spine to ascertain which tissue they personally consider to be responsible for giving the person the pain. This presenting pain may, however, just be a symptom, and the cause of the pain could be somewhere else, away from the actual site of the pain.

Dr. Ida Rolf, who invented the Rolfing soft tissue technique, states: "Where you think the pain is, the problem is not." One of my popular sayings that I impress on my students (which I consider to relate to what Dr. Rolf states) is the following:

"The only person interested in the pain is your patient; you the therapist should try to find the actual cause of the pain and not simply treat where it hurts."

It is very important that when assessing your patients, you should observe the position of the lower limb and in particular the foot and ankle complex, as a faulty foot and ankle structure can profoundly affect leg length and the natural position of the pelvis. The most common asymmetrical foot position that patients present with has to be what is commonly called an *over-pronated foot* (or pes planus), as shown in Figure 5.7.

It has been widely thought that when we actually present with a true LLD, the body will try to compensate for the longer leg through lowering the medial arch of the foot by pronating at the STJ. The action of pronation is called *tri-planar motion*

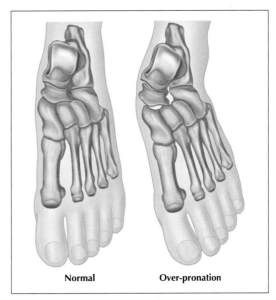

Normal   Over-pronation

Figure 5.7. Over-pronation syndrome.

and consists of three movements: dorsiflexion of the ankle, eversion, and abduction of the foot complex. The position of this increased pronation is basically the body's natural compensatory mechanism to try to "shorten" the leg because it is anatomically longer.

The plantar surface of our feet has thousands of sensory receptors that are responsible for the position of the foot; the smallest shift in weight will be enough to signal the brain to induce a compensatory reaction. On the contralateral side (shorter leg), the compensatory mechanism will cause the medial arch to adopt a supinated position (tri-planar motion of plantar flexion, inversion, and adduction). The compensatory mechanism changes the position of the arch in an attempt to lengthen the apparent shorter leg. When physical therapists assess their patients they will need to check for this compensatory pattern, because, if left unchecked, excessive foot pronation caused by an anatomically longer leg (subsequent supination of the contralateral foot as compensation) will in turn cause an internal rotation of the lower extremity and an external rotation of the contralateral lower limb. This compensatory mechanism will then have the effect of altering the whole kinetic chain from the foot all the way up to the occiput.

True LLD and the Relationship to the Pelvis

Let's continue with a "thought process" just for a moment. Now consider that your patient has an actual longer leg on the left side, which you have ascertained because of the higher position of the iliac crest and the possible compensatory pronation of the STJ on the same side, as well as the leg length appearing longer (through observation of the medial malleoli) in the supine and long sitting position. Before I continue with the discussion, just have a think to yourself about what position the innominate bone might be in if the left leg, say, is *anatomically* longer.

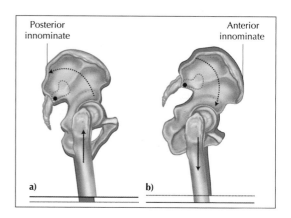

Figure 5.8. (a) Long-leg innominate compensation; (b) Short-leg innominate compensation.

The innominate rotation will naturally be coupled with a LLD as a result of the compensatory mechanisms: if you look at Figure 5.8(a), you will see that the femoral head on the long-leg side forces the innominate into a superior and posteriorly rotated position. Conversely, the innominate on the low femoral head side drops down and anteriorly rotates (Figure 5.8(b)). What we have now, therefore, is the left innominate being forced into a *posterior* rotation and the right innominate into an *anterior* rotation.

Think about what lies between the two innominate bones—yes, the sacrum. As a result of the compensatory rotation of both of the innominate bones (because of the anatomical LLD) in opposite directions to each other, a motion of the sacrum occurs—left-on-left (L-on-L) sacral torsion (Figure 5.9), which was covered in Chapter 2. Recall, a L-on-L sacral torsion means that the sacrum has rotated to the left on the left oblique axis and has side bent to the right, as it is ruled by Type I spinal mechanics (rotation and side bending are coupled to opposite sides, as established by Fryette (1918) and the law of spinal mechanics, which will be discussed in Chapter 6). This complexity of the innominate rotations that are coupled with a sacral torsion is usually depicted as a *pelvic torsion*, or even a *pelvic obliquity*, and will require

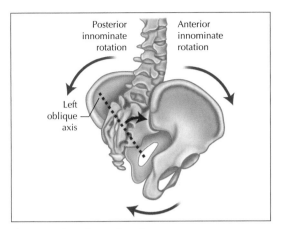

Figure 5.9. L-on-L sacral torsion.

a good understanding before a treatment plan is introduced.

True LLD and the Relationship Between the Trunk and the Head

You will notice in Figure 5.10(a) & (b) that on the left side there is a lower shoulder position on the high innominate side: this is a common finding in the case of a compensatory functional scoliosis. Some authors, however, have considered this to occur as a result of a "handedness pattern": for example, if you are left handed, the left shoulder might appear to be lower, and if you are right handed, the right shoulder might appear to be lower. I agree that the pattern of handedness is probably true, but only if the iliac crests are level; otherwise some form of scoliosis has to exist, especially if the iliac crest and shoulder positions are asymmetric.

What else do you observe in Figure 5.10(b)? If you look at what is happening to the left QL, you might assume that this muscle is being held in a shortened position because of the higher left innominate. This assumption is correct, as you can also see that the lumbar spine is side bending toward the longer left leg (concavity) and rotating toward the shorter right leg (convexity).

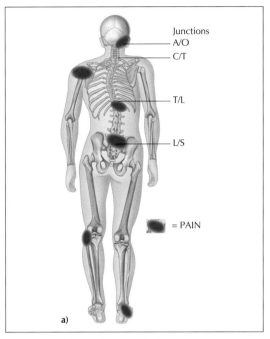

Figure 5.10. (a) Functional scoliosis compensation.

As a result of the ascending functional scoliosis, the right shoulder is higher. You might also notice a short "C" curve in the cervical spine; this will probably cause the scalenes, sternocleidomastoid (SCM), upper trapezius, and possibly the levator scapulae muscles on the right side to adopt a shortened and subsequently

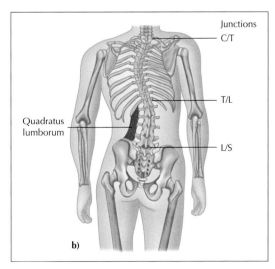

Figure 5.10. (b) Functional scoliosis compensation. Quadratus lumborum on left is short/tight.

tight position. This typical adaptation of muscular imbalance will help maintain an erect head position with the eyes level. The body will always want to be level no matter what and will do almost anything to accomplish this, through naturally adapting the position of the occipitoatlantal joint (OAJ), and in so doing can suffer enduring pain to maintain equilibrium. Common painful conditions that patients might present with are headaches, active trigger points, tinnitus, temporomandibular joint (TMJ) dysfunction, and even eye and facial pain.

LLD and the Gait Cycle

As we walk, if our gait cycle pattern has been altered because of an actual or an apparent LLD, the shorter leg will feel like it is stepping down, and the long leg will compensate by a sort of "vaulting" motion. It is almost like stepping into a small pothole with every step you take; imagine repeating this at least ten to fifteen thousand times a day—it will easily cause potential pain patterns of dysfunction! Common compensations are sometimes seen when patients are asked to walk: on the short-leg side, the patient might have a tendency to walk on their toes, and on the long-leg side, the patient may have a tendency to flex their knee, but this will depend on the discrepancy.

For the body to be an effective locomotor during the gait cycle, a well-aligned and symmetrical body is essential. When the positions of the innominate bones of the pelvis are altered by actual or apparent leg length discrepancies, it is easy to see how patients can present with pain, not only at the SIJ and lumbar spine but also everywhere else in their body that is going through a compensation pattern.

I mentioned earlier that there could be a weakness of the Gmed on one side of the body; this weakness could lead to a potential compensatory pattern for subsequent shortness issues with the tensor fasciae latae (TFL) and ITB on the other

side. If there is weakness of the Gmed, the patient can have either a *Trendelenburg* pattern of gait or a *compensatory Trendelenburg* pattern of gait (see "Standing Balance Test," later in this chapter). Whichever way you look at this, the patient is going to have an antalgic type of gait, which simply means that they will walk with some form of limp; this compensation can only cause one thing over time and that will simply be pain.

Summary of LLD Compensations to the Sacrum

- The sacrum typically *rotates* toward the *long* leg and *side bends* toward the *short* leg.
- A posterior sacrum (counter-nutation) has been found to be associated with same-side piriformis spasm.
- An anterior sacrum (nutation) has been found to be associated with same-side Gmed spasm.

Summary of LLD Compensations to the Lumbar Spine

- The lumbar spine typically *rotates* toward the side of the low sacral base/*short* leg and *side bends* toward the *long* leg.
- Facet pain due to compression is common on the concavity side (side-bending side) of the lumbar spine.
- The iliolumbar ligament can cause pain as it is stretched on the convex side of the lumbar spine and has been argued to refer pain to the groin, testicle, and medial thigh on the same side as the stretched ligament.

Summary of LLD Compensations to the Iliopsoas Muscle

- The iliopsoas muscle is generally considered to be tight on the side of the short leg. Note that a left iliopsoas muscle spasm can cause a pelvic side shift to the right, mimicking a shorter left leg.

- The iliopsoas muscle (iliacus in particular) can cause the innominate bone to compensate by rotating anteriorly on the side of the short leg, functionally causing a lengthening of that leg, while the innominate bone on the long side may do the opposite (posterior innominate rotation).
- Unilateral spasm (contraction) of the iliopsoas can create a lumbar concavity on the same side (because of side bending), with rotation to the opposite side, and potentially sets up a positive side shift on the side opposite to the spasm. It is important that the physical therapist always assesses for and treats iliopsoas spasm in the case of a suspected short leg or a positive pelvic lateral side shift.
- Iliopsoas spasm pain is generally worse on standing from a seated position, and less pain is perceived as the iliopsoas stretches out.

In summary, when looking at the level of the iliac crest, one has to determine if there is a LLD. If there is, one then has to ascertain if the dysfunction is a true discrepancy or a functional discrepancy, as the compensation pattern can change depending on the diagnosis. For example, if you find a true anatomical LLD, the innominate bone on the longer leg will normally try to compensate by rotating posteriorly, as seen in Figure 5.7 and explained earlier. Moreover, the femur and lower limb on the anatomically longer leg will follow the compensatory model by rotating medially, as seen in Figure 5.5, and the foot will try to pronate at the STJ, since the longer leg will attempt to *shorten* itself. At the same time, the actual shorter leg will compensate by supinating at the ankle mortise; this in effect can cause the tibia and femur to rotate externally and the innominate bone to rotate anteriorly as the leg tries to make itself appear *longer*.

Over-Pronation Syndrome

Let's look at another compensation model for a patient who appears to have a LLD. In this case it is a *functional* LLD, and the apparent shorter leg of

the patient exhibits an over-pronation of the STJ, rather than the true longer leg compensating by pronating to shorten itself. As a result, the body will try to compensate by causing an internal rotation of the tibia and femur (Figure 5.11(a)); this will have the effect of the innominate bone rotating anteriorly (posteriorly in a true LLD, as explained earlier), which in turn can cause an increased lumbar lordosis with subsequent lower back pain.

According to podiatrists, over-pronation syndrome is a very common pattern found in the majority of people to some extent or another. It is best identified with the patient standing barefoot. The big clue is that one arch is lower or flatter than the other: the lower arch side is over-pronating. Sometimes, both sides may be over-pronating, but one side is generally over-pronating more than the other, or one side might be normal and the other side lower.

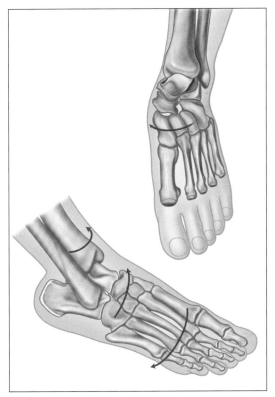

Figure 5.11. (a) A foot in over-pronation with internal tibial rotation.

It is easy to confirm the condition by simply placing one finger under the patient's arch, noting how much of your finger goes underneath, and comparing the result with the other side. Are they the same or different? If one side is noticeably lower than the other, you have found a patient with an over-pronation syndrome. Another test to confirm over-pronation is to observe the Achilles tendon from the posterior aspect: you will typically notice a bowing on the side with the lower arch.

It should be noted that over-pronation syndrome could originate not only from the foot and ankle but also from the innominate bone of that side. When the foot and ankle complex over-pronates, the innominate bone will normally rotate anteriorly. However, if we look at it the other way around, an anterior rotation of the innominate (common on the right side) can force the medial arch of the foot into an over-pronated position. This becomes a chicken and the egg situation, but that is irrelevant, as the only consideration is whatever presents itself now. In my experience, you might need to correct the innominate rotation and the over-pronation to help reduce the patient's presenting symptoms.

If you feel the pronation is attributed to the most common presentation of a right anterior innominate rotation with a compensatory left posterior innominate rotation, then you might also notice the right foot appears to be in a position of *relative* external rotation or abduction, even though the tibia is still in a position of internal rotation because of the pronation of the STJ. This is possibly caused by the anticlockwise (left) rotation of the pelvis (compared with the left foot, which appears to be in supination and relative internal rotation or adduction). As mentioned earlier, even though the foot appears to be externally rotated, the tibia is still in an overall position of internal rotation (Figure 5.11(b)).

On the side that appears to be pronated with a relative external rotation or abduction of the foot (most common on the right side; the tibia is still maintained in an internally rotated position,

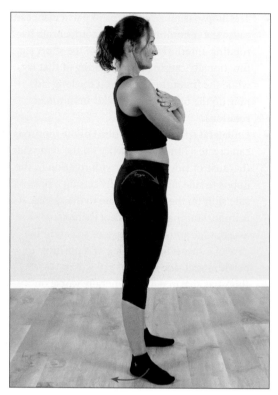

Figure 5.11. (b) External rotation/abduction of the foot and ankle with STJ pronation, commonly found with a right anterior innominate rotation.

Figure 5.11(c)), the following musculoskeletal presentations are common:

- Medial collateral ligament and medial plica
- Groin and/or medial thigh pain
- Medial tibial stress syndrome (shin splints)
- Medial ankle ligaments sprain
- Posterior tarsal tunnel syndrome/posterior tibial nerve
- Compression of the sural nerve at the lateral ankle
- Increased Q angle (valgus) and stress to the lateral compartment of the knee
- Lateral tracking of the patella
- Plantar fasciitis
- Sesamoiditis
- Achilles tendinopathy

On the side that appears to be supinated with a relative internal rotation or adduction of the foot

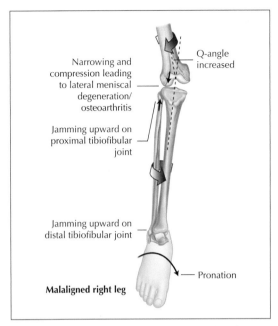

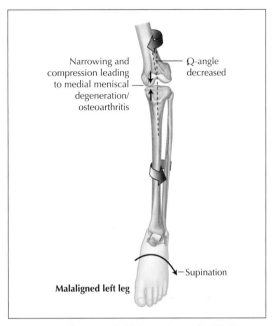

Figure 5.11. (c) Internal tibial rotation and ankle/foot with STJ pronation, commonly found with a right anterior innominate rotation.

Figure 5.11. (d) External tibial rotation and ankle/foot with STJ supination, commonly found with a posterior innominate rotation.

as compared to the other side (common on the left side; the tibia is still maintained in an externally rotated position, Figure 5.11(d)), the following musculoskeletal presentations are common:

- Strain to the hip abductors
- Greater trochanteric bursitis
- Lateral shin pain
- Lateral ankle ligaments sprain
- Nerve traction injury to the lateral femoral cutaneous and superficial peroneal nerves
- Increased pressure to the medial knee compartment due to varus position and decreased Q angle
- Traction of the lateral collateral ligament
- Tibial and metatarsal stress fractures
- Plantar fasciitis
- Morton's neuroma
- Achilles tendinopathy

You can see already that both compensatory mechanisms I have mentioned throughout this chapter have a pronation issue at the STJ; however, the *true* leg length compensation of the longer leg

forced the innominate bone to rotate *posteriorly*, whereas the *functional* LLD of the over-pronation syndrome caused the innominate bone to rotate *anteriorly*.

You can probably gather from all the information above that there can be a lot going on at the same time throughout the kinetic chain; everything that has been mentioned can affect the *length* of the leg. It is correct to assume that this area of discussion is somewhat complex, and it might be difficult to know where to start in the assessment or even in the treatment program.

In all that has been discussed above, there lies a potential solution to the jigsaw puzzle of patients' symptoms and dysfunctions. There exists what I call a *key* to unlocking the problem; the difficulty in physical therapy, however, is finding where to start and "insert the key" (excuse the expression). I can guarantee that, over the years, inexperienced therapists will have time and time again inserted the key into the wrong place, i.e. where the patient feels the pain and not where the problem lies. Recall the wise words of Dr. Ida Rolf!

During the practical components of my lectures to physical therapists attending my courses, I sometimes hear myself saying the following:

"Treat any dysfunctions that you find at the time during the treatment session, and the body will hopefully guide you onto the correct pathway."

After that statement I normally say this:

"If, however, after three or even five physical therapy sessions, the patient's symptoms are not reducing, then you the therapist will need to alter your thought process and reassess and potentially treat other areas of the patient's body that you initially felt might not be related to the cause of their presenting symptoms."

LLD and the Relationship to the Gluteal Muscles

So how does all this affect the glutes? When you have a compensation pattern, the femur not only rotates to compensate in the transverse plane (as explained earlier), but also experiences a compensatory mechanism of adduction and abduction in the frontal plane. Thus, in simple terms, if you have a lower limb that is held in an adducted position, then the abductor muscle group can be forced into a lengthened and subsequently weakened position, while the adductors will be held in a shortened and subsequently tight position. For a leg that is held in abduction, the situation is reversed.

If you look back at Figure 5.6 you will see that the left leg appears longer because of the higher left iliac crest, the innominate has rotated posteriorly, the femur has internally rotated, and the foot has pronated. In this compensation the left leg will be in a position of adduction (Figure 5.12), and consequently the right leg will be held in a position of abduction (Figure 5.13). This will have an effect

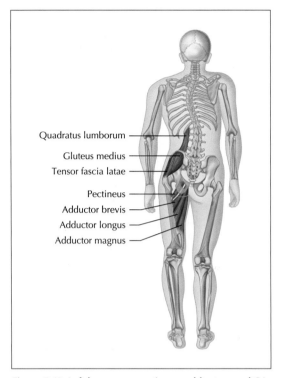

Figure 5.12. Left leg compensations—adductors and QL short and tight, with Gmed and TFL long and weak.

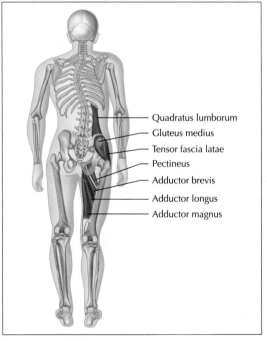

Figure 5.13. Right leg compensations—adductors and QL long and weak, with Gmed and TFL short and tight.

on the musculature of the associated areas: some of these muscles will be held in a shortened position and some in a lengthened position.

Standing Balance Test

When a patient is asked to stand on one leg and lift the opposite knee toward their waist, the physical therapist needs to observe the level of the PSIS as the patient transfers their weight to one leg. The patient should be able to shift their weight onto the stance leg (the right leg in Figure 5.14) with good muscular control of the Gmed of that leg. If the PSIS dips down on the leg that is being lifted (the left leg in Figure 5.15) rather than remaining level (Figure 5.14), it might be assumed that the Gmed on the opposite side (right side) is unable to control the movement; the patient might then have an altered pattern of gait when they go through the gait cycle (Figure 5.16). This altered gait pattern is called a *Trendelenburg gait* and is illustrated for a weak *left* Gmed in Figure 5.16.

If this dysfunctional gait is present over a prolonged period, a compensatory Trendelenburg might develop (Figure 5.17, overleaf). The reasons

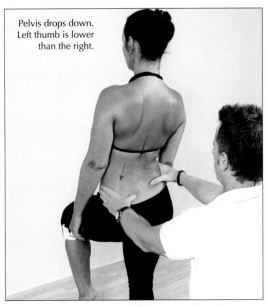

Figure 5.15. Positive test for weakness of the right Gmed—the left PSIS dips down on the left.

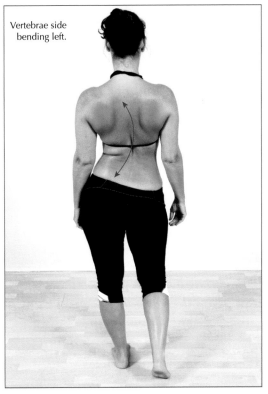

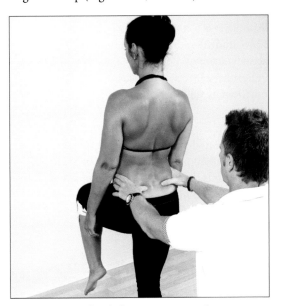

Figure 5.14. Standing balance test—normal.

Figure 5.16. Trendelenburg gait—weak left Gmed.

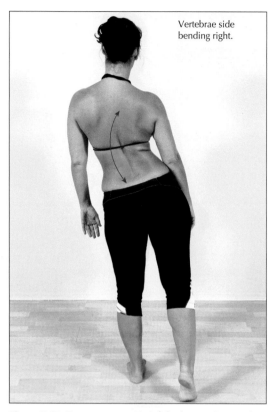

Vertebrae side bending right.

Figure 5.17. Compensatory Trendelenburg gait—weak left Gmed.

for this altered gait can be numerous to say the least, but one cause could be that one of the legs is held in an adducted position because of the shortening of the adductors (as mentioned above). This altered pattern will in turn result in a reciprocal inhibition (RI) to the antagonistic muscles: the abductors—in particular the Gmed—will now be held in a lengthened position that can then predispose the Gmed to becoming weak.

When I teach the standing balance test (Figure 5.14), I say to my students that you need to look out for three things:

1. **Position of the PSIS**
   The first, as I mentioned above, is the position of the PSIS as the patient transfers their weight from one leg to the other.

2. **Shift of the pelvis**
   The second is how much movement occurs as the patient shifts onto the weight-bearing leg; you may notice one side shifting more than the other, indicating a possible Gmed weakness.

3. **Stability on one leg**
   Finally, the third is how stable the patient is when they stand on one leg compared with the other. You will be amazed how many very fit athletes struggle to stand on one leg unaided and maintain good control. This instability could be a result of a weak Gmed, but remember also that a change in a patient's ability to stabilize might be due to a previous injury/trauma to the ankle complex, thus affecting the neurological proprioceptors in controlling the specific position.

Friel et al. (2006) conducted a study about ipsilateral hip abductor weakness after an inversion ankle sprain; their results showed that hip abduction and plantar flexion were significantly weaker on the involved side. They concluded that unilateral ankle sprains led to weaker hip abduction (Gmed), and suggested exercises to strengthen the hip abductors when developing rehabilitation protocols for ankle inversion sprains.

Schmitz et al. (2002) demonstrated through an EMG study that there was an increase in Gmed activity during sudden ankle inversion motion in healthy subjects as well as in those with functionally unstable ankles.

Hopefully, after reading this chapter, you will have some understanding of what is happening when a patient presents with musculoskeletal dysfunctions, such as LLD, over-pronation syndrome, and muscle imbalances. In the next chapter I will continue with the journey on this theme by looking at the specific movement mechanics of the spine.

The Laws of Spinal Mechanics

Spinal Mechanics: Fact or Fiction?

A medical doctor by the name of Robert Lovett was the first person (I believe) to confirm coupled spinal motions, other than the standard primary motion of flexion and extension (Lovett 1903). He believed that side bending and rotation of the spine are parts of one compound movement and cannot be dissociated: he found that a flexible rod bent in one plane could not bend in another plane without twisting. In all his experiments Lovett proved that if the spine was in a position of lordosis, it rotated in the *opposite* direction to that of the side bending motion; moreover, if the spine was in a position of kyphosis, it rotated in the *same* direction as that of the side bending motion.

He considered that only three spinal movements were possible within the vertebral column: (1) flexion; (2) extension; and (3) side bending with rotation. He also concluded that side bending, or lateral flexion, must accompany spinal rotation (i.e. the motions are coupled).

Lovett proposed that coupled motion occurs in a second plane of motion within a joint system, and is part and parcel of the primary motion. Two or more motions are considered "coupled" when it is not possible to produce one motion without inducing the second one; spinal coupling occurs because of the morphological shape of the facet joint surfaces and the connecting ligaments and spinal curvatures.

In the early 1900s the osteopath Harrison M. Fryette contributed some pioneering work on the mechanics of spinal motion. He spent many years of his life researching this topic and eventually presented a paper in 1918 on the principles of spinal motion, which was sent to the American Osteopathic Association (Fryette 1918).

Initially, Fryette's paper was poorly received and he did not gain acceptance. Many years passed before he eventually received formal recognition for his ideas. In the late 1940s Fryette was invited to the UK by Edward Hall to do a presentation on his work. Fryette spoke about what he called "The Total Osteopathic Lesion," and he had such a profound effect on Hall that his biomechanical view of spinal motion was relabeled to "Fryette's Laws of Spinal Mechanics," which up until then had been referred to only as *principles*. (Hall wrote the first article on that subject in the 1956 yearbook of The Osteopathic Institute of Applied Technique.)

A quote from Fryette:

"No intelligent scientific spinal technic can be developed that is not based on an accurate understanding of the physiological movements of the spine."

Regarding the motion of the spine, Stoddard (1962) states the following in his manual on osteopathic technique:

"Rotation of the spine is always accompanied by some degree of lateral flexion. Likewise, lateral flexion of the spine is accompanied by some degree of vertebral rotation."

How All This Came About

Fryette utilized and established correlations with a lot of the earlier work conducted by Lovett in 1903. The research methodology consisted of cadaveric study and in vivo research via the application of gummed paper stickers. These bits of sticky paper were attached to the spinous processes of the vertebrae of a small number of individuals; the results were then obtained by observing the relative spinal motion of these gummed paper stickers.

It is hard to appreciate how much the research into spinal mechanics has progressed over the last 50–100 years, from the simple observatory techniques of Fryette employing sticky paper to the use of advanced technology such as computer simulation, computerized tomography (CT scan), magnetic resonance imaging (MRI scan), and cineradiology (viewing an organ in motion with a special movie camera). We can even detect motion of the spine and pelvis by implanting gallium balls and Steinman pins.

If we were able to jump ahead into the future by, say, 100 years, it would be very interesting to see what actually changes in terms of research and technology. It goes without saying, especially as time passes, that the more we are able to visualize and research living spinal motion, the more complex and unpredictable the precise combination of individual spinal joint motion becomes for each particular area and segment of the vertebral column.

I have read numerous articles and many books by various authors over the last few years while researching the subject of spinal motion, before eventually deciding to write this particular book on the pelvis and SIJ. Those practitioners in question, who I consider to be experts in their field of manual therapy, all seem to have a slightly different opinion on spinal mechanics/motion, which I think is fine, as everyone is entitled to have an opinion. Some of the information that I have read, however, actually comes across as rather conflicting, because there currently does not appear to be any standardization in this field of study. Rather than having what we call definitive "laws of spinal motion" or "principles of spinal motion," there are substantial individual and regional variations, and, as yet, no true accurate model for predicting the behavior of the vertebral column as regards specific motion.

Koushik physio (2011) says in his website blog:

"The work of Fryette must be applauded for its longevity and insight, and celebrated as part of our osteopathic heritage and history, but the "laws" can no longer be viewed as such, nor do they serve as a viable explanation of physiological motion behavior. With all this uncertainty why do some of us still persist in promoting a model for physiological motion based on work conducted over 100 years ago?"

In one way I totally agree with what this author says. Yes, I am basically of the same mind that perhaps the work of Fryette might be outdated; however, another part of me totally disagrees with what is being said. Why, I hear you ask? Because I spend a lot of my time traveling the world, as well as the UK, teaching a variety of physical therapy courses; when these courses relate in particular to the motion of the spine, it amazes me that the majority of therapists who I come into contact with have not been taught anything about the specific motion of the vertebral column and the biomechanics of the pelvic girdle/SIJ during their own studies … and this truly disappoints me. This is true even in the case of qualified and experienced osteopaths, chiropractors, and physiotherapists.

These days, if I am honest, I have no idea of the current criteria for what is actually covered in terms of spinal motion in specific degree courses run in the UK. One thing I know for sure, however, is that there cannot be much time spent learning about this fascinating area during these undergraduate and even postgraduate courses, as otherwise my own physical therapy courses would not be as busy as they are.

I therefore now have a dilemma: I must at least teach a concept of spinal motion to my students, so the question is, do I teach a concept from Fryette that has been around for over 100 years and is considered by some to be outdated—even though some experts say Fryette's views should not be used any more? Or do I teach what is believed to be the most recent findings, as contradictory as they might be?

The answer is that I of course teach Fryette's Law, as my own personal approach to this is the following. I teach my students one way, one method, and as I have already said, I use the concept of Fryette's way of thinking about the way the spine moves. At least then, I honestly believe, after completing my course the students (including the more experienced therapists) will actually be able to get to grips with, and hopefully have a far better understanding of, the concept of Fryette's laws and the underpinning principles and concepts of spinal mechanics.

Ultimately I am more than happy that those therapists who have chosen to attend my courses will have a good initial grounding in applying the laws of Fryette, hopefully with specific relevance and application to their own private patients and athletes presenting with back or pelvic pain. Naturally, over time, things progress, especially in relation to current research methodology and technology. Therapists can themselves gradually evolve their techniques in practice as they become more experienced and knowledgeable, so they should be able to adapt very well to those ongoing changes.

Gracovetsky's "Spinal Engine Theory"

Serge Gracovetsky (1988) elaborated on a particular idea of spinal motion, which he discussed in his book *The Spinal Engine*. He considered the spine to be the "primary engine" in the role of locomotion and proposed that the legs were not responsible for gait, but were merely "instruments of expression" and extensions of the spinal engine. He argued that the spine was not a rigid lever during the gait cycle and that its ability to produce axial compression and torsion was a fundamental driving force during locomotion.

In his discussions Gracovetsky says that during heel-strike, kinetic energy is not displaced into the earth as in the pedestrian model, but efficiently transmitted up through the myofascial system, causing the spine to resonate in the gravitational field. He did not view the spine as a compressive loading system, whereby the intervertebral discs act as shock absorbers; he regarded the outer anulus fibrosus disc fibers and their accompanying facet joints as dynamic antigravity torsional springs that store and unload tensional forces to lift and propel the body in space. He also considered that the natural process of interlocking of the facet joints and intervertebral discs transmitted virtually all of the available counter-rotational pelvic torque that is needed to aid the inner and outer core muscles for locomotion.

A quote from Gracovetsky:

"The spine is an engine driving the pelvis. Human anatomy is a consequence of function.

The knee cannot be tested in isolation, as it is part of the overall function and purpose of the musculoskeletal system. The leg transfers the heel-strike energy to the spine. It is a mechanical filter. The knee is a critical part of that filter and improper energy transfer will affect spinal motion. Functional assessment of the spine ought to be part of the assessment of knee surgery."

Let's think back to the earlier concept of Lovett: it is this lumbar lateral flexion/rotation coupling that serves as the Gracovetsky spinal engine "drivetrain." For example, left lateral lumbar flexion will drive right rotation of the lumbar spine, and subsequently the SIJ and pelvis.

What I would like to do now is return to the discussion of Chapter 4 and in particular of the gait cycle, and look at this concept in a slightly different way. Some authors have considered that the biceps femoris muscle of the hamstring group, along with its connection to the posterior (deep) longitudinal sling (Figure 6.1), effectively starts the spinal engine. The biceps femoris has been likened to the *pull cord* of the spinal engine in view of its action of inducing a "force closure" mechanism in the SIJ. This closure of the SIJ will naturally lead to a subsequent transmission of force up into the osteo-articular-ligamentous tissues of the lumbosacral spine; this force will eventually continue into the muscles of the lumbar erector spinae.

EMG studies have demonstrated that the biceps femoris muscle is particularly active at the end of the swing phase of gait, through the early loading of the stance phase. During the transition from swing to stance, the heel contact phase of the gait cycle effectively closes the kinetic chain, and the biceps femoris can now perform its work in a manner that is commonly called a *closed kinetic chain*. Within the closed chain, the biceps femoris acts on its more proximal attachment within the chain, namely the pelvis. The biceps femoris attaches directly to the ischial tuberosity and also to the sacrotuberous ligament, sacrum, iliac crests,

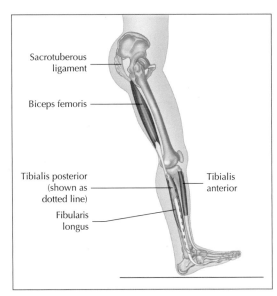

Figure 6.1. Posterior (deep) longitudinal sling.

and up through the multifidi and lumbar erector spinae (Figure 6.1).

At heel contact the ipsilateral (same side) hip and contralateral (opposite side) shoulder are in a position of flexion, which effectively preloads the posterior oblique sling (Figure 6.2(a)), specifically the ipsilateral Gmax and contralateral latissimus dorsi. This allows extra- spinal propulsion in a "sling-like" manner, with the superficial lamina of the thoracolumbar fascia serving as an intermediary between these kinetically linked muscles (Figure 6.2(b)).

The force transmitted through the osteo-articular-ligamentous structures induces "form closure" of the spinal facet joints and rotation in the lumbar spine; coupled with a lateral flexion moment, the spinal engine *initiates and selects the gears* to drive the pelvis into a forward rotation. The induced lumbar rotation effectively stores elastic energy in the spinal ligaments and the anulus fibrosus of the intervertebral discs, and it is this return of energy that drives gait.

In order to return the energy, the spine must be stabilized from above: this is accomplished via

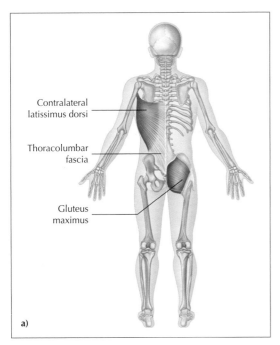

a)

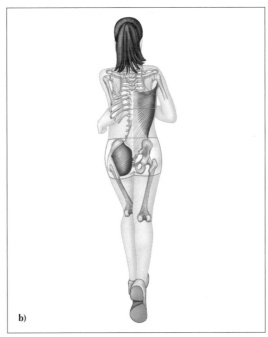

b)

Figure 6.2. (a) Posterior oblique sling.

Figure 6.2. (b) Posterior oblique sling utilized whilst running.

contralateral arm swing and trunk rotation produced by the contralateral Gmax and latissimus dorsi involvement. The coupling patterns of the spine have evolved to facilitate the return of this force. The counter-rotation is considered to be recruited directly from the spine and not from the legs.

Spinal Mechanics Explained

Each and every patient, especially from a spinal mechanics point of view, should be assessed on the basis that they are unique, especially since some people present with vertebral anomalies, which may cause abnormal physiological movement. The following information relating to spinal physiological movement is based on empirical experience rather than on scientific theory; however, it is dependable and useful in helping the budding therapist to understand what they should expect to palpate in the majority of people.

By developing good hand–eye coordination and tactile tissue tension sense, it is certainly possible to detect spinal lesions or, in modern terms, *somatic spinal dysfunctions*. These dysfunctions can be palpated as abnormal vertebral positioning; they function either statically or dynamically, while surrounding abnormal soft tissue texture is a common feature. Once the somatic spinal dysfunctions have been identified and appropriately treated, the offending vertebral segment(s) can then be re-evaluated to determine whether the treatment approach has been successful. This whole process can be demonstrated clinically, provided that the underpinning knowledge of basic spinal physiological movement has been studied and put into practice by the practitioner.

Fryette's Laws basically consist of three laws (originally known as *principles*) pertaining to spinal positioning. The first two laws were developed by Fryette in 1918, and the third law by C.R. Nelson in 1948. The laws are defined as a set of guiding principles that can be used by appropriately trained practitioners to discriminate between dysfunctions that are present within the axial skeleton.

The first two laws only relate to the thoracic and lumbar vertebrae, and the motion available is only considered to be governed by the patterns of force generated by the intervertebral discs, ligaments, and associated musculature. On the other hand, cervical spine motion, which is not classified as a motion that follows Fryette mechanics, is mainly determined by the orientation of the facet joints. We can, however, describe the cervical spine motion as Fryette-*like* mechanics because of the similarity.

Law 1: Neutral Mechanics—Type I

Neutral mechanics relates to standing or sitting in a relaxed upright position, with normal neutral spinal curves. But what is neutral? *Neutral* in the world of spinal mechanics is not defined as a single point, but rather as a range in which the weight of the trunk is borne on the vertebral bodies and intervertebral discs, and the facet joints are in an idle state.

Fryette wrote: "Neutral is defined to mean the position of any area of the spine in which the facets are idling, in the position between the beginning of flexion and the beginning of extension."

This basically means that in neutral, the facet joints are neither in a state of extension (closed) nor in a state of flexion (open)—they are simply idling or resting between these two positions.

According to Fryette, when the spine is in a *neutral* position, side bending to one side will be accompanied by horizontal rotation to the *opposite* side: this is referred to as *Type I spinal mechanics* (Figure 6.3). This first law is observed

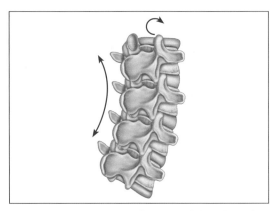

Figure 6.3. Type I spinal mechanics—side bending left, rotation right.

in what is known as a *Type I spinal dysfunction*, where more than one vertebra is out of alignment and cannot be returned to neutral by flexion or extension of the vertebrae. The group of vertebrae in question demonstrates a coupled relationship: when side bending forces are induced in a group of typical vertebrae to one side, the entire group will rotate to the *opposite* side, in other words obeying Type I or Law 1 spinal mechanics. This spinal motion will produce a convexity similar to a spinal curvature known as a *scoliosis*.

Type I (neutral) dysfunctions generally occur in groups of vertebrae, for example T1–7, and are typically seen in spinal conditions such as scoliosis. The vertebrae of a Type I dysfunction tend to compensate for a single Type II dysfunction, and are usually at the beginning or the end of the group dysfunction, although the dysfunction can sometimes be located at the apex of the curvature.

Another way of looking at Type I spinal mechanics is as follows. In the neutral position for the thoracic and lumbar spines, side bending will create a concavity to the same side as the side bend and a convexity to the side of the rotation (opposite side). For example, side bending to the left will create a concave curve on the left side of the body and a convex curve on the right side.

Note: Neutral spinal mechanics is a naturally occurring motion of the spine that is required to promote Gracovetsky's spinal engine, due to the side bending and rotation to the opposite side. Any spinal dysfunction that are present will reduce the overall efficiency of the 'engine' (spinal).

Law 2: Non-Neutral Mechanics—Type II

Fryette states that when the spine is in a position of flexion or extension, by either standing or sitting while in a forward- or backward-bent position (also known as *non-neutral*), side bending to one side will be accompanied by rotation to the *same* side: this is referred to as *Type II mechanics* (Figure 6.4).

This second law is observed in Type II spinal dysfunctions, where only one vertebral segment is restricted in motion, and becomes much worse in a position of flexion or extension. As mentioned above, there will be a coupled spinal motion, with side bending and rotation in the *same* direction when this dysfunction is present.

Let's look at this from another angle. Put simply, if the thoracic or lumbar spine is sufficiently forward or backward bent, the coupled motions of side bending and rotation of a single vertebral unit will occur in the same direction (i.e. to the same side).

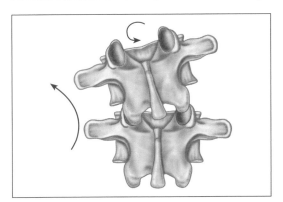

Figure 6.4. Type II spinal mechanics—side bending left, rotation left.

Type II (non-neutral) spinal dysfunctions are generally thought to occur in a single vertebral segment. However, two Type II dysfunctions can appear next to each other at the same time, but the occurrence of more than two is rare.

Law 3

According to Nelson (1948), when motion is introduced in one plane, the motion in the other two planes is modified (reduced). The third law basically sums up the first two laws: it simply states that dysfunction in one plane of motion will reduce the motion in all other planes. For example, if rotation is restricted, then side bending and flexion/extension will also be restricted.

Viewing Perspective

When assessing for spinal movement, the spine is usually viewed from behind. Generally speaking, a spinal dysfunction exists when we try to place the patient's spine in a neutral position, but this position of symmetry cannot to be achieved; the likely reason for this is a dysfunction of either a group of vertebrae or a single spinal segment.

It is possible to detect an abnormal ROM of the spine when patients perform flexion, extension, side bending, and rotation in the cardinal planes; one should be able to see if there is a restricted ROM.

The following sections detail the specific spinal mechanic motion for each of the areas of the vertebral column. I have already explained the term *neutral* (i.e. the facet joints are idling between flexion and extension), so this position is termed *neutral mechanics*. By contrast, the term *non-neutral mechanics* generally refers to either a spinal position of forward bending (flexion) or a spinal position of backward bending (extension).

1. Lumbar Spine

Neutral Mechanics: Type I

When side bending to one side, the vertebral bodies rotate to the *opposite* side.

Non-Neutral Mechanics: Type II

When side bending to one side, the vertebral bodies rotate to the *same* side.

Exceptions to the Rule: L5

In neutral mechanics, during side bending to one side L5 may rotate to either the opposite side or the same side (obeying non-neutral mechanics, even though the spine is in a relatively neutral position) whenever there is some asymmetry/ dysfunction of the sacral base or if there are facet joint anomalies present.

2. Thoracic Spine

Neutral Mechanics: Type I

When side bending to one side, the vertebral bodies rotate to the *opposite* side.

Non-Neutral Mechanics: Type II

When side bending to one side, the vertebral bodies rotate to the *same* side.

3. Cervical Spine

As mentioned earlier, spinal motion in the cervical spine is mainly determined by the orientation of the facet joints and does not come within the realm of Fryette's laws; however, we can say these mechanics are Fryette-*like*, because the motion is similar.

Occipitoatlantal Joint

The occipitoatlantal joint (OAJ) connects the occipital bone to the atlas and always follows Type I (like) mechanics: in side bending to one side, the occiput rotates to the *opposite* side, independent of whether the occiput is in a neutral or a non-neutral position (flexion or extension).

Atlantoaxial Joint: (C1/C2)

The atlantoaxial joint (AAJ), which lies between the atlas and the axis, is mainly considered to only rotate. There has been some discussion suggesting that, in either neutral or non-neutral mechanics, during side bending movements the atlas (C1) is capable of rotating to either side. Dysfunctions typically found at this level are thought to consist mainly of a rotational component.

The level of C2–C6 in the cervical spine is believed to only follow Type II (like) mechanics, in that side bending and the rotation are always coupled to the *same* side, regardless of whether the cervical spine is in a neutral position or a non-neutral position (flexion or extension).

C2–C6: Neutral Mechanics

When side bending to one side, the vertebral bodies rotate to the *same* side, i.e. Type II-*like* mechanics.

C2–C6: Non-Neutral Mechanics

When side bending to one side, the vertebral bodies rotate to the *same* side, i.e. Type II-*like* mechanics.

C7 has facet joints that are orientated in a similar way to the thoracic spine, so this spinal level will follow the classic law of Fryette.

Spinal Mechanics: Definitions

The specific position of a vertebra can be referred to in two different ways:

1. The position of the vertebra, relative to the vertebra below.
2. The direction of the motion restriction of the vertebra, relative to the vertebra below.

In other words, the same vertebral segment can be described from two different points of view.

For example, let's say T4 is fixed in an extended, side-bent right, and rotated-right position. This simply means that the T4 is fixed in a position of extension, side bend, and rotation, all to the right side, on top of the vertebra immediately below, i.e. T5. This is because the right T4 inferior facet is fixed in a *closed* position on the superior facet on T5. The motion restriction has to be in forward flexion as well as in left side bending and left rotation (opposite to the fixed position). This type of dysfunction obeys Type II mechanics, as already explained earlier; however, taking it a stage further, we would now classify the spinal dysfunction as a *T4 extension, rotation, side bend right*, or *T4 ERS(R)*, which will be discussed shortly.

In terms of diagnosing somatic spinal dysfunction, the positional diagnosis is determined and named according to the direction of the vertebra that has the easiest motion. Let's take a look at what I mean by that in more detail.

Spinal dysfunction is typically described as either *extended* or *flexed*, with a rotation and a side bending component to the same side, or possibly to the opposite side, as you will read later.

Before we define the terminology for spinal dysfunctions, we first need to confirm the presence of a spinal dysfunction by ascertaining the specific position and motion of the vertebra being tested. We can establish this by asking our patient to adopt three different positions of the vertebral column: neutral, extension, and flexion. The vertebral position through palpation simply becomes either symmetrical (level) or asymmetrical (not level) in these three positions, depending on the type of spinal dysfunction/facet restriction present at the time.

If there are no facet restrictions present, when you forward bend your spine, the left and right facet joints (top vertebra in relation to the bottom vertebra) will slide forward in a superior and anterior direction to open; conversely, when you backward bend your spine, the left and right facet joints will slide backward in an inferior and posterior direction to close. However, if the facet joints are for some reason restricted in either a flexion or an extension position, the restricted joint will now act as a pivot point, especially when performing the spinal motion of forward and backward bending.

To illustrate this, ask your patient to adopt a neutral position (normally a sitting position, for the thoracic spine) and lightly place your left and right thumbs on the T4/5 transverse process (TP). Lightly palpate for a few seconds and compare the left and right TPs to see if there is any asymmetry; if so, you have now identified the presence of a spinal dysfunction—in a very simple way, you have located a facet restriction. For instance, if the left thumb, while in contact with the left TP, appeared to palpate *shallow* (i.e. the TP feels closer to the surface of the skin), whereas the right thumb (on the right TP) palpated *deep* (i.e. the thumb traveled further to reach the right TP), this would be indicative of T4 (superior) having rotated to the left side on T5 (inferior) below (see Figure 6.5(c)).

What this does not tell you, however, is whether the *left* facet joint is fixed in a *closed* position or whether the *right* facet joint is fixed in an *open* position. That is why it is necessary to palpate the TPs in the position of spinal extension (backward bending) and spinal flexion (forward bending) in order to confirm or discount the presence of a fixed closed facet joint or a fixed open facet joint.

Let's try to look at this concept in a relatively simple way (I hope) by using the thoracic T4/5 as an example. As already discussed above, we should now know that when the patient is in a neutral position, T4 has rotated to the left side, because the left TP palpated as shallow (more prominent) and the right TP palpated as deep (less prominent). From the neutral position, we now ask our patient to forward bend, while the thumbs are still in contact with the TPs; you notice the left and right TPs in the forward-bent position become more asymmetrical (the TP on one side becomes more prominent, and the TP on the other less prominent).

Imagine just for a moment that you consider the left thumb to feel more prominent (think of it as a bump) and now the right thumb feels even deeper (less prominent); this must mean that the left facet joint is fixed in a *closed* position on the *left* side, see Figure 6.5(i). Why? When the patient forward bends, the right facet joint is free to glide anteriorly as normal, but the left facet joint is now fixed posteriorly; because the left facet cannot open normally during forward bending, the left facet joint that is fixed in a closed position becomes a pivot point. Because of this pivot, one could say that the right facet basically has to open even more during forward bending, but ends up rotating around the left fixed facet joint that cannot open; this is why the left and right thumbs appear even more asymmetric. In this case the left thumb has become more prominent (the bump increases because the left TP is fixed posteriorly) in the forward-bent position.

When you ask the patient to adopt a position of extension, the thumbs will now palpate level (symmetric), because the left facet joint is already fixed posteriorly in a closed position, and the right facet joint simply continues its natural motion of closing. The left and right thumb positions on the TPs therefore become symmetric (level) in extension (the bump on the left TP disappears), see Figure 6.5(f).

Consider now another type of dysfunction—the case where the right facet joint is fixed in an open position. When we palpate the T4/5 TP in neutral, we will still notice the left thumb is shallow (bump) and the right thumb is deeper, indicating a left rotation, see Figure 6.9(c). However, when the patient forward bends their spine, the thumbs now become symmetric (i.e. the thumbs are now level and the bump disappears), see Figure 6.9(i). By contrast, when the patient backward bends their spine, you notice that the thumbs become asymmetric (i.e. symmetry is lost in extension—the bump felt by the left thumb on the TP increases), see Figure 6.9(f). This time the left thumb actually appears more prominent (bump present), and the right thumb appears to travel deeper in the backward-bent position. Why? In a forward-bent position, both of the facet joints are able to open as normal, hence the thumbs becoming level in this position; however, in a backward-bent position of extension, because the *right* facet is fixed in an *open* position (even though it has rotated to the left side), the facet joint cannot close on the right side, but the fixed pivot point created by the right open facets keeps the right TP fixed anteriorly. Since the backward bending motion causes the left side to move more posteriorly, the left TP appears to move further into left rotation. The thumbs therefore appear asymmetric and now, in the backward-bent position, the left thumb on the left TP becomes more prominent (bump appears) than the right thumb.

Note: The above dysfunction relates to the right facet joint fixed in an open position. This is called an FRS(L) as you will read shortly.

One way of remembering these two processes, as it will help you with your own patients, is to understand the following two rules:

Rule 1: In forward bending, if the prominent TP becomes even more prominent (bump appears), then that side is fixed closed.

Rule 2: In backward bending, if the prominent TP becomes more prominent (bump appears), then the opposite side is fixed open.

Maitland (2001) offers another explanation, which might help you better understand what I am trying to say. First, you determine rotation in a neutral position. Then, keeping your thumbs on the TPs of the rotated vertebra, forward and backward bend your client, and feel and watch what happens under your thumbs. Look for the position where the bump (the posterior or prominent vertebra TP of the rotated vertebra) disappears. Maitland says that the position where the bump disappears (or vertebral derotation appears to occur) is the position in which the facets are restricted:

"If the bump disappears in forward bending, the facets are fixed in the forward-bent position, which means the facets are fixed open (flexion fixed)."

"If the bump disappears in back bending, the facets are fixed in the back bent position, which means the facets are fixed closed (extension fixed)."

We will now look at some of the typical terminology that practitioners use in their clinics, along with a few common examples of spinal dysfunctional patterns that patients might present with in your own clinic. Hopefully, once you have read all the information in this chapter, and practiced all the necessary spinal positions in order to confirm or discount the presence of either a fixed facet or an open facet, we can look at some form of treatment strategy, especially for the lumbar spine (see Chapter 13). Specific treatment for the area of the thoracic spine, however, is not covered in this text, even though I have given some examples of the assessment process. Nevertheless, one should be able to modify the treatment techniques shown for the lumbar spine in Chapter 13 and adapt/apply them to dysfunctions in the thoracic spine.

> **Definition:** An *extension, rotation, side bending (ERS) dysfunction* involves a facet joint (inferior and superior component) which is fixed in a closed position. It is classified as a *non-neutral (Type II) spinal mechanics dysfunction*.

Extension, Rotation, Side Bending Left—ERS(L)

This is a situation in which the *left* facet joint is fixed in a *closed* position.

ERS(L) refers to the orientation of an uppermost vertebra that is fixed in an extended, side-bent, and rotated position to the left side (Figure 6.5(a)).

Two examples will be considered: in the first, T4 is assumed to be fixed in a closed position on the left side on T5; in the second, L5 is assumed to be fixed in a closed position on the left side on S1. We will now test the levels of T4/5 and L5/S1 in the three positions of neutral, flexion, and extension.

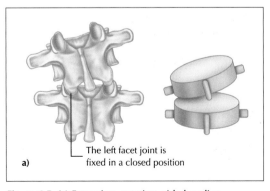

The left facet joint is fixed in a closed position

a)

Figure 6.5. (a) Extension, rotation, side bending left—ERS(L).

Neutral Position

With the patient in a neutral position, place your thumbs approximately 1" (2.5cm) lateral to the T4 and T5 spinous processes, so that the thumbs are in gentle contact with the left and right TPs (repeat the same process when you are ready to do the L5/S1 vertebrae). If there is an ERS(L) present, you will notice that the left thumb appears to be more prominent (shallow) and the right thumb appears to be

deeper in the neutral position (Figure 6.5(b–d)), indicating that the vertebra has rotated to the left side.

Extension Position

As the patient backward bends, observe the relative levels of your thumbs. You will notice that the left and right thumbs are level (Figure 6.5(e–g)).

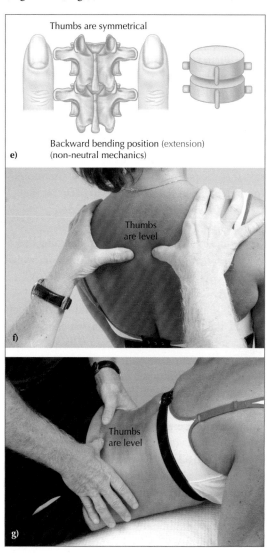

Figure 6.5. (b) Neutral position—the left thumb appears shallow and the right thumb appears deeper, indicating a left rotation of the vertebra. (c) Thoracic spine T4/5. (d) Lumbar spine L5/S1.

Figure 6.5. (e) Extension position—the left and right thumbs now appear to become level. (f) Thoracic spine T4/5. (g) Lumbar spine L5/S1.

Flexion Position

Next look at the relative positions of your thumbs as the patient forward bends. This time you will notice that the left thumb appears to become more prominent (bump appears) and that the right thumb appears to travel deeper (Figure 6.5(h–j)). This asymmetric positioning of the thumbs indicates a fixed closed facet joint on the left side.

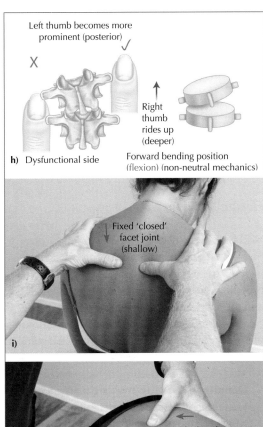

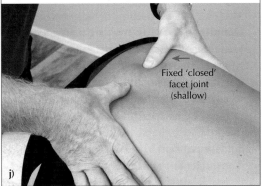

Figure 6.5. (h) Flexion position—the left thumb appears more prominent and the right thumb appears deep, indicating a fixed closed vertebra on the left side. (i) Thoracic spine T4/5. (j) Lumbar spine L5/S1.

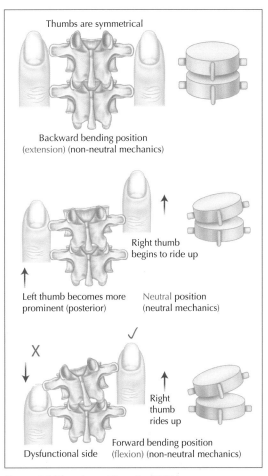

Figure 6.6. Thumb positions for ERS(L).

Extension, Rotation, Side Bending Right—ERS(R)

This is a situation in which the *right* facet joint is fixed in a *closed* position.

ERS(R) refers to the orientation of an uppermost vertebra that is fixed in an extended, side-bent, and rotated position to the right side (see Figure 6.7(a)).

Two examples will be considered: in the first, T4 is assumed to be fixed in a closed position on the right side on T5; in the second, L5 is assumed to be fixed in a closed position on the right side on S1.

We will now test the levels of T4/5 and L5/S1 in the three positions of neutral, flexion, and extension.

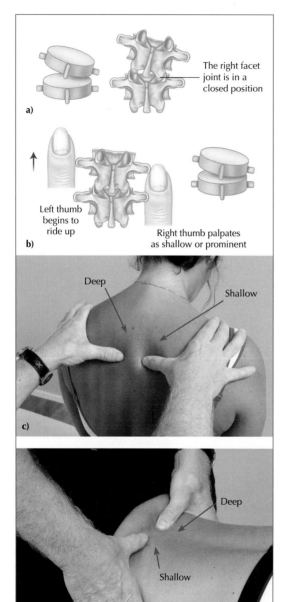

Figure 6.7. (a) Extension, rotation, side bending right— ERS(R). (b) Neutral position—the right thumb appears more prominent and the left thumb appears deeper, indicating a right rotation of the vertebra. (c) Thoracic spine T4/5. (d) Lumbar spine L5/S1.

Neutral Position

With the patient in a neutral position, place your thumbs approximately 1" (2.5cm) lateral to the T4 and T5 spinous processes, so that the thumbs are in gentle contact with the left and right TPs (repeat the same process when you are ready to do L5/S1). If there is an ERS(R) present, you will notice that the right thumb appears to be shallow and the left thumb appears to be deeper in the neutral position (Figure 6.7(b–d)), indicating a right rotation of the vertebra.

Extension Position

As the patient backward bends, observe the relative levels of your thumbs. You will notice that the left and right thumbs are level (see Figure 6.7(e–g)).

Flexion Position

Next look at the relative level of your thumbs as the patient forward bends. You will notice that the right thumb appears to become more prominent (bump appears) and the left thumb appears to travel deeper (see Figure 6.7(h–j)). This asymmetric positioning of the thumbs indicates a fixed closed facet joint on the right side.

> **Definition:** A *flexion, rotation, side bending (FRS) dysfunction* involves a facet joint which is fixed in an open position. It is classified as a *non-neutral (Type II) spinal mechanics dysfunction.*

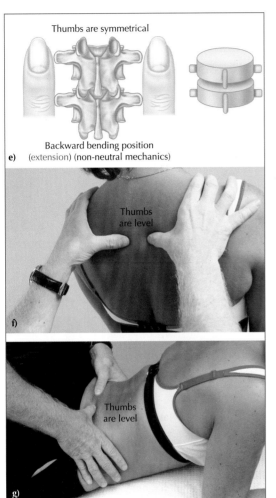

Figure 6.7. (e) Extension position—the left and right thumbs now appear to become level. (f) Thoracic spine T4/5. (g) Lumbar spine L5/S1.

Flexion, Rotation, Side Bending Left—FRS(L)

This is a situation in which the *right* facet joint is fixed in an open position.

Note that, although the dysfunction is to the *right* facet, *FRS(L)* refers to the orientation of an uppermost vertebra that is fixed in a flexed,

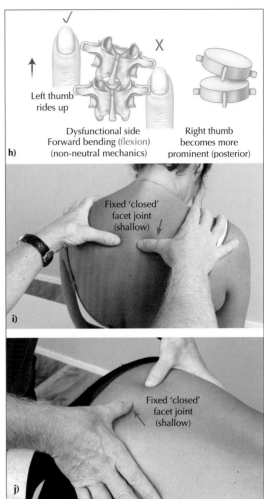

Figure 6.7. (h) Flexion position—the right thumb appears more prominent and the left thumb appears deeper, indicating a fixed closed vertebra on the right side. (i) Thoracic spine T4/5. (j) Lumbar spine L5/S1.

side-bent, and rotated position to the *left* side. It is the *right* facet, however, that is dysfunctional, because it is fixed in an open position (see Figure 6.9(a)).

We will now test the levels of T4/5 and L5/S1 in the three positions of neutral, flexion, and extension.

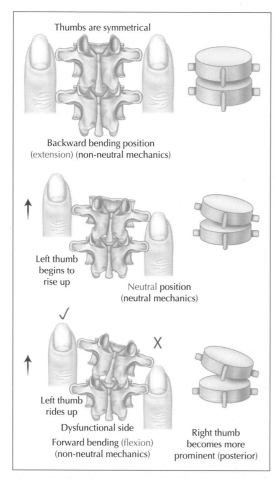

Thumbs are symmetrical

Backward bending position
(extension) (non-neutral mechanics)

Left thumb
begins to
rise up

Neutral position
(neutral mechanics)

✓

✗

Left thumb
rides up

Dysfunctional side
Forward bending (flexion)
(non-neutral mechanics)

Right thumb
becomes more
prominent (posterior)

Figure 6.8. Thumb positions for ERS(R).

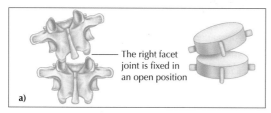

The right facet
joint is fixed in
an open position

a)

Figure 6.9. (a) Flexion, rotation, side bending left—FRS(L).

Neutral Position

With the patient in a neutral position, place your thumbs approximately 1″ (2.5cm) lateral to the T4 and T5 spinous processes, so that the thumbs are in gentle contact with the left and right TPs (repeat the same process when you are ready

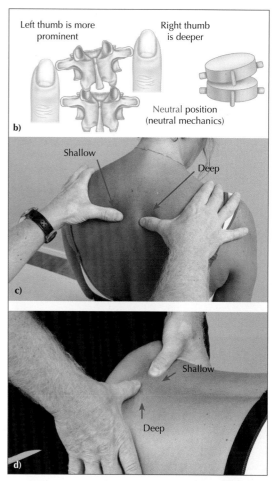

Left thumb is more
prominent

Right thumb
is deeper

Neutral position
(neutral mechanics)

b)

Shallow

Deep

c)

Shallow

Deep

d)

Figure 6.9. (b) Neutral position—the left thumb appears shallow and the right thumb appears deeper, indicating a left rotation of the vertebra. (c) Thoracic spine T4/5. (d) Lumbar spine L5/S1.

to do L5/S1). If there is an FRS(L) present, you will notice that the left thumb appears to be more prominent and the right thumb appears to be deeper in the neutral position (Figure 6.9(b–d)), indicating that the vertebra has rotated to the left side.

Extension Position

As the patient backward bends, observe the relative position of your thumbs. You will notice that the left thumb appears to become more prominent (bump appears) and the right thumb appears to travel deeper (Figure 6.9(e–g)). This asymmetric positioning of the thumbs indicates a fixed open facet joint on the right side (side opposite to rotation).

Flexion Position

Next look at the relative position of your thumbs as the patient forward bends. You will notice that the left and right thumbs are now level (Figure 6.9(h–j)).

Flexion, Rotation, Side Bending Right—FRS(R)

This is a situation in which the *left* facet joint is fixed in an open position.

Note that, although the dysfunction is to the *left* facet, *FRS(R)* refers to the orientation of an uppermost vertebra that is fixed in a flexed, side-bent, and rotated position to the *right* side. It is the

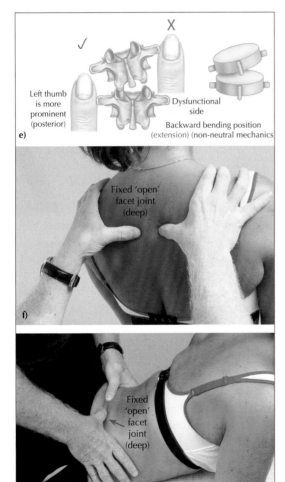

Figure 6.9. (e) Extension position—the left thumb appears more prominent and the right thumb appears deeper, indicating a fixed open facet joint on the right side. (f) Thoracic spine T4/5. (g) Lumbar spine L5/S1.

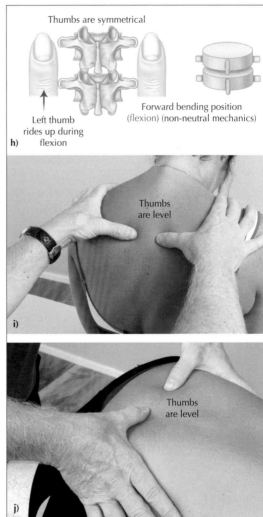

Figure 6.9. (h) Flexion position—the left and right thumbs now appear to become level. (i) Thoracic spine T4/5. (j) Lumbar spine L5/S1.

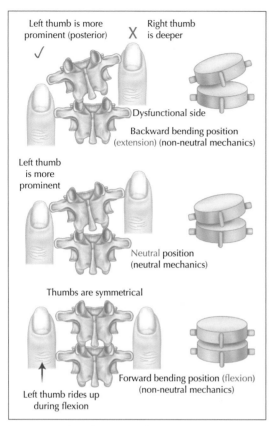

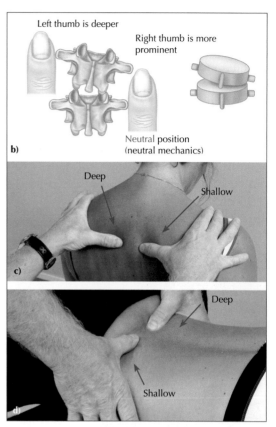

Figure 6.10. Thumb positions for FRS(L).

Figure 6.11. (b) Neutral position—the right thumb appears shallow and the left thumb appears deeper, indicating a right rotation of the vertebra. (c) Thoracic spine T4/5. (d) Lumbar spine L5/S1.

left facet, however, that is dysfunctional, because it is fixed in an open position (Figure 6.11(a)).

We will now test the levels of T4/5 and L5/S1 in the three positions of neutral, flexion, and extension.

Neutral Position

With the patient in a neutral position, place your thumbs approximately 1" (2.5cm) lateral to the

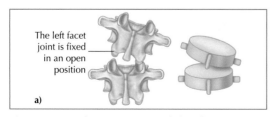

Figure 6.11. (a) Flexion, rotation, side bending right—FRS(R).

T4 and T5 spinous processes, so that the thumbs are in gentle contact with the left and right TPs (repeat the same process when you are ready to do L5/S1). If there is an FRS(R) present, you will notice that the left thumb appears to be deep and the right thumb appears to be shallow in the neutral position (Figure 6.11(b–d)), indicating that the vertebra has rotated to the right side.

Extension Position

As the patient backward bends, observe the relative position of your thumbs. You will notice that the right thumb appears to become more prominent (bump appears) and the left thumb appears to travel deeper (Figure 6.11(e–g)).

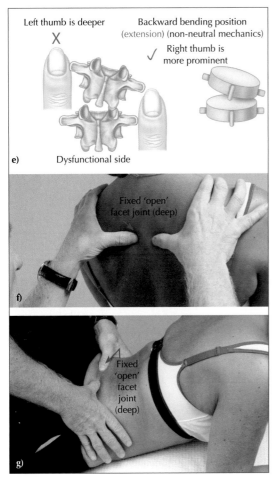

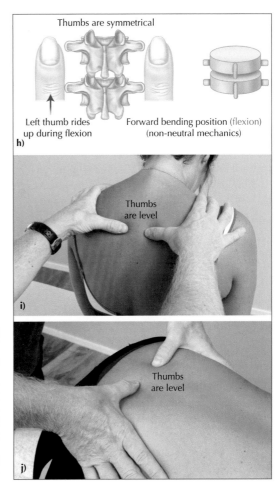

Figure 6.11. (e) Extension position—the right thumb appears more prominent and the left thumb appears deeper, indicating a fixed open facet joint on the left side. (f) Thoracic spine T4/5. (g) Lumbar spine L5/S1.

Figure 6.11. (h) Flexion position—the left and right thumbs now appear to become level. (i) Thoracic spine T4/5. (j) Lumbar spine L5/S1.

This asymmetric positioning of the thumbs indicates a fixed open facet joint on the left side (side opposite to rotation).

Flexion Position

Next look at the relative position of your thumbs as the patient forward bends. You will notice that the left and right thumbs are now level (Figure 6.11(h–j)).

Definition: A *neutral mechanics (Type I) dysfunction of a group of vertebrae (NR)*

typically involves a group of three or more vertebrae, and the side bending is considered to be the primary motion restriction, with a secondary rotational component. As explained earlier, this dysfunction produces a concavity on the same side as the side bending, and a convexity on the side of the rotation. This type of dysfunction is considered to be a compensatory group dysfunction as a result of a primary dysfunction; the primary dysfunctions are usually an FRS or ERS. The vertebrae in question side bend to one side and rotate to the opposite side.

Group Neutral Dysfunction, Rotation Left—NR(L)

This is a situation involving at least three vertebrae, which are side bent to the right and rotated to the left.

The rotation to the left is maintained throughout the range of backward bending, neutral, and forward bending (Figure 6.13). The amount of rotation may vary a little throughout this ROM, and will most likely be maximal in the neutral position.

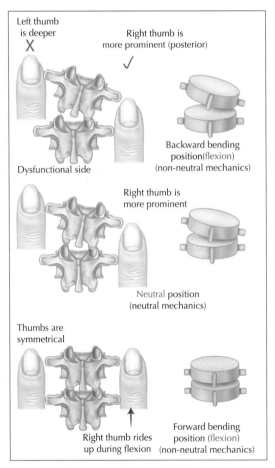

Figure 6.12. Thumb positions for FRS(R).

Group Neutral Dysfunction, Rotation Right—NR(R)

This is a situation involving at least three vertebrae, which are side bent to the left and rotated to the right.

The rotation to the right is maintained throughout the range of backward bending, neutral, and forward bending (Figure 6.14). The amount of rotation may vary a little throughout this ROM, and will most likely be maximal in the neutral position.

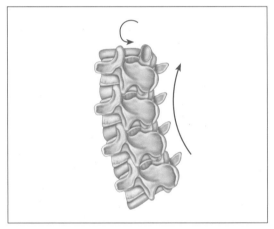

Figure 6.13. Neutral dysfunction—side bending right, rotation left—NR(L).

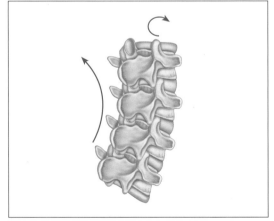

Figure 6.14. Neutral dysfunction—side bending left, rotation right—NRR

Muscle Energy Techniques and Their Relationship to the Pelvis

In later chapters you will read and learn about specific techniques that can be incorporated into a treatment plan to help correct pelvic and lumbar spine dysfunctions. I consider the techniques I will be demonstrating in this chapter to be some of the best soft tissue techniques that one can use to correct any soft tissue or spinal joint anomalies. You might have already guessed what these are—*muscle energy techniques (METs)*.

Since I discuss in this book how to treat specific dysfunctions associated with the SIJ, pelvis, and lumbar spine, I need to explain the role of METs, so that you have a better understanding of when and why to employ this type of soft tissue treatment. Physical therapists have what I call a toolbox of various techniques at their disposal, to help release and relax muscles, which will then assist the patient's body to promote the healing mechanisms. METs, first described by Fred Mitchell in 1948, are one such tool, which if used correctly can have a major influence on a patient's well-being. (The reader is referred to Gibbons (2011) for a fuller account of METs.)

Definition: *Muscle energy techniques (METs) are a form of osteopathic manipulative diagnosis and treatment in which the patient's muscles are actively used on* request, from a precisely controlled position, in a specific direction, and against a distantly applied counterforce.

METs are unique in their application, in that the patient provides the initial effort and the practitioner just facilitates the process. The primary force comes from the contraction of the patient's soft tissues (muscles), which is then utilized to assist and correct the presenting musculoskeletal dysfunction. This treatment method is generally classified as a *direct* form of technique as opposed to *indirect*, since the use of muscular effort is from a controlled position, in a specific direction, and against a distant counterforce that is usually applied by the practitioner.

Some of the Benefits of METs

When teaching the concept of METs to my students, one of the benefits I emphasize is their use in normalizing joint range, rather than in improving flexibility. This might sound counterintuitive; what I am saying is if, for example, your patient cannot rotate their neck (cervical spine) to the right as far as they can to the left, they have a restriction of the cervical spine in right rotation. The normal rotational range of the cervical spine is 80 degrees, but let's say the patient can only rotate 70 degrees to the right. This is where METs come in. After an MET has been employed on the tight restrictive muscles, hopefully the cervical spine will then be capable of rotating to 80 degrees—the patient has made all the effort and you, the practitioner, have encouraged the cervical spine into further right rotation. You have now improved the joint range to "normal." This is not stretching in the strictest sense—even though the overall flexibility has been improved, it is only to the point of achieving what is considered to be a normal joint range.

Depending on the context and the type of MET employed, the objectives of this treatment can include:

- Restoring normal tone in hypertonic muscles
- Strengthening weak muscles
- Preparing muscles for subsequent stretching
- Increasing joint mobility

Restoring Normal Tone in Hypertonic Muscles

Through the simple process of METs, we as physical therapists try to achieve a relaxation in the hypertonic shortened muscles. If we think of a joint as being limited in its ROM, then through the initial identification of the hypertonic structures, we can employ the techniques to help achieve normality in the tissues. Certain types of massage therapy can also help us achieve this relaxation effect, and generally an MET is applied in conjunction with massage therapy. I personally feel that massage with motion is one of the best tools a physical therapist can use.

Strengthening Weak Muscles

METs can be used in the strengthening of weak or even flaccid muscles, as the patient is asked to contract the muscles prior to the lengthening process. The therapist should be able to modify

the MET by asking the patient to contract the muscle that has been classified as *weak*, against a resistance applied by the therapist (isometric contraction), the timing of which can be varied. For example, the patient can be asked to resist the movement using approximately 20–30% of their maximum capability for 5–15 seconds. They are then asked to repeat the process five to eight times, resting for 10–15 seconds between repetitions. The patient's performance can be noted and improved over time.

Preparing Muscles for Subsequent Stretching

In certain circumstances, what sport your patient participates in will be determined by what ROM they have at their joints. Everybody can improve their flexibility, and METs can be used to help achieve this goal. Remember, the focus of METs is to try to improve the normal ROM of a joint.

If you want to improve the patient's flexibility past the point of normal, a more aggressive MET approach might be necessary. This could be in the form of asking the patient to contract a bit harder than the standard 10–20% of the muscle's capability. For example, we can ask the patient to contract using, say, 40–70% of the muscle's capability. This increased contraction will help stimulate more motor units to fire, in turn causing an increased stimulation of the Golgi tendon organ (GTO). This will then have the effect of relaxing more of the muscle, allowing it to be lengthened even further. Either way, once an MET has been incorporated into the treatment plan, a flexibility program can follow.

Increasing Joint Mobility

One of my favorite sayings when I teach muscle-testing courses is:

"A stiff joint can cause a tight muscle, and a tight muscle can cause a stiff joint."

Does this not make perfect sense? When you use an MET correctly, it is one of the best ways to improve the mobility of the joint, even though you are initially relaxing the muscles. This is especially the case with the use of METs to correct any dysfunctions that you find in the pelvis (see Chapter 13). The focus of the MET is to get the patient to contract the muscles; this subsequently causes a relaxation period, allowing a greater ROM to be achieved within that specific joint.

Physiological Effects of METs

There are two main effects of METs and these are explained on the basis of two distinct physiological processes:

- Post-isometric relaxation (PIR)
- Reciprocal inhibition (RI)

When we use METs, certain neurological influences occur. Before we discuss the main process of PIR/RI, we need to consider the two types of receptor involved in the stretch reflex:

- Muscle spindles, which are sensitive to change, as well as speed of change, in length of muscle fibers
- GTOs, which detect prolonged change in tension

Stretching the muscle causes an increase in the impulses transmitted from the muscle spindle to the posterior horn cell (PHC) of the spinal cord. In turn, the anterior horn cell (AHC) transmits an increase in motor impulses to the muscle fibers, creating a protective tension to resist the stretch. However, increased tension after a few seconds is sensed within the GTOs, which transmit impulses to the PHC. These impulses have an inhibitory effect on the increased motor stimulus at the AHC; this inhibitory effect causes a reduction in motor impulses and consequent relaxation. This implies that the prolonged stretch of the muscles will increase the stretching capability, because the protective relaxation of the GTOs overrides

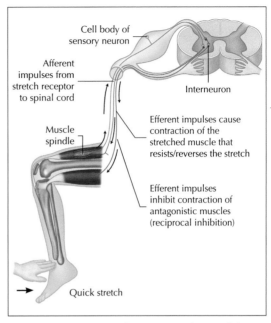

Figure 7.1. The stretch reflex arc. A quick "stretch by hand" to activate the muscle spindles.

the protective contraction due to the muscle spindles. A fast stretch of the muscle spindles, however, will cause immediate muscle contraction, and since it is not sustained, there will be no inhibitory action (Figure 7.1). This is known as the *basic reflex arc*.

PIR results from a neurological feedback through the spinal cord to the muscle itself when an isometric contraction is sustained, causing a reduction in tone of the muscle which has been contracted (Figure 7.2). This reduction in tone lasts for approximately 20–25 seconds, so you now have a perfect window of opportunity to improve the ROM, as during this relaxation period the tissues can be more easily moved to a new resting length.

When **RI** is employed, the reduction in tone relies on the physiological inhibiting effect of antagonists on the contraction of a muscle (Figure 7.2 overleaf). When the motor neurons of the contracting agonist muscle receive excitatory impulses from the afferent pathway, the motor neurons of the opposing antagonist muscle receive inhibitory impulses at the same time, which

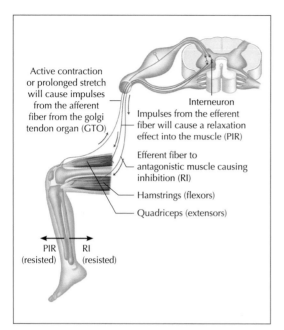

Active contraction or prolonged stretch will cause impulses from the afferent fiber from the golgi tendon organ (GTO)

Interneuron

Impulses from the efferent fiber will cause a relaxation effect into the muscle (PIR)

Efferent fiber to antagonistic muscle causing inhibition (RI)

Hamstrings (flexors)

Quadriceps (extensors)

PIR (resisted)   RI (resisted)

Figure 7.2. Post-isometric relaxation (PIR) and reciprocal inhibition (RI).

prevent it contracting. It follows that contraction or extended stretch of the agonist muscle must elicit relaxation or inhibit the antagonist; however, a fast stretch of the agonist will facilitate a contraction of the agonist.

In most applications of METs, the point of bind, or just short of the point of bind, is the preferred position in which to perform an MET. Clearly, an MET is a fairly mild form of stretching compared with other techniques, so one can assume its use is therefore more appropriate in the rehabilitation process. It should be borne in mind that most problems with muscle shortening will occur in postural muscles. Since these muscles are composed predominantly of slow-twitch fibers, a milder form of stretching is perhaps more appropriate.

MET Procedure

- The patient's limb is taken to the point where resistance is felt, i.e. the point of bind. It can be more comfortable for the patient if you

ease off to a point slightly short of the point of bind in the affected area that you are going to treat, especially if these tissues are in the chronic stage.

- The patient is asked to isometrically contract the muscle to be treated (PIR) or the antagonist (RI), using approximately 10–20% of the muscle's strength capability against a resistance that is applied by the therapist. The patient should be using the agonist if the method of approach is PIR; this will release the tight, shortened structures directly. (See the PIR example below.)

- If the RI method of MET is used, the patient is asked to contract the antagonist isometrically; this will induce a relaxation effect in the opposite muscle group (agonist), which would still be classified as the *tight* and *shortened* structures. (See the RI example below.)

- The patient is asked to slowly introduce an isometric contraction, lasting between 10 and 12 seconds, avoiding any jerking of the treated area. This contraction, as explained above, is the time necessary to load the GTOs, which allows them to become active and to influence the intrafusal fibers from the muscle spindles. This has the effect of overriding the influence from the muscle spindles, which inhibits muscle tone. The therapist then has the opportunity to take the affected area to a new position with minimal effort.

- The contraction by the patient should cause no discomfort or strain. The patient is told to relax fully by taking a deep breath in, and as they breathe out, the therapist passively takes the specific joint that lengthens the hypertonic muscle to a new position, which therefore normalizes joint range.

- After an isometric contraction, which induces a PIR, there is a relaxation period of 15–30 seconds; this period can be the perfect time to stretch the tissues to their new resting length.

- Repeat this process until no further progress is made (normally three to four times) and hold the final resting position for approximately 25–30 seconds.

- A period of 25–30 seconds is considered to be enough time for the neurological system to lock onto this new resting position.
- This type of technique is excellent for relaxing and releasing tone in tight, shortened soft tissues.

A refractory period (the brief period needed to restore the resting potential) of about 20 seconds occurs with RI; however, RI is thought to be less powerful than PIR. Therapists need to be able to use both approaches, because the use of the agonist may sometimes be inappropriate owing to pain or injury. Since the amount of force used with an MET is minimal, the risk of injury or tissue damage will be reduced.

MET Method of Application

"Point of Bind" (or "Restriction Barrier")

In this chapter the word "bind" is mentioned many times. The *point of bind*, or *restriction barrier*, occurs when resistance is first felt by the palpating hand/fingers of the therapist. Through experience and continual practice, the therapist will be able to palpate a resistance of the soft tissues as the affected area is gently taken into the position of bind. This position of bind is *not* the position of stretch—it is the position just before the point of stretch. The therapist should be able to feel the difference and not wait for the patient to say when they feel a stretch has occurred.

Acute and Chronic Conditions

The soft tissue conditions that are treated using METs are generally classified as either *acute* or *chronic*, and this tends to relate to tissues that have had some form of strain or trauma. METs can be used for both acute and chronic conditions. *Acute* involves anything that is obviously acute in terms of symptoms, pain, or spasm, as well as anything that has emerged during the previous three to four weeks. Anything older and of a less obviously acute nature is regarded as *chronic* in determining which variation of MET is suitable.

If you feel the presenting condition is relatively acute (occurring within the last three weeks), the isometric contraction can be performed at the point of bind. After the patient has contracted the muscle isometrically for the duration of 10 seconds, the therapist then takes the affected area to the new point of bind.

In chronic conditions (persisting for more than three weeks), the isometric contraction starts from a position just before the point of bind. After the patient has contracted the muscle for 10 seconds, the therapist then goes through the point of bind and encourages the specific area into the new position.

PIR versus RI

How much pain the patient is presenting with is generally the deciding factor in determining which method to initially apply. The PIR method is usually the technique of choice for muscles that are classified as *short* and *tight*, as it is these muscles that are initially contracted in the process of releasing and relaxing.

On occasion, however, a patient may experience discomfort when the agonist, i.e. the shortened structure, is contracted; in this case it would seem more appropriate to contract the opposite muscle group (antagonist), as this would reduce the patient's perception of pain, but still induce a relaxation in the painful tissues. Hence, the use of the RI method, using the antagonists, which are usually pain free, will generally be the first choice if there is increased sensitivity in the primary shortened tissues.

When the patient's initial pain has been reduced by the appropriate treatment, PIR techniques can be incorporated (as explained earlier, PIR uses an isometric contraction of the tight shortened structures, in contrast to the antagonists being used in the RI method). To some extent, the main factor in deciding the best approach is whether the sensitive tissue is in the acute stage or in the chronic stage.

After having used PIR and RI on a regular basis, I have found that the best results for lengthening the hypertonic structures are achieved with PIR (provided the patient has no pain during this technique). However, once I have performed the PIR method, if I feel more ROM is needed in the shortened tight tissue, I bring into play the antagonists using the RI method for approximately two more repetitions, as explained in the RI example below. This personal approach for my patients has had the desired effect of improving the overall ROM.

PIR Example

To illustrate the PIR method of MET treatment, we are now going to apply the procedure to the adductor pollicis muscle (*pollicis* relates to the thumb, or pollex). You might consider it more appropriate to demonstrate how METs work by means of an example related to the pelvis; however, I wanted the therapist to be able to practice the technique on themselves first, so that they can better understand the MET concept. Once the technique has been understood and subsequently practiced using this simple example, the therapist will then be ready to tackle more complex METs with the aim of helping to restore function to the pelvis.

Place your left (or right) hand onto a blank piece of paper and, with the hand open as much as possible, draw around the fingers and the thumb (Figure 7.3).

Remove the paper and actively abduct the thumb as far as you can, until a point of bind is felt. Next, place the fingers of your right hand on top of the left thumb and, using an isometric

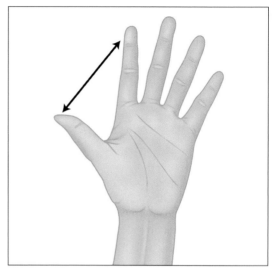

Figure 7.3. The distance between the thumb and finger is measured.

contraction, *adduct* your thumb against the downward pressure of the fingers, so that an isometric contraction is achieved (Figure 7.4). After applying this pressure for 10 seconds, breathe in, and on the exhalation passively take the thumb into further *abduction* (but do not force the thumb). Repeat this sequence two more times and on the last repetition,

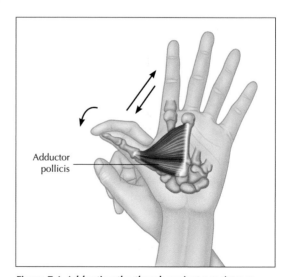

Adductor pollicis

Figure 7.4. Adducting the thumb against a resistance applied by the opposite hand (PIR method).

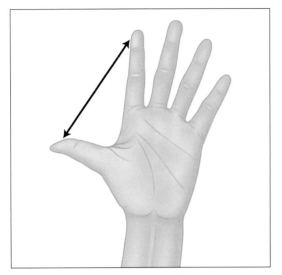

Figure 7.5. The hand redrawn after the MET treatment using PIR and RI.

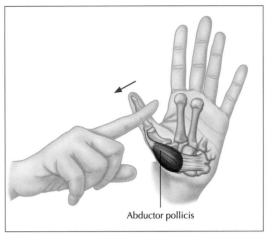

Abductor pollicis

Figure 7.6. Abducting the thumb against a resistance applied by the opposite hand (RI method).

maintain the final resting position for at least 20–25 seconds.

Now place your hand back on the piece of paper and draw around it again (Figure 7.5); hopefully you will see that the thumb has abducted further than before.

RI Example

To apply the RI method, follow the same procedure as for the PIR method, i.e. go to the point of bind by still abducting the thumb. From this position of bind, instead of *adducting* the thumb (PIR) against a resistance, perform the opposite movement and *abduct* your thumb (using the abductor pollicis brevis/longus muscle) against a resistance (Figure 7.6). After applying this pressure for 10 seconds, breathe in, and on the exhalation passively take the thumb into further *abduction* (again, do not force the thumb). Repeat this sequence one or two more times and on the last repetition, maintain the final resting position for at least 20–25 seconds.

As before, place your hand back on the piece of paper and draw around it again (Figure 7.5); hopefully you will see that the thumb has abducted further than previously.

METs and the Muscles of the Pelvis

The muscles that I consider to be specifically related to the position of the pelvis and lumbar spine are:

- Iliopsoas
- Rectus femoris
- Adductors
- Hamstrings
- Tensor fasciae latae (TFL) and iliotibial band (ITB)
- Piriformis
- Quadratus lumborum (QL)

I am going to show you how to assess for each of these muscles, which have a natural tendency to shorten and subsequently become tight. After the testing procedure has been explained, I will demonstrate specific METs to encourage these short/tight muscles to lengthen, so that we can assist and hopefully normalize the dysfunctional position.

Iliopsoas

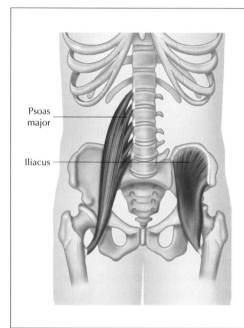

Origin
Psoas major: TPs of all the lumbar vertebrae (L1–L5). Bodies of the twelfth thoracic and all lumbar vertebrae (T12–L5). Intervertebral discs above each lumbar vertebra.

Iliacus: Superior two-thirds of the iliac fossa. Anterior ligaments of the lumbosacral and SIJs.

Insertion
Lesser trochanter of the femur.

Action
Main flexor of the hip joint. Assists in lateral rotation of the hip. Acting from its insertion, it flexes the trunk, as in sitting up from the supine position.

Nerve
Psoas major: Ventral rami of lumbar nerves (L1–L4).

Iliacus: Femoral nerve (L2–L4).

Figure 7.7. (a) Origin, insertion, action, and nerve innervation of the iliopsoas.

Assessment of the Iliopsoas

It is important that we are able to assess for relative shortness within the hip flexor group, as Grieve (1983) says that an increased tension in the iliopsoas muscle is felt to be one of the main reasons for the recurrence of malalignment syndrome, even after the alignment of the pelvis has been corrected.

Schamberger (2013) points out that it is common to find more tension/tenderness in the left iliopsoas than in the right side. One reason for this might be that the left SIJ may actually become hypermobile as a result of the increased stress imposed if the right SIJ becomes "locked" (as a result of a right anterior innominate with a compensatory left rotated posterior innominate) or becomes hypomobile for other reasons. The left iliopsoas would contract in an attempt to stabilize the now hypermobile left SIJ.

Modified Thomas Test

To test the right hip, the patient is asked to lie back on the edge of a couch while holding onto their left knee. As they roll backward, the patient pulls their left knee as far as they can toward their chest (Figure 7.7(b)). The full flexion of the hip encourages full posterior rotation of the innominate bone and helps to flatten the lordosis.

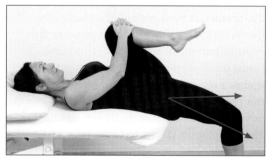

Figure 7.7. (b) The right knee is below the level of the hip, indicating a normal length of the iliopsoas.

From this position, the therapist looks at where the patient's right knee lies, relative to the right hip. The position of the knee should be just below the level of the hip; Figure 7.7(b) demonstrates a normal length of the right iliopsoas.

In Figure 7.8 the therapist demonstrates with their arms the position of the right hip compared with the right knee. You can see that the hip is held in a flexed position, which confirms the tightness of the right iliopsoas in this case.

With the patient in the modified Thomas test position, the therapist can apply an abduction of the hip (Figure 7.9), and an

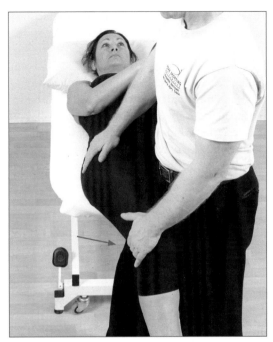

Figure 7.10. Restricted hip adduction, indicating a tight TFL/ITB.

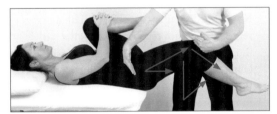

Figure 7.8. A tight right iliopsoas is confirmed. A tight rectus femoris can also be seen here.

adduction of the hip (Figure 7.10). A ROM of 10–15 degrees for each of these is commonly accepted to be normal.

If the hip is restricted in abduction, i.e. a bind occurs at an angle of less than 10–15 degrees, the muscles of the adductor group are held in a shortened position; if the adduction movement is restricted, the TFL and the ITB are held in a shortened position.

MET Treatment of the Iliopsoas

To treat the right side, the patient adopts the same position as in the modified Thomas test above. The patient's left foot is placed into the therapist's right side and pressure is applied by the therapist to induce full flexion of the patient's left hip. Stabilizing the patient's right hip with their right hand, the therapist puts their left hand just above the patient's right knee. The patient is asked to flex their right hip against the therapist's resistance for

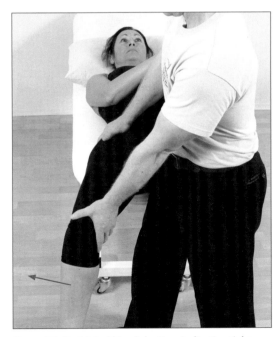

Figure 7.9. Restricted hip abduction, indicating tight adductors.

10 seconds (Figure 7.11); this specific contraction of the iliopsoas muscle will induce a PIR.

Following the isometric contraction, and during the relaxation phase, the therapist slowly applies a downward pressure. This will cause the hip to passively go into extension and will induce a lengthening of the right iliopsoas (Figure 7.12). Gravity will also play a part in this technique, by assisting in the lengthening of the iliopsoas.

Alternatively, it is possible to contract the iliopsoas from the flexed position (Figure 7.13). This is normally used if the original method of activating the iliopsoas causes discomfort to the patient. Allowing the hip to be in a more flexed position will slacken the iliopsoas, which will assist in its contraction and help reduce the discomfort.

The patient is asked to flex their right hip against a resistance applied by the therapist's left hand

(Figure 7.13). After a 10-second contraction, and during the relaxation phase, the therapist lengthens the iliopsoas by taking the hip into an extended position (Figure 7.14(a)).

Tip: The psoas major is also known as filet mignon, which is a piece of beef taken from the tenderloin. A bilateral shortness of the psoas major can cause the pelvis to anteriorly tilt, in turn causing the lumbar spine to adopt a position of hyperlordosis and drawing the sacrum into a position of increased nutation. This can result in compression of the facet joints, leading to lower back pain.

Note: If full sit-ups are performed on a regular basis (not recommended), the iliopsoas is predominantly the muscle being used. Repeated sit-ups will make the iliopsoas stronger and tighter, and result in weakness of the abdominals; this can maintain a patient's lower back pain.

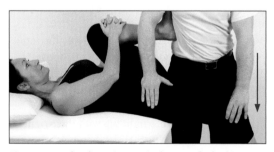

Figure 7.11. The patient flexes their right hip against resistance from the therapist's left hand, while the hip is being stabilized by the therapist's right hand.

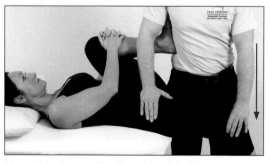

Figure 7.13. The patient resists hip flexion from a flexed position.

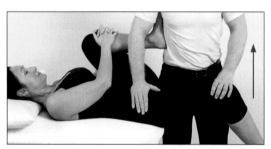

Figure 7.12. The therapist passively extends the hip to lengthen the iliopsoas, with the assistance of gravity.

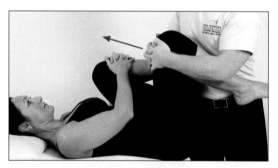

Figure 7.14. (a) Lengthening of the right iliopsoas.

To prove the involvement of the iliopsoas (during the sit-up motion), have your patient lie on their back with their knees bent. Hold the patient's ankles and ask them to dorsiflex their ankles while you resist the movement. This will stimulate the anterior chain musculature, including the iliopsoas, which is part of this chain. The patient then performs the full sit-up movement (Figure 7.14(b)) (most fit individuals will be able to do many sit-ups).

To deactivate or switch off the iliopsoas, the patient is asked to plantar flex their ankles (instead of dorsiflexing them), or to squeeze their glutes. Either of these actions stimulates the posterior chain musculature, causing the iliopsoas to switch off, as activation of the gluteal muscles results in a relaxation of the iliopsoas through RI. When the patient is now asked to perform the sit-up, the movement will prove to be impossible, confirming that the iliopsoas is generally the prime mover in a full sit-up (Figure 7.14(c)).

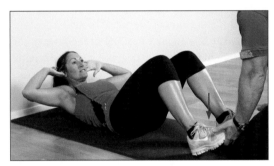

Figure 7.14. (b) Dorsiflexion assists the activation for the contraction of the iliopsoas (switch on).

Figure 7.14. (c) Plantar flexion or activating the glutes assists the deactivation for the contraction of the iliopsoas (switch off).

Rectus Femoris

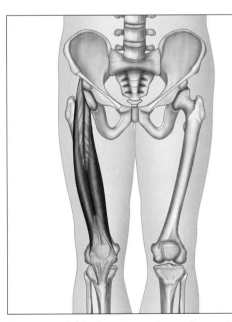

Origin
Straight head (anterior head): AIIS.

Reflected head (posterior head): Groove above the acetabulum (on the ilium).

Insertion
Patella, then via the patellar ligament to the tuberosity of the tibia.

Action
Extends the knee joint and flexes the hip joint (particularly in combination movements, such as in kicking a ball). Assists iliopsoas in flexing the trunk on the thigh. Prevents flexion at the knee joint as the heel strikes the ground during walking.

Nerve
Femoral nerve (L2–L4).

Figure 7.15. Origin, insertion, action, and nerve innervation of the rectus femoris.

Assessment of the Rectus Femoris

Modified Thomas Test

This test is an excellent way of identifying shortness not only in the rectus femoris but also in the iliopsoas as explained earlier. To test the right rectus femoris, the patient adopts the position in Figure 7.16, in which they are holding onto their left leg. The patient is asked to pull their left knee toward their chest, as this will posteriorly rotate the innominate bone on that side; this will be the test position. From this position, the therapist looks at the position of the patient's right knee and right ankle. The angular position of the knee to the ankle should be about 90 degrees; a normal length of the right rectus femoris is shown below.

In Figure 7.17 the therapist demonstrates the position of the right knee compared with the right

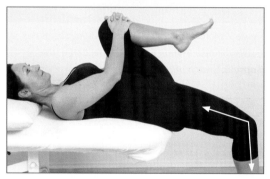

Figure 7.16. To test the right rectus femoris, the patient lies on the couch and holds onto their left leg. A normal length of the rectus femoris is shown.

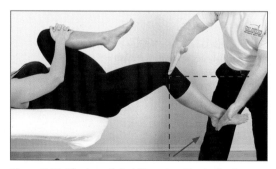

Figure 7.17. The knee is held in extension, indicating a tight rectus femoris.

ankle. Here, the lower leg is seen to be held in a position of extension, which confirms the tightness of the right rectus femoris. You will also notice the position of the hip—it is held in a flexed position. This indicates a tightness of the iliopsoas and was discussed earlier.

MET Treatment of the Rectus Femoris

The patient is asked to adopt a prone position, and the therapist passively flexes the patient's right knee until a bind is felt. At the same time, the therapist stabilizes the sacrum with their right hand, which will prevent the pelvis from rotating anteriorly and stressing the lower lumbar spine facet joints.

> **Note:** If you consider the patient to have an increased lumbar lordosis, a pillow can be placed under their stomach. This will help flatten the lordosis and can reduce any potential discomfort.

From the position of bind, the patient is asked to extend their knee against a resistance applied by the therapist (Figure 7.18), as this contraction will induce a PIR in the rectus femoris muscle.

After a 10-second contraction, and during the relaxation phase, the therapist encourages the knee into further flexion, which will lengthen the rectus femoris (Figure 7.19).

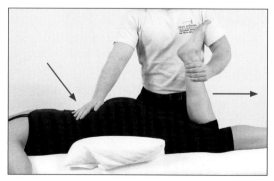

Figure 7.18. The patient extends their knee while the therapist applies resistance.

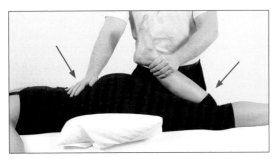

Figure 7.19. The therapist passively flexes the patient's knee to lengthen the rectus femoris while stabilizing the lumbar spine.

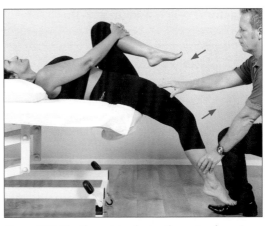

Figure 7.20. The therapist palpates the rectus femoris, and the patient extends their knee against a resistance.

Alternative MET Treatment of the Rectus Femoris

Some patients may find that the previous MET for the rectus femoris puts a strain on their lower back. An alternative and possibly a more effective MET for the rectus femoris is based on the modified Thomas test position.

The patient adopts the position of the modified Thomas test as described earlier. The therapist controls the position of the patient's right thigh, and slowly and passively flexes the patient's right knee toward their bottom. A bind will be reached very quickly in this position, so take extra care when performing this technique for the first time.

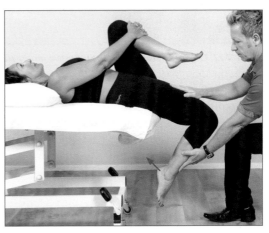

Figure 7.21. The therapist passively flexes the patient's knee to lengthen the rectus femoris.

From the position of bind, the patient is asked to extend their knee against a resistance applied by the therapist (Figure 7.20). After the 10-second contraction, and during the relaxation phase, the therapist passively takes the knee into further flexion (Figure 7.21). This is a very effective way to lengthen a tight rectus femoris.

Tip: Bilateral hypertonicity of the rectus femoris will cause the pelvis to adopt an anterior tilt, resulting in lower back pain due to the L5 facet joints being forced into a lordotic (extended) position.

If one side (typically the right side) of the rectus femoris muscle is held in a shortened position, this will have the effect of pulling the innominate bone into an anteriorly rotated position, with relative counter-nutation of the sacrum to the same side.

Adductors

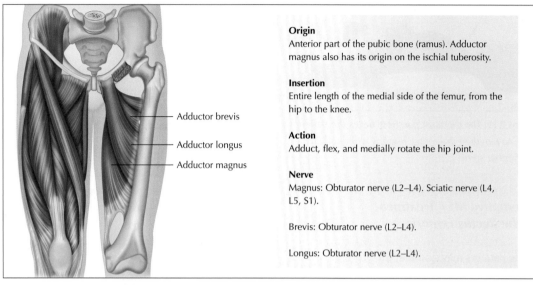

Origin
Anterior part of the pubic bone (ramus). Adductor magnus also has its origin on the ischial tuberosity.

Insertion
Entire length of the medial side of the femur, from the hip to the knee.

Action
Adduct, flex, and medially rotate the hip joint.

Nerve
Magnus: Obturator nerve (L2–L4). Sciatic nerve (L4, L5, S1).

Brevis: Obturator nerve (L2–L4).

Longus: Obturator nerve (L2–L4).

Figure 7.22. Origin, insertion, action, and nerve innervation of the adductors.

Assessment of the Adductors

Hip Abduction Test

To test the left side, the patient adopts a supine position on the couch. The therapist takes hold of the patient's left leg and passively abducts the hip while palpating the adductors with their right hand (Figure 7.23). When they feel a bind, the position is noted. The normal ROM for passive abduction is 45 degrees; if the range is less than this, a tight left adductor group is indicated.

However, there is an exception to the rule. If the ROM is less than 45 degrees, it could be that the medial hamstrings are restricting the movement of passive abduction. To differentiate between the short adductors and the medial hamstrings, the knee is flexed to 90 degrees (Figure 7.24); if the range now increases, this indicates shortness in the medial hamstrings.

In summary, to identify if the hamstrings are the restrictive factor, the therapist passively flexes the knee and then continues with the passive

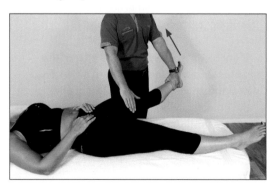

Figure 7.23. The therapist abducts and palpates the adductors for bind.

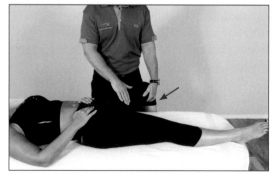

Figure 7.24. The knee is bent to isolate the short adductors.

abduction. If the ROM improves, the hamstrings are the restrictive tissues and not the short adductors.

> **Note:** The term short adductor refers to all of the adductor muscles that attach to the femur, the exception being the gracilis. This particular muscle attaches to a point below the knee, on the pes anserinus (goose foot) area of the medial knee, and acts on the knee as well as on the hip.

MET Treatment of the Adductors

One of the most effective ways of lengthening the adductors (short) is to utilize an MET from the position (Figure 7.25(a–b)). The patient adopts a supine position with their knees bent and heels together; the hips are slowly and passively taken

into abduction by the therapist until a bind is felt in the adductors.

From the position of bind, the patient is asked to adduct their hips against a resistance applied by the therapist, to contract the short adductors.

After a 10-second contraction, and during the relaxation phase, the hips are passively taken into further abduction by the therapist (Figure 7.26(a–b)).

> **Tip:** Overactivity of the adductors will potentially result in a weakness inhibition of the abductor muscles, in particular the Gmed. This can result in a Trendelenburg pattern of gait (see Chapter 5).

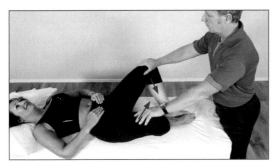

Figure 7.25. (a) The patient adducts their legs against resistance from the therapist.

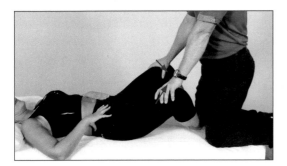

Figure 7.25. (b) Alternative position—the therapist kneels on the couch as the patient adducts their legs against resistance from the therapist.

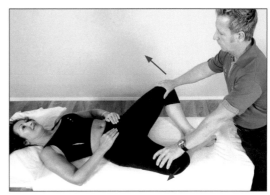

Figure 7.26. (a) The therapist lengthens the adductors.

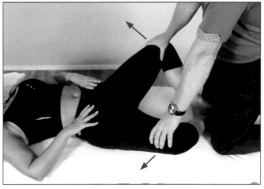

Figure 7.26. (b) Alternative position—the therapist lengthens the adductors.

Hamstrings

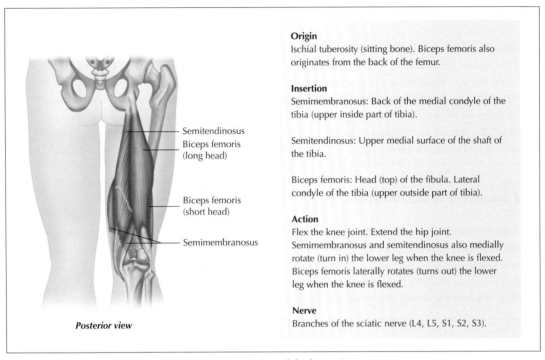

Origin
Ischial tuberosity (sitting bone). Biceps femoris also originates from the back of the femur.

Insertion
Semimembranosus: Back of the medial condyle of the tibia (upper inside part of tibia).

Semitendinosus: Upper medial surface of the shaft of the tibia.

Biceps femoris: Head (top) of the fibula. Lateral condyle of the tibia (upper outside part of tibia).

Action
Flex the knee joint. Extend the hip joint. Semimembranosus and semitendinosus also medially rotate (turn in) the lower leg when the knee is flexed. Biceps femoris laterally rotates (turns out) the lower leg when the knee is flexed.

Nerve
Branches of the sciatic nerve (L4, L5, S1, S2, S3).

Semitendinosus
Biceps femoris (long head)

Biceps femoris (short head)

Semimembranosus

Posterior view

Figure 7.27. Origin, insertion, action, and nerve innervation of the hamstrings.

General Assessment of the Hamstrings

Hip Flexion Test

This test helps to provide the practitioner with an overall impression of the general length of the hamstring muscles. The patient lies in a supine position with both legs extended. The therapist passively guides the patient's left hip into flexion until a point of bind is felt. The normal ROM is anywhere between 80 and 90 degrees; less than 80 degrees indicates that the hamstrings are held in a shortened position. However, "neural tension" of the sciatic nerve and a specific hamstring injury can also restrict the ROM (flexion) of the hip joint.

As you can see in Figure 7.28(a), the patient has a normal ROM in their hamstrings. Anything less than 80–90 degrees would be classified as *short* (Figure 7.28(b)).

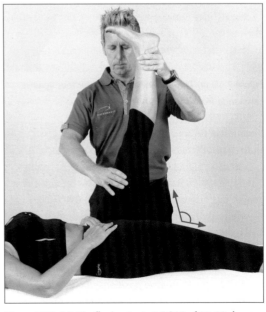

Figure 7.28. (a) Hip flexion test. A ROM of 80–90 degrees is normal.

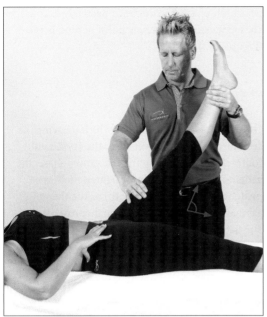

Figure 7.28. (b) Hip flexion test. A ROM of 45 degrees is demonstrated here, indicating short hamstrings.

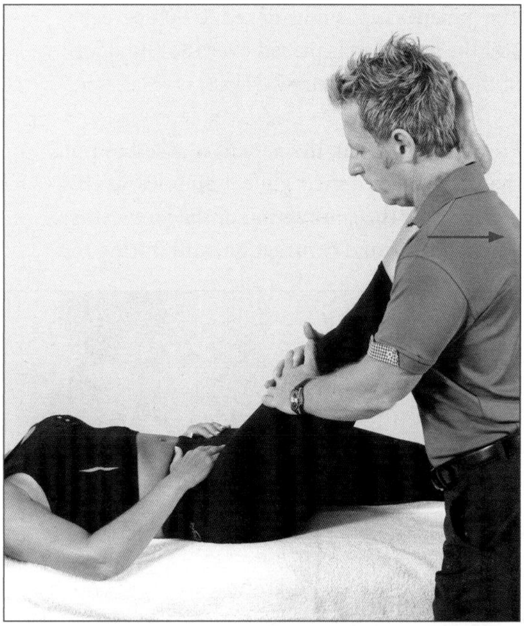

Figure 7.29. The patient pushes their right leg down against the therapist's shoulder.

MET Treatment of the Hamstrings (Non-Specific)

The following technique is very good for lengthening the hamstrings as a group; later in this chapter we will see how to specifically target the medial and lateral hamstrings.

The therapist adopts a standing posture and passively controls the patient's right leg into hip flexion until a bind is felt in the hamstrings. From this position, the patient's lower leg is placed on the therapist's right shoulder (Figure 7.29).

The patient is asked to push down against the therapist's shoulder for 10 seconds. After the contraction of the hamstrings, and during the relaxation phase, the therapist passively takes the right leg into further flexion (Figure 7.30).

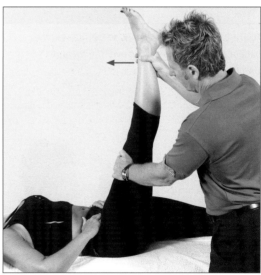

Figure 7.30. The therapist passively takes the hip into further flexion.

Alternative MET for the Insertion of the Hamstrings

This technique is very good for lengthening the insertion component of the hamstrings.

The patient's hip is now flexed to 90 degrees and the lower leg is placed over the shoulder of the therapist (Figure 7.31).

From this position, the patient is asked to pull their heel toward their gluteal muscles, as this will activate the contraction of the hamstrings. After a 10-second contraction, and during the

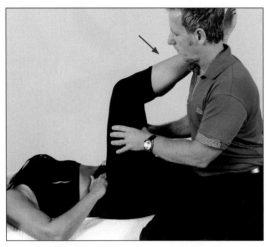

Figure 7.31. With the hip flexed to 90 degrees, the patient places their lower leg over the therapist's shoulder.

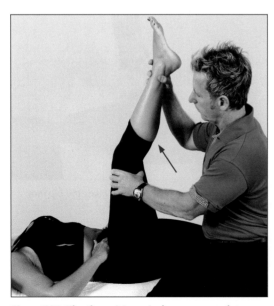

Figure 7.32. The therapist passively encourages knee extension to lengthen the hamstrings.

relaxation phase, the therapist passively encourages knee extension until a new point of bind is felt (Figure 7.32).

RI Method

The patient is asked to contact the hamstrings as described above; however, after the 10-second contraction, and during the relaxation phase, the patient is asked to slowly straighten their knee (which was flexed to start with) as the therapist passively takes the knee into further extension. The patient will be contracting their quadriceps as they straighten the knee actively; this will induce an RI effect in the hamstrings, allowing a more effective and safe lengthening to occur.

Assessment of the Medial Hamstrings (Semitendinosus and Semimembranosus)

After conducting a general assessment of the hamstrings, if the ROM is less than 80 degrees, we can conclude that there is a soft tissue restriction present within the hamstring muscle group. However, the assessment does not tell us which aspect of the hamstrings is the tighter structure.

With specific testing it is possible to identify the individual components of the hamstring muscles that are responsible. The following tests can be incorporated into the assessment to help differentiate muscle length anomalies in the medial hamstrings from those in the lateral hamstrings.

In order to investigate whether the semi-tendinosus/semimembranosus is the restrictive tissue, the medial hamstrings are isolated as follows. The patient's leg is controlled by the therapist, who applies an external rotation and abduction, while at the same time the hip is passively flexed (Figure 7.33(a–b)). The point of bind is noted; if the ROM is less than that in the original test, the medial hamstrings can be assumed to be the shortened muscles.

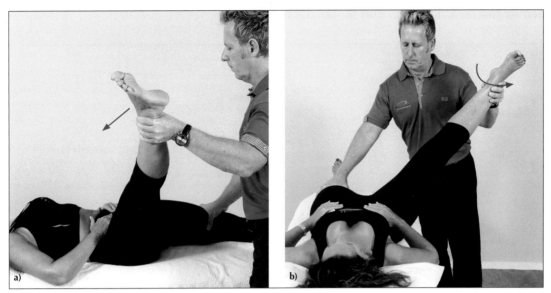

Figure 7.33. (a) To specifically identify the medial hamstrings as the restrictive tissue, the patient's leg is externally rotated and abducted while the hip is passively flexed. (b) Alternative view of the test position.

Assessment of the Lateral Hamstrings (Biceps Femoris)

This specific test will isolate the biceps femoris. The therapist applies an internal rotation and adduction, while the patient's leg is taken into passive flexion (Figure 7.34(a–b)). If the motion feels restrictive, the therapist needs to determine whether the ROM is less than that in the original hip flexion test; if it is, the lateral hamstring of the biceps femoris can be identified as the short tissue.

Tip: Remember, the medial and lateral hamstrings might need treating individually rather than together.

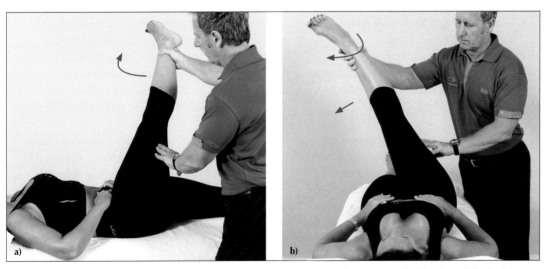

Figure 7.34. (a) To test the biceps femoris, the therapist applies an internal rotation and adduction while the leg is taken into passive flexion. (b) Alternative view of the test position.

Tensor Fasciae Latae (TFL) and Iliotibial Band (ITB)

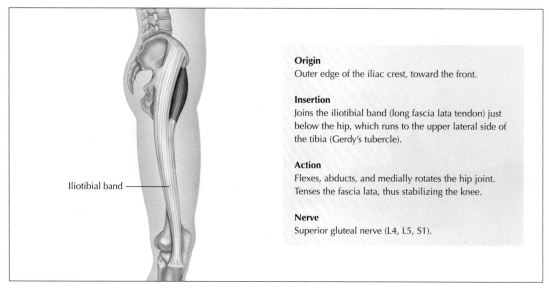

Iliotibial band

Origin
Outer edge of the iliac crest, toward the front.

Insertion
Joins the iliotibial band (long fascia lata tendon) just below the hip, which runs to the upper lateral side of the tibia (Gerdy's tubercle).

Action
Flexes, abducts, and medially rotates the hip joint. Tenses the fascia lata, thus stabilizing the knee.

Nerve
Superior gluteal nerve (L4, L5, S1).

Figure 7.35. Origin, insertion, action, and nerve innervation of the TFL/ITB.

Assessment of the TFL and ITB

Ober's Test

An orthopedic surgeon by the name of Frank Ober wrote an article called "Back strain and sciatica" (Ober 1935a) and first described this test in 1937. He discussed the relationship of a contracted TFL muscle and the ITB to lower back pain and sciatica.

The patient is asked to adopt a side-lying position, and the therapist (with the assistance of the patient) places the patient's shoulder, hip, and knee in alignment (Figure 7.36(a)).

When the therapist feels that the patient has sufficiently relaxed, they slowly bend their own knees (as in a half squat) while maintaining control of the patient's left knee as it is lowered to the couch. If the knee is seen to drop below the level of parallel, the TFL/ITB is classified as *normal* (Figure 7.36(b)); if the thigh remains (or drops only slightly below) parallel, the TFL/ITB is classified as *short* (Figure 7.36(c)).

Note: If there is perceived shortness within the TFL and ITB, the leg will remain relatively abducted, but the hip will naturally want to "fall" into hip flexion with internal rotation as the therapist lowers the leg (Figure 7.36(d)). If this is allowed to happen as the leg approximates the couch, one could mistakenly assume the length of the TFL and ITB to be normal, but a tight TFL/ITB will take the hip into this dysfunctional position. It is therefore important to be very diligent when controlling the patient's leg during the test and not allow the hip to flex and internally rotate.

Please bear in mind the following: when Ober's test is positive, we naturally assume that the TFL and ITB are short and subsequently tight, and that the treatment protocol is to "stretch" and/or perform manual therapy techniques to encourage lengthening of the ITB. However, research has now shown that altering the length of the ITB through manual therapy is next to impossible: according to Chaudhry et al. (2008), a change

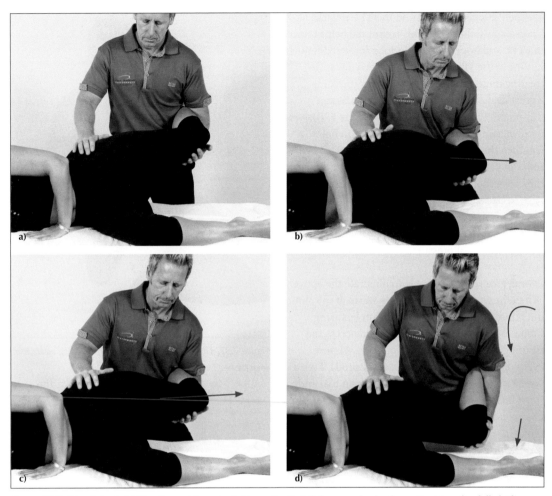

Figure 7.36. Ober's test: (a) The therapist controls the patient's left knee and asks the patient to relax fully before the knee is lowered toward the couch; (b) a normal length of the TFL/ITB, indicated by the knee dropping down; (c) a tight TFL/ITB, indicated by the knee remaining where it is; (d) allowing the hip to "fall" into hip flexion and internal rotation can lead to the incorrect conclusion of a normal ITB/TFL.

in length of the ITB by only 1% will require approximately 1 ton (925kg) of pressure. Hence, there is little chance of actually causing any significant deformation to the ITB and making it less tight through manual therapy and stretching techniques.

A study by Tenney et al. (2013), however, demonstrated that the activation of the abdominals and hamstring muscles in subjects who experience lumbopelvic pain (with a positive Ober's test) led to an improvement in the position of the pelvis,

and subsequently to an overall improvement in the results of Ober's test.

MET Treatment of the TFL and ITB

I consider the following MET an appropriate procedure to be included within a treatment plan, as I feel that it will assist in some way to alter the "tone" of the TFL muscle, rather than altering the length of the connective tissue component, i.e. the ITB. It makes a lot more sense to me to use the PIR effect of METs on the TFL muscle, as I personally believe that this technique helps relax the TFL and hopefully will induce some reduction in tone in the ITB. This is my preferred way of treating these structures, rather than spending a great deal of time performing deep massage techniques (generally called *stripping* the ITB), or advocating the use of a foam roller, to help lengthen the ITB. Techniques of this type (foam roller in particular) may not actually be doing what they have supposedly been designed for in the past, because the soft tissue structure of the ITB (as already discussed) has been shown through research not to change in length by even 1% using almost one ton of pressure.

Let me give you an example to illustrate the above. When the weather is particularly warm at my clinic in Oxford, and especially when I am lecturing, I tend to look out of the window and across the running track to a small area of grass. Almost every day (only when the weather is good), I see a young man spending anywhere between two and three hours rolling his legs using a foam roller. He has been given the nickname "Roller Dave" for obvious reasons, and I have even questioned him on why he does this to his legs. He simply says to me that his therapist recommends doing that every day to *release* his ITBs … I will leave that thought process with you! I am sure some of the students who have attended my courses in Oxford will be smiling when they read about Roller Dave, as they too have undoubtedly seen him rolling his legs many times!

Anyway, back to the treatment protocol. The patient adopts a supine position, and the therapist crosses the patient's flexed left leg over the right leg. The therapist controls the patient's left knee with their right hand and holds onto the patient's right ankle with their left hand. The patient's right leg is then placed into an adducted position until a bind is felt. From the position of bind, the patient is asked to abduct their right leg against a resistance applied by the therapist (Figure 7.37).

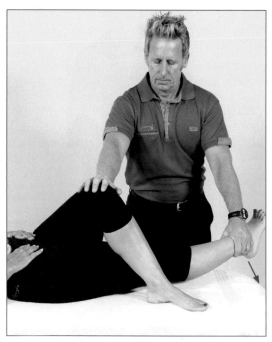

Figure 7.37. The patient abducts their right leg against a resistance.

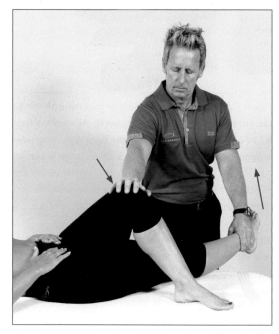

Figure 7.38. (a) The patient's left knee is stabilized, while the therapist adducts the right leg, lengthening the TFL muscle.

After a 10-second contraction, and during the relaxation phase, the therapist passively takes the patient's right leg into further adduction (Figure 7.38(a)). This will encourage a lengthening of the right TFL and may possibly have an effect on the ITB as well (albeit small).

If you look at Figure 7.38(b), the patient has adopted a side-bent position to the left; this will encourage a lengthening of the right QL muscle as well as a lengthening of the TFL and ITB.

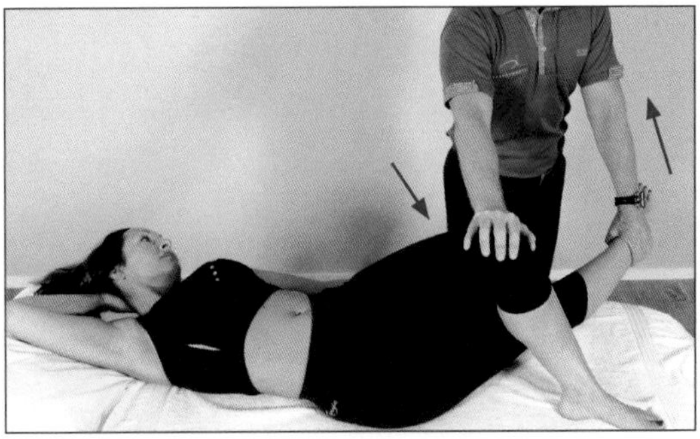

Figure 7.38. (b) The patient side bends to the left, while the therapist adducts the right leg, lengthening the QL and TFL muscles.

Piriformis

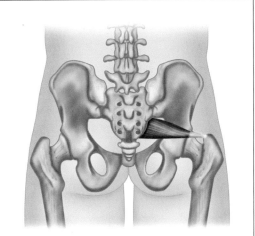

Origin
Internal (front) surface of the sacrum S2–S4.

Insertion
Greater trochanter (top) of the femur.

Action
Laterally rotates and extends the hip joint. Abducts the thigh when the hip is flexed. Helps hold the head of the femur in its socket.

Nerve
Ventral rami of the lumbar nerve (L5) and the sacral nerves (S1, S2).

Figure 7.39. Origin, insertion, action, and nerve innervation of the piriformis.

Observation Assessment of the Position of the Hip

The initial assessment for the relative length of the piriformis muscle is by observation. The patient is asked to adopt the supine position, and the patient's lower limbs are observed from the cephalic end of the couch. The focus of attention will be on the relative position of the foot.

As you can see in Figure 7.40 overleaf, the patient's left foot appears to be further away from the midline than the right foot. The actual movement has come from the hip, which is in a position of external rotation. This possibly relates to a shortened piriformis on the left side.

The piriformis is a very important muscle regarding sacral torsions, because of its attachment onto the anterior surface of the sacrum. Since its pull is in a diagonal direction, the muscle can rotate the sacral base posteriorly and downward relative to the innominate bone. This motion can then cause a wedging against the innominate, resulting in a loss of mobility of the SIJ, and consequently hypomobility of the joint.

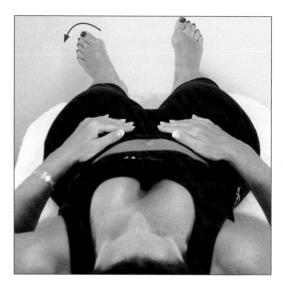

Figure 7.40. The left leg is held in an externally rotated position.

Passive Assessment of the Piriformis

In order to look at the position of the hip to help us decide whether the piriformis is held in a shortened position, we ask the patient to adopt a prone position. One of the patient's knees is flexed to 90 degrees, and the hip is passively controlled by the therapist and allowed to internally rotate. This is repeated with the other knee flexed to 90 degrees. The side that has the least ROM possibly indicates relative shortness of the corresponding piriformis (Figure 7.41).

Another way of assessing the relative length of the piriformis is as follows. The patient is asked to adopt a prone position with both of their knees bent, and then let their legs "flop out"; this will induce internal rotation of the hip joints.

From the cephalic position of the patient, the therapist observes the position of the lower limb, which appears to be asymmetric on one side (Figure 7.42). One can assume that the patient's left side is the dysfunctional side, as the hip is in a position of external rotation. In this case, internal rotation of the hip is restricted, which means that the piriformis on that side is held in a shortened position.

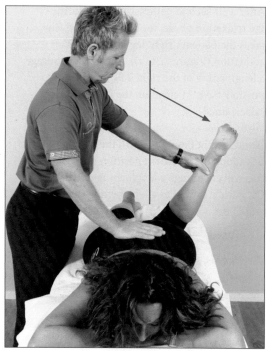

Figure 7.41. The left hip is passively taken into internal rotation to assess for shortness of the piriformis.

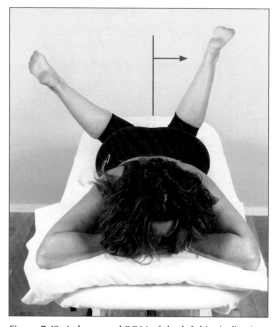

Figure 7.42. A decreased ROM of the left hip, indicating a short left piriformis.

MET Treatment of the Piriformis

The patient adopts the position of the test as described above, but with the right leg straight and the left knee bent. The therapist makes sure that the pelvis/sacrum is stabilized with their right hand, while controlling the patient's left leg with their left hand. The patient's left leg is passively taken into internal rotation until the position of bind is felt, and the patient is asked to contract the piriformis by pulling their leg against resistance applied by the therapist's left hand. This will induce an external rotation of the hip joint (Figure 7.43).

After a 10-second contraction of the piriformis, and during the relaxation phase, the therapist takes the patient's left hip into further internal rotation. This will lengthen the piriformis (Figure 7.44).

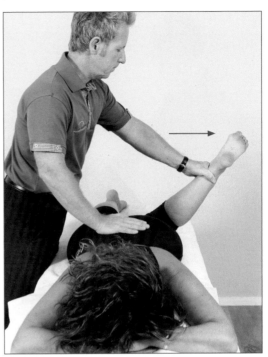

Figure 7.44. The therapist lengthens the piriformis while stabilizing the lumbar spine.

Alternative MET Technique for the Piriformis

Technique 1

This time the patient is asked to adopt a supine position, and the therapist passively takes the patient's left leg and crosses it over the right leg. Controlling the movement of the patient's left innominate with their right hand, the therapist applies pressure to the patient's left knee, passively inducing adduction of the hip to the point of bind.

The patient is asked to abduct their left leg (the piriformis is an abductor), while the therapist resists the movement (see Figure 7.45 overleaf).

After a 10-second contraction, and during the relaxation phase, the therapist passively takes

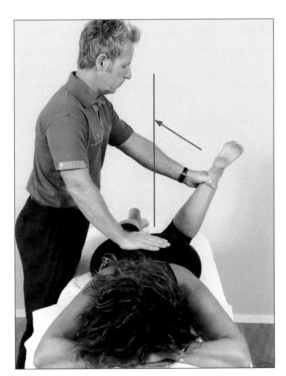

Figure 7.43. The patient is asked to pull their left leg across their body against a resistance. The therapist stabilizes the lumbar spine with the right hand.

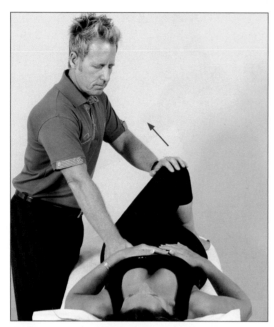

Figure 7.45. Technique 1: from the point of bind, the patient abducts against the pressure applied by the therapist in the direction of the arrow.

the patient's left leg into further adduction (Figure 7.46).

Technique 2

This is my preferred way of lengthening the piriformis muscle.

Controlling the patient's left leg, the therapist tries to encourage flexion of the hip, while at the same time externally rotating the hip with some adduction. This technique will place the piriformis into a position of relative bind, but will need fine-tuning by the therapist and feedback from the patient to finally achieve the optimum position. From this finely tuned position of bind, the patient is asked to push their knee away, into the abdomen of the therapist. This will induce a contraction of the piriformis (Figure 7.47).

After a 10-second contraction, and during the relaxation phase, the therapist passively encourages

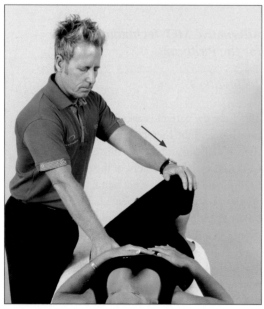

Figure 7.46. Technique 1: the therapist takes the patient's left leg into further adduction and stabilizes the innominate/lumbar spine with the right hand.

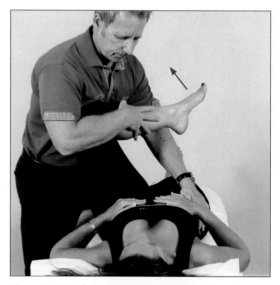

Figure 7.47. Technique 2: this technique will need fine-tuning to get to the optimum position. From the position of bind the patient is asked to push their knee away.

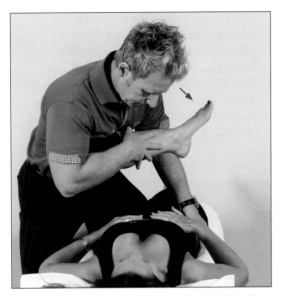

Figure 7.48. Technique 2: using their chest and hand, the therapist encourages further external rotation and adduction of the patient's left hip.

the hip into further external rotation while applying some hip flexion/adduction (Figure 7.48).

Tip: The sciatic nerve of one in five of the population (20%) passes through the piriformis muscle. This can result in buttock and leg pain, but generally no back pain is present, so make sure you eliminate disc/lumbar spine pathology from your hypothesis.

Note: It is considered that after 60 degrees of hip flexion, the piriformis changes from an external rotator to an internal rotator—this is because of its anatomical attachments. If you look closely at Figure 7.48, this is the reason why the patient's left hip is placed in an externally rotated position. This will now lengthen the piriformis, as the left hip has exceeded 60 degrees of flexion.

Quadratus Lumborum (QL)

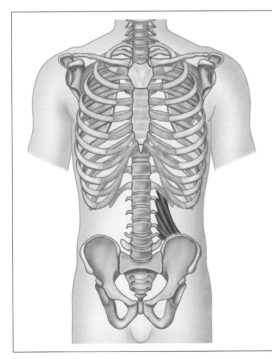

Origin
Iliac crest. Iliolumbar ligament (the ligament from L4/5 to the ilium).

Insertion
12th rib. TPs of the upper four lumbar vertebrae (L1–L4).

Action
Laterally flexes vertebral column. Fixes the 12th rib during deep respiration (e.g. helps stabilize the diaphragm of singers exercising voice control). Helps extend the lumbar spine component of the vertebral column and gives it lateral stability.

Nerve
Ventral rami of the subcostal nerve and upper three or four lumbar nerves (T12, L1, L2, L3).

Figure 7.49. Origin, insertion, action, and nerve innervation of the QL.

Assessment of the QL

In my experience I find that the standing side flexion test is relatively good for indicating tightness of the QL.

The patient stands upright and maintains a neutral position of the lumbar spine. From the standing position, the patient is asked to side bend to the left, and at the same time slide their left hand down the outside of their left leg (Figure 7.50). When the position of bind is reached (this is felt by the therapist palpating the right side of the QL as the patient side bends to the left), the patient's left middle finger should be in contact with the head of the fibula on the left side.

If the middle finger is close or touches the fibula head on the left side, the QL on the right (contralateral) side is classified as *normal*; if there is a restriction, the QL on the right is classified as *tight*.

Note: This test is not conclusive for determining shortness of the QL, as many other lumbar spine factors will affect the overall result. For example, any intervertebral lumbar disc pathology or facet joint restriction/pain will be affected during this test and will give the therapist a false-positive result.

MET Treatment of the QL

PIR Method

The patient is asked to adopt the shape of a banana on the couch: this is achieved by the patient assuming a side-lying supine position, with their right hand placed underneath their head, and their right leg over their left leg. The left leg overlies the edge of the couch (Figure 7.51).

Once the patient has adopted this position, the therapist places their right hand under the head of the patient and cradles the right axilla. The left hand of the therapist stabilizes the patient's left pelvis.

From this position, the patient is asked to side bend to the right against the resistance applied to their axilla by the therapist's right hand (Figure 7.52). This will induce a PIR method of contraction in their right QL.

After a 10-second contraction, and during the relaxation phase, the therapist induces further side bending to the left, which will lengthen the QL on the right side.

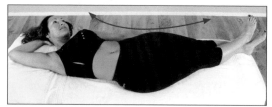

Figure 7.51. The patient's right QL is taken to the point of bind by assuming the "banana" position.

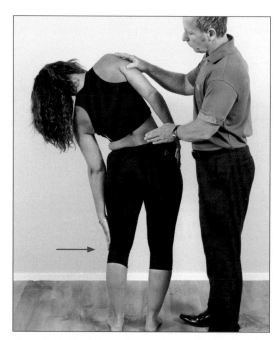

Figure 7.50. The left hand approximates the head of the fibula if the right QL is of normal length.

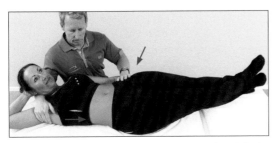

Figure 7.52. The patient side bends to the right while the therapist's left hand stabilizes the patient's left pelvis.

Reciprocal Inhibition (RI) Method

The position of the patient and the procedure are similar to those explained for the PIR method, the only difference being that when the therapist encourages the new position of bind, the patient is asked to reach their left hand toward their left leg (Figure 7.53). This will induce a contraction of the left QL and cause the right QL to relax through RI, allowing a lengthening to occur.

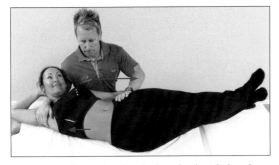

Figure 7.53. The patient is asked to slowly side bend to the left as the therapist guides the motion. This induces an RI effect in the right QL.

Alternative MET for the QL

For an alternative MET for the QL, the patient is placed in a side-lying position, with their left leg off the side of the couch (Figure 7.54). The therapist stabilizes the lower ribs (attachment of the QL) with their right hand and controls the patient's left leg with their left hand. The patient is asked to abduct their left leg against the resistance applied by the therapist's left hand; this will induce a PIR contraction of the left QL muscle.

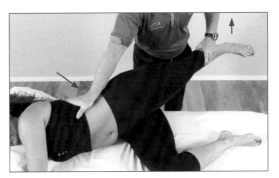

Figure 7.54. The patient abducts their left leg, while the therapist's right hand stabilizes the lower ribs.

After a 10-second contraction, and during the relaxation phase, the therapist slowly and passively takes the patient's left leg into further adduction while stabilizing the patient's lower back (Figure 7.55). This will lengthen the QL on the left side.

> **Tip:** The QL can become overactive and subsequently shorten if the contralateral (opposite) Gmed is weak. It can also be strained by overreaching to one side, for example to the right; in this case, the strain sustained to the left side will result in a protective spasm of the left QL. If the left QL becomes shortened, it will appear as if an iliosacral upslip (see Chapter 12) has occurred on the left side of the innominate bone.

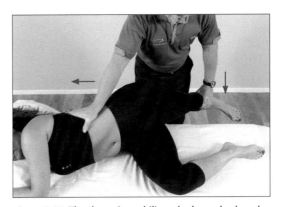

Figure 7.55. The therapist stabilizes the lower back and gently applies cephalic pressure to the 12th rib with their right hand while encouraging adduction of the left leg.

The Hip Joint and Its Relationship to the Pelvis

Almost every time I give a lecture on the areas of the pelvic girdle, hip, and groin, or even on the knee and ankle joint complex, I always hear myself saying the following to my students:

"If one has an underlying pathology within the complexity of the hip joint, then this will eventually become a potential site for pain and dysfunction in distant sites of the body, especially in certain areas of the pelvis and lower back, and even in the knee joint and lower limb."

After saying this I tend to remind the students of the famous words of Dr. Ida Rolf:

"Where the pain is, the problem is not."

This chapter will hopefully highlight those wise words of Dr. Rolf, which relate to not focusing our treatment where the pain is (i.e. the patient's presenting symptoms). We as physical therapists (who I call "detectives of therapy") should try to isolate the underlying cause of a patient's presenting pain and try not to simply "rub where it hurts."

I have seen a great many patients who have presented to the clinic with what has been defined or classified as the typical presentation of SIJ pain, mainly because the presenting pain is located in this particular area of the pelvis. At my sports injury and back pain clinic at the University of Oxford, I must have seen thousands of patients presenting with ongoing pain in the lumbar spine, lateral hip, groin, buttocks, adductor muscles, and hamstring muscles, as well as in the knee joint and lower limb; the underlying cause of their pain, however, is to be found in a completely different structure/tissue/source than the area of the body that suffers the pain.

Now when you read this, I don't want you to jump to any conclusions on the basis of what I have just said. I am not saying that every time your patient presents with pain somewhere in their body the primary cause of their symptoms relates to this specific chapter about the hip joint. However, occasionally it may well be that some underlying pathology located within the hip joint complex is actually the *key* to unlocking the patient's presenting symptoms. The focus of this chapter is naturally biased toward the hip joint, so the extra knowledge you will gain from reading it will potentially provide some of the answers to the questions you might have been asking yourself about your own patients, or even about some of the issues regarding your own presenting symptoms.

This chapter in itself will hopefully guide you along the right pathway. The extra information you will gain through reading it should at least assist you in providing the correct management strategy for your patients: this can be through either treating using manual therapy techniques or possibly even giving you the confidence to refer patients to a specialist for a second opinion.

The assessment processes that I will be demonstrating below will help you formulate an accurate hypothesis of what might be the underlying causative factor responsible for maintaining your patient's presenting symptoms. That is why I always like to "screen" the hip joints of almost every patient who walks through the clinic door—I personally want to make sure that there are no underlying pathological changes within this joint, especially when patients present with pain located in the areas of the pelvic girdle, lumbar spine, knee joint, and so on.

Hip Joint Anatomy

As I am sure you are aware, the hip joint (iliofemoral joint) is classified as a *synovial ball and socket joint*. This joint consists of the head of the femur articulating with the socket (acetabulum) of the pelvic girdle, which is made up of three bones—the ilium, ischium, and pubis. Because of the multiaxial motion that is possible at the hip joint, it will not come as a surprise that it is one of the most mobile joints of the body. Given its inherent architecture of a deep acetabulum (socket), however, the joint has a great deal of stability as well as mobility (Figure 8.1).

The motion possible at the hip joint can vary between individuals, but the normal ranges are:

- flexion: 0–130 degrees
- extension: 0–30 degrees
- internal rotation: 0–35 degrees
- external rotation: 0–45 degrees
- abduction: 0–45 degrees
- adduction: 0–25 degrees

As already explained in previous chapters, the pelvic girdle is capable of anterior and posterior rotation/tilt, while at the same time the lumbar spine is either flexing or extending. All pelvic girdle rotations/tilts/motions actually result from motion at one or more locations—the left hip, the right hip, or the lumbar spine. It is not essential for movement to occur in all three of these areas; however, motion must exist in one of them for the pelvis to rotate.

Table 8.1 highlights specific motion at the pelvic girdle and the associated motions of the lumbar spine and hip joints.

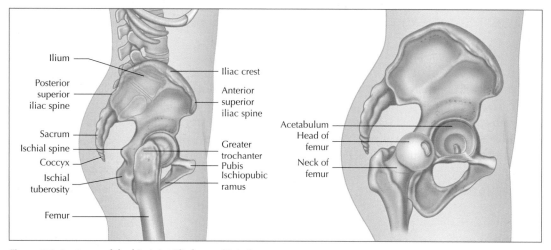

Figure 8.1. Anatomy of the hip joint (iliofemoral joint).

Table 8.1. Pelvic, hip, and lumbar motion guidelines.

Pelvic motion/rotation	Lumbar spine motion	Right hip motion	Left hip motion
Anterior tilt	Extension	Flexion	Flexion
Posterior tilt	Flexion	Extension	Extension
Left lateral shift	Left side bending	Abduction	Adduction
Right lateral shift	Right side bending	Adduction	Abduction
Left transverse rotation	Right transverse rotation	External rotation	Internal rotation
Right transverse rotation	Left transverse rotation	Internal rotation	External rotation

Screening the Hip Joint

With regard to screening, or assessing, the hip joint, I tend to have a few simple diagnostic tests that will either confirm or discount the presence of associated pathology within the joint:

1. Passive ROM for external rotation
2. Passive ROM for internal rotation
3. Passive ROM for flexion
4. Quadrant test
5. FABER test
6. FAIR test
7. Thomas test and modified Thomas test

These tests are simply used as guidelines in screening for any underlying pathology that might be associated with the hip joint. Remember, this book is all about the pelvis, not about the hip joint. Nevertheless, one needs to make sure that the hip joint in itself is not responsible, or even partly responsible, for dysfunction and pain in the pelvic girdle or lumbar spine regions. The tests I will be demonstrating for the hip joint are taken from my own experiences of treating thousands of patients, so much so that I have included some of my own thoughts on the way one might apply some of the tests. There are numerous other tests that can be used to screen the hip joint, but that will be the choice of the therapist at that time in their own clinic with their own patients; as I have said already, the tests I am demonstrating here have been selected on the basis of my own personal experience and preferences.

The specific passive ROM tests given in this chapter for screening the hip joints for pathology are used in particular for identifying the awareness one would feel through one's hands at the end range of the joint that is being tested; this technique is called the *joint end feel*. The end feel of a joint is basically the quality of movement that is perceived by the therapist at the very end of the available ROM. The joint end feel can reveal a great deal about the nature of various pathologies located within the joint that is being tested.

There are four common classifications of what is considered to be a "normal" joint end feel (or joint end range) and which are typically present within any synovial joint:

- Soft end feel, e.g. knee flexion
- Hard end feel, e.g. elbow extension
- Muscular end feel, e.g. hip flexion (hamstrings)
- Capsular end feel, e.g. external rotation of the shoulder joint

When you are assessing your patients/athletes, and especially when you are performing the passive ROM tests, you may experience (through your hands) a different type of joint end feel to what has already been described as a "normal end feel." In this case you can assume that there is what is called a *pathological end feel* present within the architecture of the joint; this positive test should be noted down, and further investigation, or even a referral to a specialist, might subsequently be necessary.

Please remember that patients have two legs and one should perform a comparison between the two, just to make sure that an actual pathology is indeed present. For example, if you passively take the patient's *left* hip into full flexion, with a range of at least 130 degrees being achieved with no pain or stiffness, and your patient is comfortable at the end of the available range, then one can assume that this movement is normal and no pathology is present. Suppose, on the other hand, only around 110 degrees of flexion or less can be achieved when the same movement (flexion) is performed on the *right* hip, and the end range of the joint also becomes particularly painful and/or feels restrictive to your patient (especially in the groin area); in addition, you perceive a "harder end feel" during the movement. From these findings, you can safely say that the ROM of the right hip is not normal; moreover, because of the restrictive/painful barrier, the end feel would be classified as *pathological*, meaning that the test is positive and further investigation is required.

Just a word of caution: in the past I have assessed relatively young patients who have actually demonstrated restrictions in some of the passive ROM tests for both of their hip joints; however, because the motion and the ROM are the same on both sides, we would still regard this movement as being normal in terms of ROM.

Another thing to consider when a hip joint has restricted internal/external rotation is the possibility that this is caused by a pelvic dysfunction. For instance, suppose a patient has a right anterior innominate rotation (the most common dysfunction): *internal* rotation of the *right* hip will usually be limited, compared with the left side, and *external* rotation of the *left* hip will be limited, compared with the right side. If the patient has a suspected *left* anterior innominate rotation, the opposite will be found: a *left* internal rotation restriction and a *right* external rotation restriction.

Rotational restrictions of the hip joint can occur when pelvic dysfunctions are present, even though the total passive ROM in internal/external rotation for each hip joint will be very similar. What I mean by that is the following. Take the case of a patient presenting with the most common malalignment syndrome of a right anterior innominate rotation, with a compensatory left posterior innominate rotation. Because of the pelvic malalignment, the right hip is restricted to, say, only 25 degrees (35 degrees is classified as *normal*) on testing passive internal rotation, and it has an increased range of 55 degrees (45 degrees is classified as *normal*) on testing passive external rotation; this gives a total ROM of 80 degrees. The left hip, however, demonstrates an increased range of 55 degrees for internal rotation, but a limited range of only 25 degrees for external rotation, thus also giving a total ROM of 80 degrees.

The discrepancy between the two hip joints on passive testing arises mainly because of the altered malalignment position of the right and left innominate bones, which has a direct relationship to the position of the adjacent hip joint. Because of this relationship, a change in the position of the innominate bone will have a direct effect on the position of the corresponding acetabulum (hip).

On realignment of the pelvis, one usually finds an improvement in ROM to the extent that the findings for the rotational components for both the left and right hips are normal/equal, even if the total ROM remains the same (i.e. 80 degrees in this case). Pelvic corrections can, however, be very effective in improving overall hip ROM, provided there are no underlying structural pathologies present within the hip joint (corrections for pelvic girdle dysfunctions are explained in Chapter 13).

1. Passive ROM for External Rotation

The therapist passively flexes the patient's hip and knee to 90 degrees (I call it the 90/90 position), as shown in Figure 8.2(a); one hand is placed over the knee and the other hand at the ankle. The hip joint is then passively taken into external rotation. A normal joint end feel range of 45 degrees should be achieved (Figure 8.2(b)).

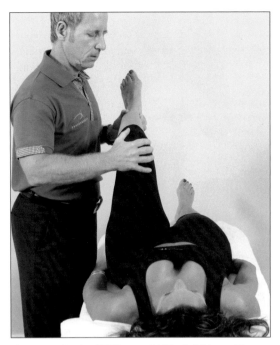

Figure 8.2. Passive ROM tests: (a) The left hip and knee are passively taken into 90 degrees of flexion—the 90/90 position.

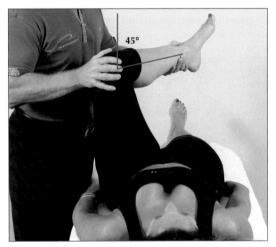

Figure 8.2. (b) The left hip is passively taken into external rotation through a normal range of 45 degrees.

2. Passive ROM for Internal Rotation

The therapist passively flexes the patient's hip and knee to 90 degrees (as above), with one hand placed over the knee and the other hand

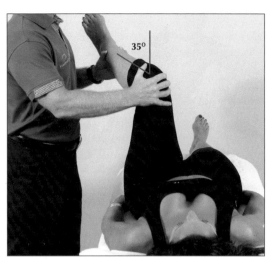

Figure 8.2. (c) The left hip is passively taken into internal rotation through a normal range of 35 degrees.

at the ankle. The hip joint is then passively taken into internal rotation. A normal joint end feel range of 35 degrees should be achieved (Figure 8.2(c)).

3. Passive ROM for Flexion

The hip joint is passively taken into full hip flexion. A normal joint end feel range of 130 degrees should be achieved (Figure 8.2(d)).

> **Note:** You can see from Figure 8.2(e) overleaf that the right leg has lifted off

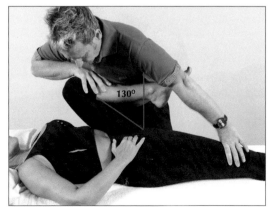

Figure 8.2. (d) The left hip is passively taken into flexion through a normal range of 130 degrees.

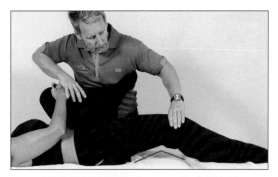

Figure 8.2. (e) The right hip is seen to be held in flexion, indicating a short iliopsoas muscle (Thomas test).

the couch during the movement; this potentially indicates a relative shortness of the right iliopsoas muscle. This test is also known as the Thomas test and is utilized to look for a fixed flexion deformity of the hip joint, normally caused by a tight iliopsoas.

4. Quadrant Test

The quadrant test is designed to assess the inner and outer quadrants of the hip joint. The therapist passively flexes the patient's hip to

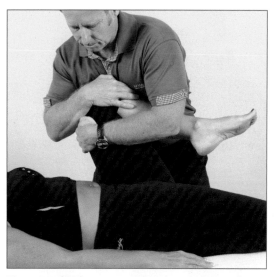

Figure 8.3. (b) The outer quadrant is tested through abducting and compressing.

90 degrees; one hand is placed over the knee and the other hand at the ankle. Next, the therapist applies a force longitudinally through the long axis of the femur (Figure 8.3(a)). The therapist then *abducts* (with compression) the hip in order to assess the *outer* quadrant (Figure 8.3(b)), and

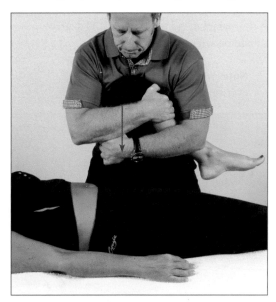

Figure 8.3. Quadrant test: (a) The left hip is compressed in neutral (90 degrees).

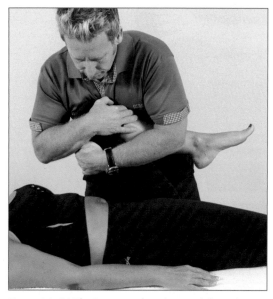

Figure 8.3. (c) The inner quadrant is tested through adducting and compressing.

adducts the hip (with compression) to assess the *inner* quadrant (Figure 8.3(c)).

If there were any underlying pathology located within the hip joint, this test would be positive, as indicated by the motion becoming resistant, as well as the patient perceiving some form of discomfort or even pain.

5. FABER Test

The FABER test (or Patrick's test, named after Hugh Talbot Patrick) relates to the specific motion of **f**lexion, **ab**duction, and **e**xternal **r**otation.

The therapist places the patient's hip into a position of flexion, abduction, and external rotation (Figure 8.4). The presence of a restriction or pain might indicate a pathological change within the hip joint or possibly a pelvic (SIJ) dysfunction, especially if this motion is particularly painful to the SIJ. Let's look at an example. If you notice that the left side is restricted or painful (to the groin or lateral hip), while trying to simply place your patient into the FABER position of flexion, abduction, and external rotation, then this could be caused by a pathological condition within

the left hip joint. Alternatively, the restriction/pain could actually be related to the right-side innominate being held in a position of anterior rotation and showing a positive FABER test on the left side; in this case a correction of the right anterior innominate (see Chapter 13) might improve the overall interpretation of the FABER test on the left side. However, if an innominate correction makes no difference whatsoever to the FABER position, one can assume that there is either an actual musculoskeletal issue present within the hip joint, or the SIJ is implicated (if there is pain in the area of the posterior part of the pelvis, near to the PSIS); both of these pathological conditions would require further investigation.

6. FAIR Test

The FAIR test stands for **f**lexion, **a**dduction, and **i**nternal **r**otation and is commonly used to identify piriformis syndrome (this test is also known as the *FADIR test*—**f**lexion, **ad**duction, **i**nternal **r**otation).

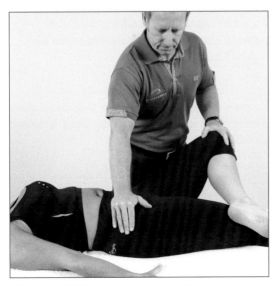

Figure 8.4. FABER test: testing the left hip.

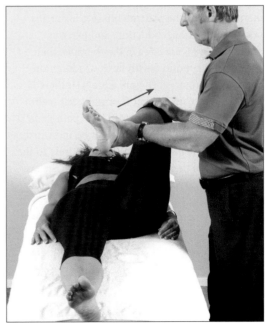

Figure 8.5. FAIR test: (a) Starting position for testing the left hip.

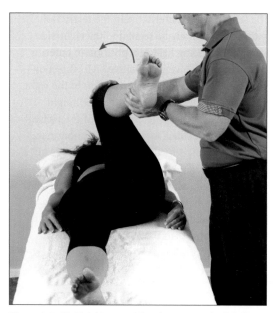

Figure 8.5. (b) Finishing position for testing the left hip.

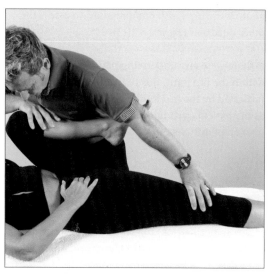

Figure 8.6. Thomas test: (a) A normal length of the right iliopsoas, as indicated by the posterior part of the hip in contact with the couch.

For the particular motion I will be demonstrating, however, I have modified the test to rule out any underlying pathology within the hip joint.

The patient adopts a supine position and the therapist places the patient's hip into a starting position of flexion, abduction, and external rotation (see Figure 8.5(a)); the therapist then continues the motion, with flexion, adduction, and internal rotation (Figure 8.5(b)). If there is a restriction or pain present (normally felt within the groin area) during this test, then pathological changes within the hip joint might be indicated. However, if the patient perceives pain only to the central part of their buttocks, and not to the area of the groin, then the piriformis muscle would be implicated.

7. Thomas Test and Modified Thomas Test

Thomas Test

This test is used to look for a *fixed flexion deformity* of the hip joint and the relationship to the apparent shortness of the hip flexors and in particular of the iliopsoas muscle.

The patient is asked to lie on their back on the couch and hold onto their left knee. As the patient rolls backward, they pull their left knee as far as they can toward their chest (the therapist can assist with this motion if needed), as shown in Figure 8.6(a). The full flexion of the hip encourages full posterior rotation of the innominate bone and helps to flatten the lumbar lordosis. A normal length of the iliopsoas, and a negative test, will be found where the right posterior thigh stays in actual contact with the couch (Figure 8.6(a)).

A fixed flexion deformity, potentially caused by shortness of the right iliopsoas, is indicated if the patient's right hip has lifted off the couch, as shown by the arrow in Figure 8.6(b).

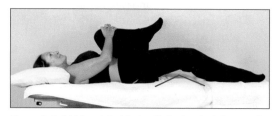

Figure 8.6. (b) The right hip is off the level of the couch, indicating a shortness of the iliopsoas.

Modified Thomas Test

You may recall that this test was demonstrated in Chapter 7 on METs; however, it is important to mention the test again, as I believe it is very relevant, especially as the specific muscles tested (iliopsoas/rectus femoris) will have a direct effect on the hip joint as well as on the pelvis.

The modified Thomas test is used to test for relative shortness of the iliopsoas, rectus femoris, adductors, and TFL/ITB. I always point out to my students that the iliopsoas muscle in particular (out of all the muscles mentioned) is always involved in one way or another in any pathological changes to the hip joint, as well as being an integral part of the functionality of the pelvis and lumbar spine.

To test the right hip, the patient is asked to lie back on the edge of a couch while holding onto their left knee. As they roll backward, the patient pulls their left knee as far as they can toward their chest (Figure 8.7(a)). The full flexion of the hip encourages full posterior rotation of the innominate bone and helps to flatten the lumbar lordosis. In this position, the therapist looks at where the patient's right knee lies, relative to the right hip. The position of the knee should be just below the level of the hip; Figure 8.7(a) demonstrates a normal length of the right iliopsoas and rectus femoris.

In Figure 8.7(b) the therapist is demonstrating with their arms the position of the right hip compared with the right knee. You can see that the hip is held in a flexed position, which confirms the tightness of the right iliopsoas in this case. A tight rectus femoris muscle can also be seen, because the knee is held in extension.

With the patient in the modified Thomas test position, the therapist can apply an abduction of the hip (Figure 8.8), and an adduction of the hip (Figure 8.9 overleaf). A ROM of 10–15 degrees for each of these is commonly accepted to be normal.

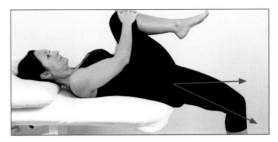

Figure 8.7. Modified Thomas test: (a) The right knee is below the level of the hip, indicating a normal length of the iliopsoas and rectus femoris.

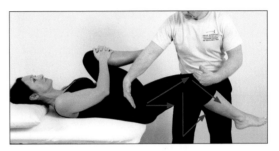

Figure 8.7. (b) A tight right iliopsoas is confirmed. Because the knee is held in extension, a tight rectus femoris is also evident.

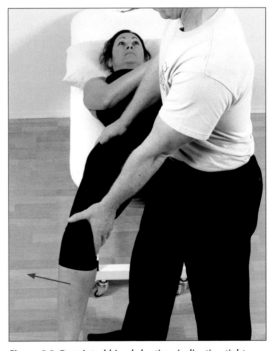

Figure 8.8. Restricted hip abduction, indicating tight adductors.

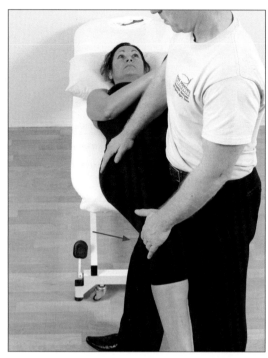

Figure 8.9. Restricted hip adduction, indicating a tight ITB/TFL.

If the hip is restricted in *abduction*, i.e. a bind occurs at an angle of less than 10–15 degrees, the *adductor* muscles are held in a shortened position; if the *adduction* movement is restricted, the *ITB* and the *TFL* are held in a shortened position.

Hip Joint Pathology

Mitchell et al. (2003) carried out a study entitled "Hip joint pathology: Clinical presentation and correlation between magnetic resonance arthrography, ultrasound, and arthroscopic findings in 25 consecutive cases." They discussed that the hip joint is becoming increasingly recognized as a source of groin pain as well as buttock and lower back pain.

In their study they found that *all* of the subjects' hips had undergone an arthroscopy at some stage, and that they had some underlying pathology;

furthermore, 72% of the patients examined reported pain in the lumbar spine and also in the groin area. Some of the patients, however, presented with pain in the buttocks (36%), lateral side of knee (20%), thigh (16%), hamstring (12%), and sciatic nerve (16%), and even in the area of the abdomen (8%).

Those authors mentioned that, although back pain is a very common musculoskeletal symptom, a possible cause of the back pain seen with hip joint pathology is the close association of the psoas muscle with the anterior surface of the hip joint.

The only consistently positive clinical test result was a restricted and painful hip quadrant compared with the contralateral hip (the pain in this test could be in the groin, lateral hip, buttock, or lower back). It should be noted that a painful hip quadrant can also arise from some other local pathology (such as a psoas bursitis or tendinopathy), and that a tight hip quadrant can arise from tight gluteal muscles. A positive FABER test result was found in 88% of the subjects examined, with pain usually in the lateral hip, but occasionally in the groin or buttock. The differential diagnosis of a positive FABER test result is SIJ pathology, especially if it refers to the contralateral buttock.

The conclusion was that hip pathology, particularly acetabular labral pathology (68% diagnosed with labral tears), might be more common than had previously been thought. In those patients with chronic groin and lower back pain, especially where there is a history of an acute injury, a high index of suspicion should be maintained. Clinical signs of a painful, restricted hip quadrant and a positive FABER test result should suggest magnetic resonance (MR) arthrography in the first instance, and the consideration of hip arthroscopy if positive.

Acetabular Labral Tear

The *acetabular labrum* is a ring of fibrocartilage that connects around the rim of the acetabulum; its main function is to help deepen the socket to assist in preventing dislocations. It is similar to the glenoid labrum located within the shoulder joint.

Some patients and athletes (mostly women) who I have seen have torn the labrum mainly through a rotatory type of sporting motion, e.g. aerobics, skiing, or hockey. However, I have also come across a lady who tore her right acetabular labrum (Figure 8.10) by forcefully trying to pull her wellington boot out of the mud when it got stuck. There are other types of injury mechanism, such as a fall; as discussed in the case study later, this trauma caused the person in question to sustain a tear of the labrum.

Patients generally tend to have some discomfort in the area of the groin. This is not always true, however—some have pain in all sorts of places (think back to the Mitchell research article), and one would not even consider the hip joint to be the responsible structure in those cases.

It has been said that patients who have an acetabular labral tear do not get diagnosed for

at least 18 months to two years; I believe the likely reason for this is that the majority of physical therapists have difficulty in confirming the tear. This must also be true of me, especially in my clinic at Oxford, as the majority of patients who I consider to be presenting with a suspect labral tear have had pain, as well as a restricted motion of the hip joint, for well over a year. What I have also noticed in the past is that most of my patients diagnosed with an acetabular labral tear are female.

I remember once discussing with a patient on the telephone the pain she was suffering around the hip and groin areas. The next bit may sound rather strange, but while I was chatting to her I asked her to lie on the floor on her back and bring her knee all the way toward her chest on her non-symptomatic side. She reported back, saying that the movement was no problem and that no pain or stiffness was felt. I then asked her to repeat the same movement on the symptomatic side; this time she said it was a struggle to perform the movement without pain, and her groin area was particularly stiff. I told her to go for an MRI scan of her hip joint, as I said it was probably a labral tear. My theory of her hip problem was correct, as she emailed me a few weeks later to tell me the news and to also say that she was being scheduled for an arthroscopy to resolve the tear.

A clicking sensation and even a locking type of feeling in the groin area are some of the symptoms that patients have mentioned to me. I strongly believe that the longer the labral tear is left (without treatment), the more the hip joint will accumulate deterioration and permanent damage, e.g. osteoarthritis, especially later on in life.

Case Study

An osteopath friend of mine asked me if I could have a look at her, as she was suffering from pain that she felt was located in the right lower part of her buttock, near to the area of the ischial tuberosity. However, she also mentioned that

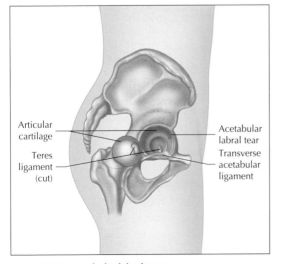

Articular cartilage

Teres ligament (cut)

Acetabular labral tear

Transverse acetabular ligament

Figure 8.10. Acetabular labral tear.

sometimes she would feel the pain in other areas of her body, for example to the upper part of her right hamstrings; at other times, she would feel the pain in the central aspect of her right buttock. Weirdly, on yet another day, the pain was felt in the greater trochanter of her right hip—very confusing or what?

The history was very important, as the initial injury sustained occurred well over four months previously. It happened while she was running and she fell on some ice, landing heavily on the right side of her body; she said it was a nasty fall, because at the time, she experienced a lot of pain, and there was substantial bruising around the right hip and thigh.

She rested for a week or so, but every time she went for a run she felt pain in one of the four areas that I have already mentioned. She had consulted a few practitioners during that time and received various opinions on the diagnosis. Some said the pain originated from a disc prolapse, while others said it was caused by a hamstring tendinopathy, piriformis syndrome, trochanteric and ischial bursitis, a sacrotuberous ligament sprain, and even facet joint syndrome, to name but a few conditions. She had an MRI scan of her lumbar spine and pelvis, but nothing of relevance was found.

I must admit that when I palpated the potential sites of pain, the areas of the ischial tuberosity, sacrotuberous ligament, piriformis, and trochanteric bursa were particularly tender. One might suspect any of these structures to be responsible for her pain; I even considered that the lumbar spine might be responsible, as after initially screening her hip joint, I found nothing of concern at the time of the examination.

A few weeks passed, and after a long run of approximately 10 miles (16km), the patient felt pain in her groin and started to run with a limp because of the discomfort. Her GP was a little

frustrated, as the MRI of her lumbar spine and pelvis confirmed no pathology was present, so a local corticosteroid was injected into the hip joint, just to see if the symptoms would change. The pain seemed to reduce almost immediately, especially over the following few days; she was therefore scheduled for an MR arthrogram of her hip joint, and a *posterior labral tear* of the acetabulum was eventually diagnosed. The labral tear was quite substantial, so an arthroscopy was performed and the labrum repaired. The patient is now able to run with no pain in any of the areas initially reported as problematic.

This case study hopefully reinforces Dr. Ida Rolf's words regarding not treating where the pain is. If the area of the above patient's presenting pain had been treated, then without a doubt she would not have gotten any better unless she had simply rested completely from running, which in this case she definitely did not want to do.

Femoroacetabular Impingement

Another pathological problem associated with the hip joint that I have come across many times in my patients is a condition called *femoroacetabular impingement (FAI)*. This condition can also be responsible for causing a referred type of pain to various sites of the body, similarly to the presenting symptoms of an acetabular labral tear.

The words "femoroacetabular impingement" relate to an area of entrapment between the femur (thigh bone) and the acetabulum (socket). This is a condition whereby some of the soft tissues around the hip joint are being compressed (impinged), and this pathology is generally considered to be caused by abnormally shaped bones at this joint. Because of the altered shape, the femur and the acetabulum do not fit together perfectly, hence the reason why they start to rub against each other and cause damage in the joint.

With femoroacetabular impingement, bone spurs tend to develop around the femoral head (ball) and/or along the acetabulum (socket) of the hip bone. The extra bone overgrowth causes these bones to rub against each other, rather than gliding smoothly. Over time, this can result in the tearing of the labrum and the breakdown of articular cartilage, which can eventually cause degenerative changes that can later lead to osteoarthritis.

Types of FAI

There are three main types of FAI: cam, pincer, and combined cam and pincer.

1. Cam-Type FAI

Cam-type FAI is generally more frequent in men than in women. With this condition the femoral head is not as round as it naturally should be and cannot rotate smoothly inside the acetabulum. A bump forms on the edge of the femoral head that can have the appearance of a "pistol grip" (Figure 8.11). As a result of this extra growth of bone spur, increased shearing-type forces are placed on the articular cartilage and also on the acetabular labrum.

2. Pincer-Type FAI

A pincer-type impingement occurs more often in women than in men. In this case an extra bone growth extends out over the normal rim of the acetabulum (Figure 8.12). As a result of this pincer-type impingement, the labrum can be forcefully compressed and subsequently torn under the prominent rim of the acetabulum.

3. Combined Cam-Type and Pincer-Type FAI

Combined impingement just means that both the pincer and the cam types are present simultaneously (Figure 8.13 overleaf).

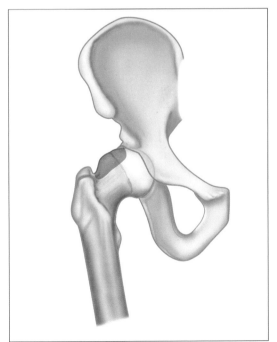

Figure 8.11. Cam-type impingement.

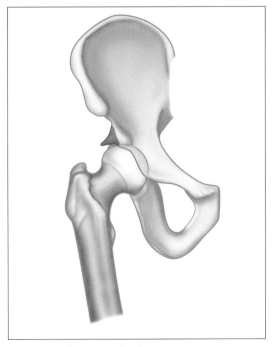

Figure 8.12. Pincer-type impingement.

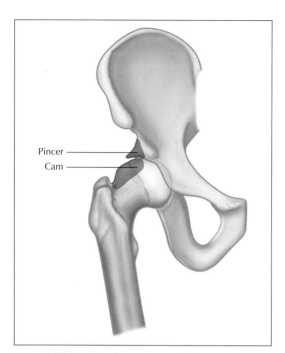

Pincer
Cam

Figure 8.13. Combined cam-type and pincer-type impingement.

With femoroacetabular impingement, patients tend to have pain initially in their groin; this is normally associated with symptoms of clicking, locking, or catching, especially when chronic impingement has resulted in an acetabular labral tear. When a labral tear and FAI both exist at the same time, the presenting symptoms tend to get worse, usually with prolonged periods of standing, sitting, or walking, but particularly with pivotal movements on the affected leg. Because of the chronicity of the condition, secondary problems naturally tend to be present: for example, some patients may limp because of the pain and stiffness, and some may present a *Trendelenburg sign*. Other patients can experience ongoing pain in their buttocks, lower back, and SIJs, as well as in their thighs and knees.

The Gluteal Muscles and Their Relationship to the Pelvis

This book is obviously focused on the pelvic girdle and the sacroiliac joint; however, I think I ought to mention the role of the glutes in this text, as these specific muscles are a core component of the overall function and stability of the pelvic girdle.

The objectives of this chapter are to look at the specific relationship of the gluteal muscles to the area of the pelvis, and how any dysfunction that might be present within the pelvic girdle can cause a misfiring or potential weakness inhibition of the activation of the gluteal musculature.

For this chapter I will concentrate on the anatomy, function, assessment, and relationship to the pelvis of only the gluteus medius (Gmed) and gluteus maximus (Gmax) muscles.

Gluteus Medius (Gmed)

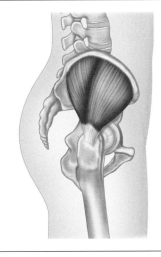

Origin
Outer surface of the ilium, inferior to the iliac crest, between the posterior gluteal line and the anterior gluteal line.

Insertion
Oblique ridge on the lateral surface of the greater trochanter of the femur.

Action
Upper fibers: Laterally rotate and may assist in abduction of the hip joint.

Anterior fibers: Medially rotate and may assist in flexion of the hip joint.

Posterior fibers: Laterally rotate and extend the hip joint.

Nerve
Superior gluteal nerve (L4, L5, S1).

Figure 9.1. Origin, insertion, action, and nerve innervation of the Gmed.

Function of the Gmed

If you think back to Chapter 4 just for a moment, you may recall that when we initiate standing on one leg, we activate what is called the *lateral sling system*; as already explained, this system consists of the Gmed, Gmin, adductors on the ipsilateral side (same side), and the QL on the contralateral side (opposite side), as shown in Figure 9.2.

Potential weakness in the Gmed probably results from the overactivation of other muscles, because of the compensation process (which will be discussed below). Patients who present with weakness in their Gmed, particularly in the posterior fibers, tend to have overactive adductor muscles and ITB through the connection with the TFL; the piriformis can also play an overactive role if the Gmed posterior fibers are shown to be weak.

The Gmed is thought of as the muscle that is *key* to dynamic pelvic stability. For example, in my experience, patients who like to run for pleasure, or even competitively, and who have poor dynamic pelvic stability because of a possible weakness of the Gmed, will tend to shorten their stride length; they will adopt a more shuffling type of

pattern, thereby reducing the ground reaction force at heel contact and decreasing the amount of muscle control required for maintaining pelvic posture.

Assessment of the Gmed

Whenever I look at patients who present with knee, lower lumbar spine, or pelvic pain, part of my assessment process includes checking the strength of the gluteal muscles and in particular the Gmed. In this chapter, as well as discussing the functional roles of this muscle and the Gmax and their relationships to the pelvis, I will also include the hip abduction and hip extension firing pattern tests, which are used for determining the correct muscle firing sequences of the hip abductors/extensors (including the Gmed/Gmax muscles).

In my opinion, the Gmed (and also the Gmax) should be assessed for every single patient and athlete who presents with pain in the areas of the lumbar spine and pelvis, and even in the lower and upper limbs. Many athletes present to my clinic with running-related overuse types of injury to the lower limb as well as to the trunk, and the

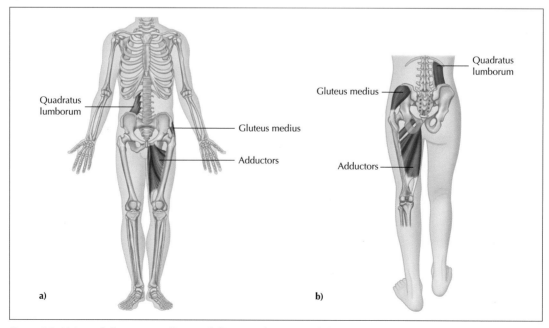

Figure 9.2. (a) Lateral sling system. (b) Lateral sling muscles activated during the gait/walking cycle.

majority of them also present with what I consider to be poor Gmed or Gmax (or both) function. I have come to the conclusion that the strength and control of these muscles is probably the most important overall component in achieving a biomechanically efficient pattern, especially in sports like running. This is not so surprising when you consider that during running you are always either completely in the air or dynamically balanced on one leg. All physical therapist practitioners should be able to assess and restore the function of both the Gmed and the Gmax.

Let's take a closer look at the anatomy of the Gmed: the muscle attaches to the entire length of the iliac crest, to the external ilium between the posterior and anterior gluteal lines, to the gluteal fascia, to the posterior border of the TFL, and to the overlying ITB. The Gmed is divided into three distinct portions—anterior, middle, and posterior—which collectively form a broad conjoined tendon that wraps around, and inserts onto, the greater trochanter of the femur. The more vertical anterior and middle portions of the Gmed appear to be in a better position for abducting the hip than the more horizontal posterior portions.

As mentioned above, the Gmed contains a posterior fiber component in its structure as well as an anterior component; it is the posterior fibers that we as therapists are concerned with. The Gmed posterior fibers work in conjunction with the Gmax, and these two muscles in particular control the position of the hip into an external rotation, which helps to align the hip, knee, and lower limb as the gait cycle is initiated.

As an example, consider a patient who is asked to walk while the therapist observes the process. When the patient puts their weight on their *left* leg at the initial contact phase of the gait cycle, the Gmed is responsible in part for the stability mechanism acting on the lower limb; this will also assist in the overall alignment of the lower limb. The patient continues with the gait cycle and now enters the stance phase. Contraction of the left Gmed in this phase of the gait cycle is responsible in part for

allowing abduction; think of it as a hitching type of motion to the *right* hip, even though the *left* Gmed is contracting. The right side of the hip is then seen to start to lift slightly higher than the *left* side. This process is very important, as it allows the *right* leg to lift a small distance off the floor and will naturally allow the *swing* motion of the right leg during the swing phase of the gait cycle.

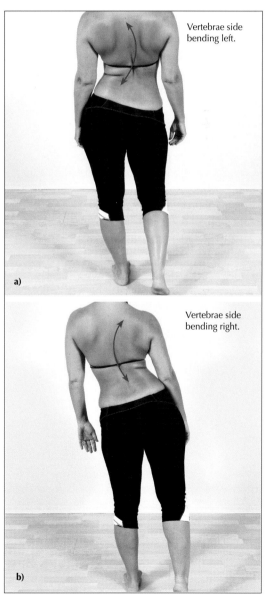

Vertebrae side bending left.

Vertebrae side bending right.

a)

b)

Figure 9.3. (a) Trendelenburg gait. (b) Compensatory Trendelenburg gait.

If there is any weakness in the *left* Gmed, the body will respond in one of two ways during the gait cycle: either the pelvis will tip down on the contralateral side to the stance leg (*right* in this case), giving the appearance of a Trendelenburg pattern of gait (see Figure 9.3(a)); or a compensatory Trendelenburg pattern will be adopted, in which the patient will be observed to shift their whole trunk excessively to the weaker hip (see Figure 9.3(b)).

Gmed weakness will not only have implications for the overall stability of the pelvic girdle and lumbar spine, but also have an effect all the way down the kinetic chain, from heel contact to the mid-stance phase. A weakness of the Gmed can cause:

- Trendelenburg or compensatory Trendelenburg pattern of gait
- Lumbar spine pathology and sacral torsions
- Hypertonicity in the contralateral (opposite side) QL
- Hypertonicity in the ipsilateral (same side) piriformis and TFL muscles and the ITB
- Excessive adduction and internal rotation of the femur
- Drifting of the knee into a valgus or possibly varus position, causing a patella mal-tracking syndrome
- Internal rotation of the lower limb (tibia), relative to the position of the foot
- Increased weight transfer to the medial aspect of the foot
- Excessive pronation of the subtalar joint (STJ)

As you can see from the above list of consequences of a weakness in the function of the Gmed, an athlete/patient is at continual risk of any sports-related injury condition that is somehow caused by increased side bending/rotation of the lumbar spine (potentially because of Trendelenburg gait patterns), as well as by other biomechanical effects to the kinetic chain. An increased lumbar motion of side bending, coupled with rotation (normally to the opposite side), will subsequently cause the sacrum to rotate and side bend in directions opposite to the motion of the lumbar spine; as a result, a forward sacral torsion might now exist, for example a L-on-L or a R-on-R, as explained in Chapter 2.

The weakness of the Gmed can also cause prolonged over-pronation of the STJ, resulting in conditions such as patellofemoral pain syndrome, medial tibial stress syndrome (shin splints), plantar fasciitis, or Achilles tendinopathy.

Hip Abduction Firing Pattern Test

To check the firing sequence on the left side, the patient adopts a side-lying posture with both legs together and their left leg on top. In this sequence, three muscles will be tested: Gmed, TFL, and QL. The therapist palpates the QL muscle by placing their right hand lightly on the muscle. Next, to palpate the Gmed and TFL, the therapist places their finger on the TFL and their thumb on the Gmed (Figure 9.4(a) and (b)).

The patient is asked to lift their left leg into abduction, a few inches from their right leg, while

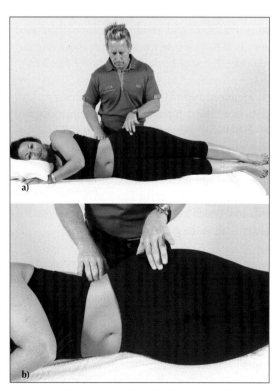

Figure 9.4. (a) Palpation of the QL, Gmed, and TFL. (b) Close-up of the hand position.

the therapist notes the firing sequence (Figure 9.5). It is important to check for any compensatory or cheating recruitment. The idea of this test is that the patient must be able to abduct their hip without: (1) hitching the left side of their pelvis (hip hitching would mean they were activating the left QL muscle); (2) falling into an anterior pelvic tilt; or (3) allowing their pelvis to tip backward.

The correct firing sequence should be Gmed, followed by TFL, and finally QL at around 25 degrees of pelvis elevation. If the QL or the TFL fires first, this indicates a misfiring sequence, potentially resulting in adaptive shortness of these muscles.

Once we have ascertained the firing sequence for hip abduction, we have to decide on the next step. Most patients feel that they need to strengthen the weak Gmed muscle by going to the gym, especially if they have been told this muscle is weak, and they do lots of side-lying abduction exercises. The difficulty in strengthening the apparent weak Gmed muscle is that this particular exercise will not, I repeat *not*, strengthen the Gmed, especially if the TFL and QL are the dominant abductors. The piriformis will also get involved, as it is a weak abductor, which can cause a pelvic/sacroiliac dysfunction, further complicating the underlying issue.

So the answer is to initially postpone the strengthening of the Gmed and focus on the shortened/tight tissues of the adductors, TFL, and QL. In theory, by lengthening the tight tissues through METs as explained in Chapter 7, the lengthened and weakened tissue will become shorter and automatically regain its strength. If, after a period of time (two weeks has been recommended), the Gmed has not regained its strength, specific and functional strength exercises for this muscle can be added.

Gmed "Anterior Fibers" Strength Test

To test the anterior fibers of the left Gmed, the patient adopts a side-lying posture with their left leg uppermost. The therapist palpates the patient's Gmed with their right hand, and the patient is asked to raise their left leg into abduction, a few inches away from the right leg, and hold this position isometrically to start with. Placing their left hand near the patient's knee, the therapist applies a downward pressure to the leg. The patient is asked to resist the pressure (Figure 9.6); if they are able to do so, the anterior fibers of the Gmed are classified as *normal*.

Gmed "Posterior Fibers" Strength Test

In testing the left side, to put more emphasis on the posterior fibers of the Gmed, the therapist controls the patient's left hip into slight extension and external rotation (see Figure 9.7).

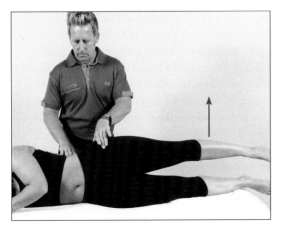

Figure 9.5. As the patient abducts their left hip, the therapist notes the firing sequence.

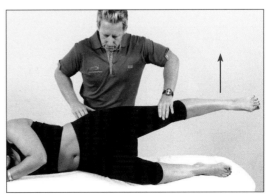

Figure 9.6. The patient abducts their left hip against resistance from the therapist.

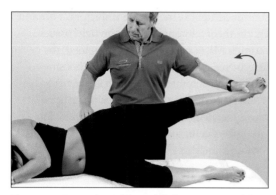

Figure 9.7. External rotation and slight extension of the hip, which emphasizes the posterior fibers of the Gmed.

The therapist applies a downward pressure as before (Figure 9.8); if the patient is able to resist this external force, the Gmed posterior fibers are classified as *normal*. If you want to assess muscular endurance as opposed to strength, ask the patient to hold the abducted leg and maintain the position for at least 30 seconds.

Recall, from the earlier discussion of the role of the Gmed during the gait cycle, that a weakness of the Gmed can cause either a Trendelenburg or a compensatory Trendelenburg pattern of gait. Think about this, and the possible consequences of this weakness, for a second! As you step onto your left leg, the lateral sling has to come into play: the left Gmed is the main muscle responsible for the control of the height of the right side of the pelvis as you try to stabilize on the left leg. If the Gmed muscle on the left is weak, the pelvis will dip (to the right) as you bear weight. The dipping action

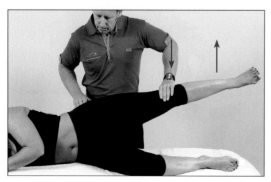

Figure 9.8. The therapist applies a downward pressure to the patient's abducted hip.

will typically cause the lumbar spine to side bend (to the left) and rotate to the right (Type I spinal mechanics) and the facet joints on the left side, as well as the intervertebral disc and the exiting nerve root, to compress, resulting in pain. This side bending motion to the left can also cause the iliolumbar ligament on the right side of the spine, as well as other structures such as the joint capsule of the facet joints, to be placed in a stretched position, which can also be a source of pain (local or referred).

I also mentioned sacral torsion earlier—if the left Gmed muscle is weak, then because of the side bending of the lumbar spine to the left and rotation to the right, the effect will be to cause an opposite motion to the sacrum; thus, the sacrum will side bend to the right and rotate to the left, as in a L-on-L sacral torsion.

Let's look at another example. If the left Gmed is weak, the opposite (right) side QL will compensate and work harder as it tries to take on the role of the weak muscle. This increased compensatory pattern will over time cause an adaptive shortening of the right QL, which can result in the formation of trigger points and subsequently lead to pain.

Case Study

Consider the following scenario: a patient presents to the clinic with pain located in the right lower side of their lumbar spine/superior ilium (QL area), which is exacerbated especially by walking/running for a certain length of time. After palpating the right side of the patient's lower back/QL area, the physical therapist says the muscle is tight and proceeds to release the trigger points that might have developed within. A contract/relax type of technique, such as an MET, might then be used to encourage normality of the length of the QL. The patient and therapist are very happy with the treatment, as most of the presenting symptoms have now subsided. However, as the patient walks the 10-minute journey back to their car the QL pain resumes—why? Because a weak left Gmed is forcing the right QL to work a lot harder than it has been designed to do, and the therapist has only treated the presenting symptoms and not the underlying cause! Remember the wise old words of Dr. Rolf—where the pain is, the problem is not!

Please note that any pelvic dysfunction found in your patient or athlete (as outlined in Chapter 12) can also be one of the main underlying causative factors for the presentation of a weakness/inhibition of the gluteal musculature. The malalignment position of the pelvis can be the key to the problem, as this dysfunction can naturally induce an overcompensatory mechanism in other muscles of the body. This is because the altered pelvic position can now cause a misfiring sequence in the specific activation of the gluteal muscles, rather than these muscles simply being weak and misfiring because of the antagonistic muscles being held in a shortened and tightened position.

In terms of treatment, this suggests that the gluteal muscles will not resume their normal firing sequence capability, or even develop their inherent strength, until the pelvis has been realigned. One might find that the gluteal muscles resume their normal firing sequence and regain their strength simply by realigning the position of the pelvis. After the correction of the pelvic girdle, it is recommended to lengthen the antagonistic muscles (but only if you feel it is still appropriate), before promoting strength-based exercises for these muscles.

Let's quickly recap the above. The first thing I suggest is to correct any presenting pelvic dysfunctions (Chapter 13). Next, if you still find short antagonistic muscles, I would suggest lengthening these through METs (Chapter 7). Finally, I recommend simple strength-based outer core exercises, to encourage and maintain the realigned position of the pelvis (Chapter 3).

Gluteus Maximus (Gmax)

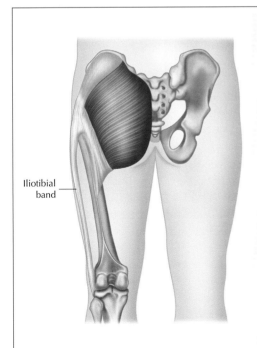

Origin
Outer surface of the ilium behind the posterior gluteal line and a portion of the bone superior and posterior to it. Adjacent posterior surface of the sacrum and coccyx. Sacrotuberous ligament. Aponeurosis of the erector spinae.

Insertion
Deep fibers of the distal portion: Gluteal tuberosity of the femur.

Remaining fibers: Iliotibial band of the fasciae latae.

Action
Assists in adduction of the hip joint. Through its insertion into the iliotibial band, helps to stabilize the knee in extension.

Upper fibers: Laterally rotate and may assist in abduction of the hip joint.

Lower fibers: Extend and laterally rotate the hip joint (forceful extension, as in running or standing up from sitting). Extend the trunk.

Nerve
Inferior gluteal nerve (L5, S1, S2).

Iliotibial band

Figure 9.9. Origin, insertion, action, and nerve innervation of the Gmax.

Function of the Gmax

From a functional perspective, the Gmax performs several key roles in controlling the relationship between the pelvis, trunk, and femur. This muscle is capable of abducting and laterally rotating the hip, which helps to control the alignment of the knee with the lower limb. For example, in stair climbing, the Gmax will laterally rotate and abduct the hip to keep the lower limb in optimal alignment, while at the same time the hip extends to carry the body upward onto the next step. When the Gmax is weak or misfiring, the knee can be seen to deviate medially and the pelvis can also be observed to tip laterally.

The Gmax also has a role in stabilizing the SIJs and has been described as one of the force closure muscles. Some of the Gmax fibers directly attach to the sacrotuberous ligament and the thoracolumbar fascia, which is a very strong,

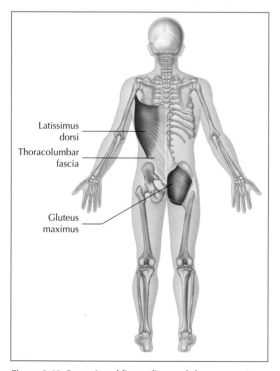

Latissimus dorsi

Thoracolumbar fascia

Gluteus maximus

Figure 9.10. Posterior oblique sling and the connection with the latissimus dorsi.

non-contractile connective tissue that is tensioned by the activation of muscles connecting to it. One of the connections to this fascia is the latissimus dorsi, and the Gmax forms a partnership with the contralateral (opposite) latissimus dorsi via the thoracolumbar fascia— this partnership connection is known as the *posterior oblique sling* (Figure 9.10), which was discussed in Chapter 3. This sling increases the compression force to the SIJ during the weight-bearing single-leg stance in the gait/walking cycle.

Misfiring or weakness in the Gmax reduces the effectiveness of the posterior oblique sling; this will predispose the SIJs to subsequent injury. The body will then try to compensate for this weakness by increasing tension via the thoracolumbar fascia by in turn increasing the activation of the contralateral latissimus dorsi. As with any compensatory mechanism, "structure affects function" and "function affects structure." This means that other areas of the body are affected: for example, the shoulder mechanics are altered, since the latissimus dorsi has attachments on the humerus and scapula. If the latissimus dorsi is particularly active because of the compensation, this can be observed as one shoulder appearing lower than the other during a step-up or a lunge type of motion.

As explained in Chapter 4, the Gmax plays a significant role in the gait cycle, working in conjunction with the hamstrings. Just before heel-strike, the hamstrings will activate, which will increase the tension to the SIJs via the attachment on the sacrotuberous ligament. This connection assists in the self-locking mechanism of the SIJs for the weight-bearing cycle. The interval of the gait cycle from heel-strike to mid-stance is where the tension in the hamstrings should decrease through the natural anterior rotation of the innominate, as well as through the slackening of the sacrotuberous ligament. The activation of the Gmax now increases while that of the hamstrings decreases in order to initiate the action of hip extension.

The Gmax significantly increases the stabilization of the SIJs during the early and mid-stance phases through the attachments of the posterior oblique sling.

Weakness or misfiring in the Gmax will cause the hamstrings to remain active during the gait cycle in order to maintain stability of the SIJs and the position of the pelvis. The resultant overactivation of the hamstrings will subject them to continual and abnormal strain.

As I mentioned earlier, the focus of this chapter is to look at what happens to the function of the pelvis when the glutes become weakened through inhibition; we looked at the Gmed earlier, so in this section we will concentrate on the Gmax. This phasic muscle has a tendency to follow a trait of becoming weakened if the antagonistic muscles have become short and tight or if there are any underlying pelvic malalignments. However, the Gmax can also test weak if there is a neurological disorder, such as a herniated disc (Chapter 10), affecting the L5 and S1 nerve root (which innervates the Gmax muscle). Any type of hip joint pathology—for example an acetabular labral tear (Chapter 8) or joint capsulitis—can also cause an inhibition weakness in the Gmax.

The main muscles that can potentially cause a weakness inhibition in the Gmax are the iliopsoas, rectus femoris, and adductors, as they all are classified as *hip flexors*, which are the antagonistic muscles to the hip extension action of the Gmax.

The assessment of the iliopsoas and other associated shortened antagonistic muscles using the modified Thomas test has already been discussed in Chapter 7. Once that assessment has been fully understood, you will need to normalize the tight and shortened antagonistic muscles by the use of METs. After mastering and applying these advanced techniques, the physical therapist will be able to incorporate them into their own treatment modality, with the aim of encouraging

the lengthening of the tight tissues. This will then promote a normal neutral position of the pelvis and lumbar spine, and in turn hopefully have the effect of "switching" the weakened Gmax back on.

Assessment of the Gmax

In this section I will discuss the hip extension firing pattern test, which is used for determining the correct firing order of the hip extensors (including the Gmax muscle). The aim of the test is to ascertain the actual firing sequence of a group of muscles, to ensure that all are firing correctly, just like the cylinders of an engine. A misfiring pattern will commonly be found in athletes and patients.

Figure 9.11 shows the correct firing pattern in hip joint extension. The normal muscle activation sequence is:

- Gmax
- Hamstrings
- Contralateral lumbar extensors
- Ipsilateral lumbar extensors
- Contralateral thoracolumbar extensors
- Ipsilateral thoracolumbar extensors

The hip extension firing pattern test is unique in its application. Think of yourself as a car with six cylinders in your engine: basically that is what your body is—an engine. The engine has a certain way of firing and so does your body. For example, the engine in a car will not fire its individual cylinders in the numerical order 1–2–3–4–5–6; it will fire in a predefined optimum sequence, say 1–3–5–6–4–2. If we have our car serviced and the mechanic mistakes two of the spark plug leads and puts them back incorrectly, the engine will still work but not very efficiently; moreover, it will eventually break down. Our bodies are no different: in our case, if we are particularly active but have a misfiring dysfunction, our bodies will also break down, ultimately causing us pain.

Hip Extension Firing Pattern Test

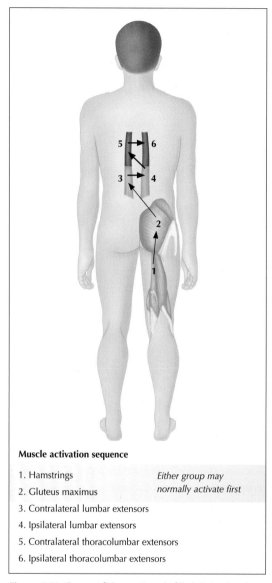

Muscle activation sequence

1. Hamstrings
2. Gluteus maximus
3. Contralateral lumbar extensors
4. Ipsilateral lumbar extensors
5. Contralateral thoracolumbar extensors
6. Ipsilateral thoracolumbar extensors

Either group may normally activate first

Figure 9.11. Correct firing pattern in hip joint extension.

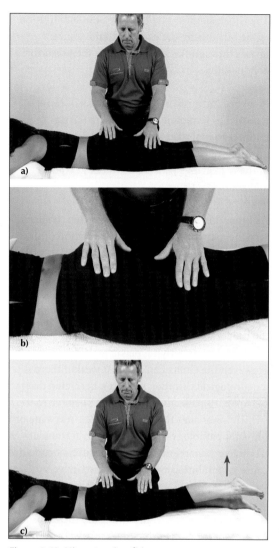

Figure 9.12. Hip extension firing pattern—sequence 1: (a) The therapist lightly palpates the patient's left hamstrings and Gmax; (b) Close-up view of the therapist's hand position; (c) The patient lifts their left leg off the couch.

Sequence 1

The therapist places their fingertips lightly on the patient's left hamstrings and left Gmax (Figures 9.12(a) and (b)), and the patient is asked to lift their left leg 2" (5cm) off the couch (Figure 9.12(c)). The therapist tries to identify which muscle fires first and notes the result of this first sequence (Table A1.1 in Appendix 1 can be used for this).

Sequence 2

The therapist places their thumbs lightly on the patient's erector spinae, and the patient is asked to lift their left leg 2" off the couch (Figure 9.13(a)

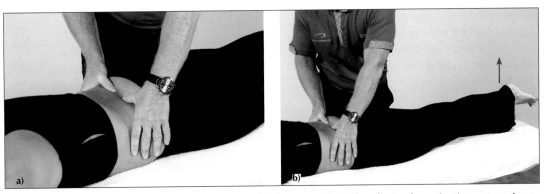

Figure 9.13. Hip extension firing pattern—sequence 2: (a) The therapist lightly palpates the patient's erector spinae; (b) The patient lifts their left leg off the couch.

and (b)). The therapist identifies and notes (in Table A1.1 in Appendix 1) which erector muscle fires first.

Sequences 1 and 2 are then repeated with the right leg, and the results recorded

(in Table A1.2 in Appendix 1). Having done this, the therapist can determine whether or not the muscles are firing correctly. The firing pattern should be: (1) Gmax, (2) hamstrings, (3) contralateral erector spinae, and (4) ipsilateral erector spinae.

Table 9.1. Hip extension firing pattern—left side.

	1st	2nd	3rd	4th
Gluteus maximus	○	○	○	○
Hamstrings	○	○	○	○
Contralateral erector spinae	○	○	○	○
Ipsilateral erector spinae	○	○	○	○

Table 9.2. Hip extension firing pattern—right side.

	1st	2nd	3rd	4th
Gluteus maximus	○	○	○	○
Hamstrings	○	○	○	○
Contralateral erector spinae	○	○	○	○
Ipsilateral erector spinae	○	○	○	○

If, when palpating in sequence 1, the Gmax is found to fire first, you can safely say that this is correct. The same applies in sequence 2: if the contralateral erector spinae contracts first, this is also the correct sequence.

However, if you feel that the hamstrings are number 1 in the sequence, or that the ipsilateral erector spinae is number 1 and the Gmax is not felt to contract, you can deduce that this is a misfiring pattern. If the misfiring dysfunction is not corrected, the body (like the engine) will start to break down and a compensatory pattern of dysfunction will be created.

In my experience, I have found that in a lot of patients, the hamstrings and the ipsilateral erector spinae are typically first to contract and the Gmax is fourth in the sequence. In these cases the erector spinae and the hamstrings will become the dominant muscles in assisting the hip in an extension movement. This can cause excessive anterior tilting of the pelvis, with a resultant hyperlordosis, which can lead to inflammation of the lower lumbar facet joints.

> **Note:** The firing patterns of muscles 5 and 6 have not been discussed in this chapter, because we need to make sure that the correct firing order of muscles 1–4 is established. I also find that when the muscle 1–4 firing sequence has been corrected, the firing pattern of muscles 5 and 6 is generally self-correcting and tends to follow the normal firing pattern sequence.

Another factor that can affect firing order is a previous injury. Bullock-Saxton et al. (1994) investigated the timing of the posterior trunk and leg muscles during hip extension firing, and the influence of a previous ankle sprain on the firing order. Those authors found a significant difference in the onset of Gmax activity (delayed onset) in the group with ankle sprain history compared with the control group.

Gait Cycle Continued

A weak or misfiring Gmax might lead to the creation of several compensatory patterns. First of all, let's look at the case where a patient has a weak Gmax, potentially caused by weakness inhibition, commonly known as *reciprocal inhibition (RI)*, through the antagonistic tightness of the iliopsoas, rectus femoris, and adductors. This soft tissue tightness of the anterior muscles will limit the amount of extension of the hip joint during the gait cycle. As compensatory reactions the innominate bone will be forced to rotate more into an anterior position, and the contralateral innominate will be forced to rotate further into a posterior position. The hamstrings, and in particular the biceps femoris, will be part of the compensation pattern by assisting the increased anterior rotation of the innominate as a result of the weakness of the Gmax. Sahrman (2002) suggested that if the hamstrings are dominant because of inhibition of the Gmax, an anterior shear of the trochanter could be palpated during the prone leg extension.

This now gets a little complex (but has already been explained in previous chapters), as the bit in between the two innominate bones, i.e. the sacrum, will now have to rotate and side bend a bit more than normal because of the increased innominate rotation. The sacrum will now have to compensate by increasing its torsion (rotate one

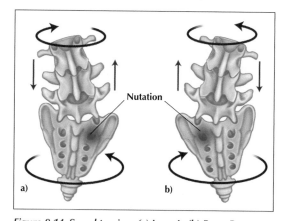

Figure 9.14. Sacral torsion: (a) L-on-L; (b) R-on-R.

way and side bend the other) in one direction; this will be either a L-on-L sacral torsion (left rotation on the left oblique axis), as shown in Figure 9.14(a), or a R-on-R sacral torsion (right rotation on the right oblique axis), as shown in Figure 9.14(b). The lumbar spine will also have to compensate by potentially counter-rotating a bit more in the opposite direction to the sacrum, as shown in the two figures.

There is a natural rotation of the sacral and lumbar spines during the gait cycle; however, because of the increased innominate rotation, the sacrum and lumbar spines have no choice but to compensate as well. In between the lumbar spine and the sacrum (L5 and S1) there lies an intervertebral disc (Chapter 10); imagine now this disc being "torqued" between the two spinal segments. This action will have a negative effect on the disc—it is like squeezing water out of a sponge, and discs do not like that type of increased motion!

One way of potentially correcting the misfiring sequence is as follows. Through muscle length testing (modified Thomas test), we need to first determine which muscles are actually held in a shortened position; METs (Chapter 7) and specific myofascial release techniques (see Gibbons (2014) for demonstrations of these) can then be used to treat and normalize these shortened and tight tissues.

Remember what I talked about earlier: any underlying malalignment position of the pelvic girdle can be another causative factor in the weakness inhibition of the Gmax. Bear that in mind, especially when trying to correct the misfiring sequence.

Thoracolumbar Fascia and Its Relationship to the Gmax and Pelvis

The thoracolumbar fascia is a thick, strong sheet of a ligamentous type of connective tissue,

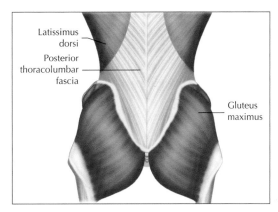

Figure 9.15. The thoracolumbar fascia and the connection to the Gmax.

which connects with, and covers, the muscles of the trunk, hips, and shoulders. The normal function of the Gmax will be to exert a pulling action on the fascia, thereby tensing its lower end (Figure 9.15); you can see from the diagram that there is a connection between the Gmax and the contralateral latissimus dorsi muscle by means of the posterior layer of the thoracolumbar fascia. Both of these muscles conduct the forces contralaterally (i.e. to the opposite side) during the gait cycle (via the posterior oblique sling), which then causes increased tension through the thoracolumbar fascia. This function is very important for rotation of the trunk and for force closure stabilization of the lower lumbar spine and the SIJ.

There is also a co-contraction of the deeper muscles of lumbar stability—i.e. the TVA and the multifidus. These muscles co-contract when you move a limb and were discussed in Chapter 3. As far as I am aware, there has been nothing published recently about the TVA and multifidus being specifically triggered by engagement of the Gmax. However, I personally believe that the TVA muscle definitely responds to Gmax contraction, and I suspect that the multifidus does too, as they all have an association with the sacrotuberous ligament of the pelvis (either directly or indirectly), which assists in force closure of the SIJ.

Case Study

This case study, I hope, emphasizes that the relationship of the glutes to the SIJ is the key link in the patient's presenting symptoms.

The patient was a 34-year-old woman and a physical trainer for the Royal Air Force. She presented to the clinic with pain near the superior aspect of her left scapula (Figure 9.16). The pain would come on four miles (6.5km) into a run, forcing her to stop because it was so intense. The discomfort would then subside, but quickly return if she attempted to start running again. Running was the only activity that caused the pain. Her complaint had been ongoing for eight months, had worsened over the past three, and was starting to affect her work. There was no previous history or related trauma to trigger the complaint.

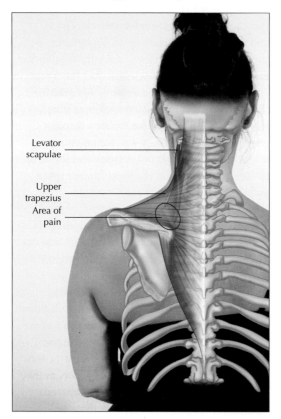

Levator scapulae

Upper trapezius

Area of pain

Figure 9.16. Diagram of the patient's painful area—left superior scapula.

After seeing different practitioners, who all focused their treatment on the upper trapezius, she visited an osteopath who treated her cervical spine and rib area. The treatments she had received were biased toward the application of soft tissue techniques to the affected area, namely the trapezius, levator scapulae, sternocleidomastoid (SCM), scalenes, and so on. The osteopath had also used manipulative techniques on the facet joints of her cervical spine—C4/5 and C5/6. METs and trigger point releases were used in a localized area, which offered relief at the time but made no difference when she attempted to run more than four miles. She had not undergone any scans (e.g. MRI or X-ray).

Taking a Holistic Approach

Let's now assess the case study patient globally rather than locally, remembering that the pain only comes on after running four miles.

When I see a new patient for the first time, no matter what the presenting pain is, I normally assess the pelvis for position and movement, as I consider this area of the body in particular to be the "foundation" for everything that connects to it. I often find in the clinic that when I correct a dysfunctional pelvis, my client's presenting symptoms tend to settle down. However, when I assessed this particular patient, I found her pelvis was level and moving correctly.

I then went on to test the firing patterns of the Gmax (explained earlier), which I often do with patients and athletes who participate in regular sporting activities. However, I only test the firing pattern sequence once I feel that the pelvis is in its correct position; the logic here is that you often get a positive result of the muscle misfiring when the pelvis is slightly out of position.

With the patient in question, I found a bilateral weakness/misfiring of the Gmax, but the firing on the right side seemed a bit slower than on her left side. As I had not found any dysfunction in the pelvis, I pursued this line of approach a little further.

Before we continue I would like to put a few questions to you to think about:

- How does a weakness of the Gmax on the right side cause pain in the left trapezius?
- Is there a link between the Gmax and the trapezius, and if so, how is this possible?
- What can be done to correct the issue?
- What has happened to cause it in the first place?

Gmax Function

Remember from earlier, the Gmax operates mainly as a powerful hip extensor and a lateral rotator, but it also plays a part in stabilizing the SIJ by helping it to force close while going through the gait cycle. Some of the Gmax muscular fibers attach to the sacrotuberous ligament, which runs from the sacrum to the ischial tuberosity, and this ligament has been termed the *key ligament* in helping to stabilize the SIJ.

Linking it All Together

So what do we know? We know that the right side of the patient's Gmax is slightly slower in terms of its firing pattern and that this muscle plays a role in the force closure process of the SIJ. This tells us that if the Gmax cannot perform this function of stabilizing the SIJ, then something else will assist in stabilizing the joint. The left latissimus dorsi is the synergist that helps stabilize the right Gmax (see Figure 9.10) and, more importantly, the SIJ. As the patient participates in running, every time her right leg contacts the ground and goes through the gait cycle, the left latissimus dorsi is over-contracting. This causes the left scapula to depress, and the muscles that resist the downward

depressive pull will be the upper trapezius and the levator scapulae. Subsequently, these muscles start to fatigue; for the patient in question, this occurs at approximately four miles, at which point she feels pain in her left superior scapula.

Treatment

You might think the easy way to treat the weakness in the Gmax is to simply prescribe strength-based exercises. However, in practice this is not always the correct solution, as sometimes the tighter antagonistic muscle is responsible for the apparent weakness. The muscle in this case is the iliopsoas (hip flexor), and its shortening can result in a weakness inhibition of the Gmax. My answer to this puzzle was to lengthen the patient's right iliopsoas muscle (Chapter 7) to see if it promoted the firing activation of the Gmax, while at the same time introducing simple strength exercises for the Gmax.

Prognosis

I advised the patient to abstain from running and to get her partner to assist in lengthening the iliopsoas, rectus femoris, and adductors using METs (Chapter 7) twice a day. Strength and stability exercises for the outer core muscles (Chapter 3) were also advised once daily until the follow-on treatment. I reassessed her 10 days later and found the firing sequence of the Gmax to be normal in the hip extension firing pattern test, and a reduction in the tightness of the associated iliopsoas, rectus femoris, and adductors. Because of these encouraging results, I advised her to run as far as felt comfortable. I was not sure if my treatment was going to correct the problem, but she reported that she had no pain during or after a six-mile (10km) run. The patient is still pain free and continues to regularly use the strengthening exercises for the Gmax and the lengthening techniques for the short/tight muscles.

Conclusion

This case study demonstrates that very often the underlying cause of a condition or problem may not be local to where the symptoms/pain presents, which means that all avenues need to be fully considered.

I hope that the information from this case study has intrigued you enough to continue reading. I would like to think that when you next assess and treat one of your patients, you will look at them in a slightly different way to what you normally would.

_____

I think of this book (and all the books I have written) as taking you on what I call a *jigsaw puzzle journey*—if you stick with it, the picture will eventually become a lot clearer.

After reading this chapter and the above case study, you should have a better understanding of the situation that if the glutes are weak or misfiring, their function (the Gmax's in particular) of tensing the thoracolumbar fascia is reduced, which will cause a natural overactivation of the contralateral latissimus and the ipsilateral multifidus. A weakness inhibition of the Gmax and Gmed will over-stimulate other compensatory mechanisms throughout the whole of the kinetic chain, all of which will naturally in some way or other have an effect on the functionality and stability of the pelvis.

The Lumbar Spine and Its Relationship to the Pelvis

The aim of this chapter is to give the reader an insight into some of the skeletal pathologies that can manifest in the lumbar spine, as well as the potential underlying causes. Let me give you an example: a patient presents to your clinic with localized pain in the muscles of the lumbar erector spinae. On examination you find that the right innominate bone is fixed in an anteriorly rotated position (the most common), which could be caused by an overactivation and subsequent shortness of the right iliopsoas and rectus femoris muscles (as demonstrated in Chapter 7 by the modified Thomas test). The origin of the rectus femoris muscle is on the AIIS of the ilium; because of this attachment, the muscle can naturally "pull" the innominate bone in an anterior and inferior direction. This fixed anterior position of the innominate can cause an inhibition (switching-off) weakness in the right Gmax and was explained in more detail in Chapter 9.

If the Gmax becomes inhibited because of the anteriorly rotated position of the right innominate bone, it will not be able to provide the correct activation sequence when a hip extension action is demanded by the patient (e.g. in walking or running); the lumbar spine erector muscle will be one of many areas that will start to overcompensate for this inhibition weakness of the Gmax (see Chapter 9). In time, an overcompensatory mechanism of the lumbar spine erector musculature in particular will cause the patient to feel tightness in the lower back, as well as potential pain.

There are many different options for treating this particular pelvis dysfunction. One way (and which works very well for me personally) is to utilize a soft tissue method, namely an MET, to normalize the iliopsoas and rectus femoris (this technique is demonstrated in Chapter 7 on METs), in addition to performing a specific MET to correct the anterior position of the innominate (see Chapter 13 on treatment of the pelvis). After having normalized both the muscles and the innominate, you would retest the Gmax firing; if the Gmax is still inhibited, a corrective firing pattern sequence can be initiated to promote the reactivation of the glutes. (For more information on glutes activation and correction, the reader is referred to Gibbons (2014).)

It would be logical to first correct (see Chapters 11 and 12) any/all of the pelvis dysfunctions (iliosacral, sacroiliac, and symphysis pubis) that are found, before continuing, assessing, and treating dysfunction of the lumbar spine (unless the spinal rotation is the primary dysfunction). Perhaps think about why I say this, before reading any further.

Hopefully, you will come to the conclusion that it is essential to address any issues with an underpinning structure before tackling problems in other areas that depend on that structure. For example, I regard the pelvis as being similar to the foundations that are laid before building a house; we would not want to build on top of the foundations if they were not level. I try to use the same analogy when I look at and assess the lumbar spine area. If the pelvis is not level to start with, then the lumbar spine cannot be level either; this area of the spinal column will therefore automatically compensate in some way through changing its natural spinal curvatures, which could result in functional/structural scoliosis. This unnatural positional change to the lumbar spine as a compensation mechanism can only lead to one thing, and you will easily guess what that is— pain, of course!

I am convinced that most of the spinal pathologies discussed in this chapter are a direct or indirect consequence of the overall position and stability integration of the pelvic girdle. It is very difficult, however, to prove this, especially since I haven't been able to find any recent clinical research to back up what I am saying. What I have stated has to be correct in one way or another, however, because the *fundamental foundation* (i.e. the pelvis) must be the main area of compensation for all of the various types of dysfunction that might be present within the body; this will have a direct knock-on effect on the entire kinetic chain, and the lumbar spine is clearly part of that compensatory chain mechanism.

Let's be a little realistic here for a moment. By the time a patient who presents with what might be diagnosed as a *specific* or *non-specific* back pain comes to see you, they probably already have some spinal pathology present. The patient might also have had confirmation of their spinal pathology by an MRI scan, X-ray, or some other diagnostic measures. Put simply, what I am saying in the above statement is therefore the following: the patient's presenting spinal pathology already *exists*, even before they walk through your clinic door!

Of the thousands of patients I have seen as a practicing sports osteopath and sports therapist, I can probably count on one hand those who have consulted me for an initial osteopathic assessment and treatment to actually *prevent* the onset of spinal and pelvic pathology, or indeed any other structural and soft tissue ailment. Let me reiterate what I mean by that. I believe that 99.9% of the patients and athletes who have visited my clinic *already* have a presentation of symptoms of pain/dysfunction somewhere in their body, and more than likely have some underlying form of spinal or pelvic dysfunction/pathology already present—and this is even before we have been formally introduced.

Lumbar Spine Anatomy

There are five individual spinal segments that make up the lumbar vertebrae, and each vertebra comprises the following structures (Figure 10.1):

- Vertebral body
- Spinous process
- Transverse process (TP)
- Superior/inferior facet joint
- Intervertebral foramen
- Spinal canal
- Lamina
- Pedicle
- Intervertebral disc: nucleus pulposus/anulus fibrosus

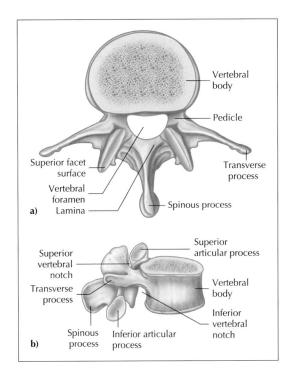

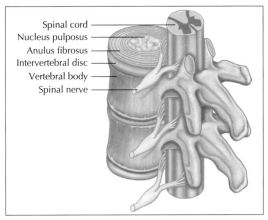

Figure 10.2. Anatomy of the lumbar spine and the intervertebral discs.

Figure 10.1. General anatomy of a lumbar vertebra (L3); a) superior view, b) lateral view.

Intervertebral Discs

Between adjacent lumbar vertebrae there is a structure known as an *intervertebral disc*; in total we have 23 of these soft tissue structures in the human vertebral column. A disc is made up of three components: a tough outer shell, called the *anulus fibrosus*; an inner gel-like substance in the center, called the *nucleus pulposus*; and an attachment to the vertebral bodies, called the *vertebral end plate* (Figure 10.2). As we get older, the center of the disc starts to lose water content, a process that will naturally make the disc less elastic and less effective as a cushion or shock absorber.

Nerve roots exit the spinal canal through small passageways between the vertebrae and the discs: such a passageway is known as an *intervertebral foramen*. Pain and other symptoms can develop when a damaged disc pushes into the spinal canal or nerve roots—a condition commonly referred to as a *herniated disc*.

Disc Herniation

Herniated discs are often referred to as *bulging discs, prolapsed discs*, or even *slipped discs*. These terms are derived from the nature of the action of the gel-like content of the nucleus pulposus being forced out of the center of the disc. Just to clarify, the disc itself does not slip; however, the nucleus pulposus tissue that is located in the center of the disc can be placed under so much pressure that it can cause the anulus fibrosus to herniate or even rupture (Figure 10.3). The severity of the disc herniation may cause the bulging tissue to press against one or more of the spinal nerves, which can cause local and referred pain,

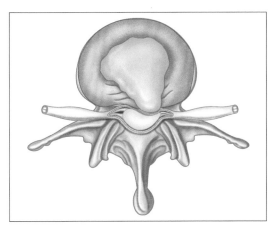

Figure 10.3. Disc herniation.

numbness, or weakness in the lower back, leg, or even ankle and foot. Approximately 85–95% of lumbar disc herniations will occur either at the lumbar segments L4–L5 or at L5–S1; the nerve compression caused by the contact with the disc contents will possibly result in perceived pain along the L4, L5, or S1 nerve root pathway (Figure 10.4).

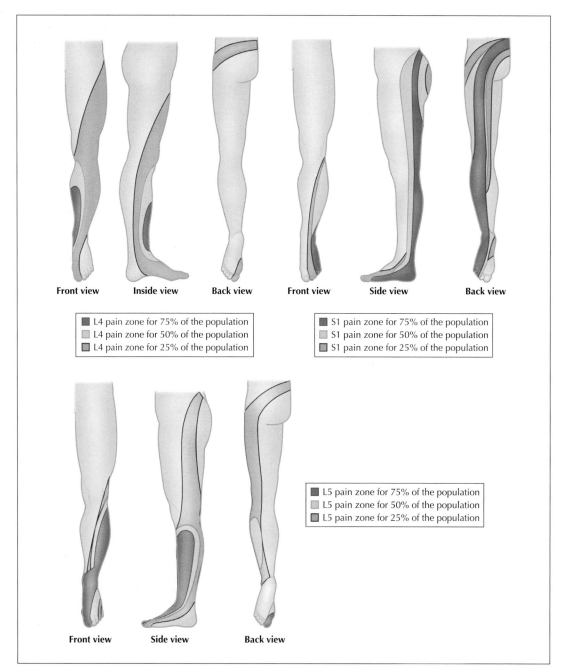

Figure 10.4. Dermatome pathway of pain for L4, L5 and S1 nerve root.

Degenerative Disc Disease

Degenerative disc disease (DDD) tends to be linked to the aging process and refers to a syndrome in which a painful disc can cause associated chronic lower back pain, which can radiate to the hip region (Figure 10.5). The condition generally occurs as a consequence of some form of injury to the lower back and the associated structures, such as the intervertebral discs. A sustained injury can cause an inflammatory process and subsequent weakness of the outer substance of the disc (anulus fibrosus), which will then have a pronounced effect on the inner nucleus pulposus. This reactive mechanism will create excessive movement, because the disc can no longer control the motion of the vertebral bodies that are located above and below the disc. This excessive movement, combined with the natural inflammatory response, will produce chemicals that will irritate the local area, which will commonly produce symptoms of chronic lower back pain.

DDD has been shown to cause an increase in the number of clusters of chondrocytes (cells that form the cartilaginous matrix and consist mainly of collagen) in the anulus fibrosus (consisting of fibrocartilage). Over a prolonged period of time the inner gelatinous nucleus pulposus can change to fibrocartilage, and it has been shown that the outer anulus fibrosus can become damaged in areas that allow some of the nucleus material to herniate through, causing the disc to shrink and eventually leading to the formation of bony spurs called *osteophytes*.

Unlike the muscles in the back, the discs of the lumbar spine do not have a natural blood supply and therefore cannot heal themselves; the painful symptoms of DDD can therefore become chronic, eventually leading to further problems, such as discal herniation, facet joint pain, nerve root compression, spondylolysis (defect of the pars interarticularis), and spinal stenosis (narrowing of the spinal canal).

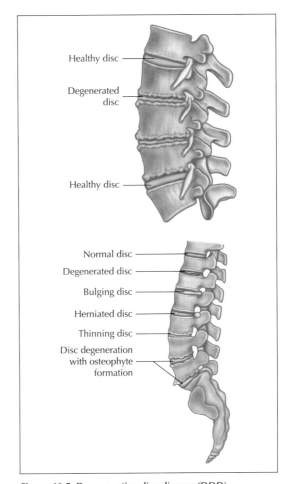

Figure 10.5. Degenerative disc disease (DDD).

Facet Joints

Located within the lumbar spine are the facet joints (anatomically known as the *zygapophyseal joints*); these structures can be responsible for provoking a lot of pain. The facet joints lie posterior to the vertebral body, and their role is to assist the spine in performing movements such as flexion, extension, side bending, and rotation. Depending on their location and orientation, these joints will allow certain types of motion but restrict others: for example, the lumbar spine is limited in rotation, but flexion and extension are freely permitted. In the thoracic spine, rotation and flexion are freely permitted; extension, however, is limited by the facet joints (but also by the ribs).

Each individual vertebra has two facet joints: the *superior articular facet*, which faces upward and works similarly to a hinge, and the *inferior articular facet* located below it. The L4 inferior facet joint, for example, articulates with the L5 superior facet joint.

Like all other synovial joints in the body, each facet joint is surrounded by a capsule of connective tissue and produces synovial fluid to nourish and lubricate the joint. The surfaces of the joint are coated with cartilage, which helps each joint to move (articulate) smoothly. The facet joint is highly innervated with pain receptors, making it susceptible to producing back pain.

Facet Joint Syndrome/Disease

Facet joints have a tendency to slide over each other, so they are naturally in constant motion with the spine; like all types of weight-bearing joint, they can simply wear out and start to degenerate over time. When facet joints become irritated (the cartilage can even tear), this will cause the bone of the joint underneath the facet joint to start producing osteophytes, leading to facet joint hypertrophy, which is the precursor of *facet joint syndrome/disease* (Figure 10.6) and eventually leads to a condition called *spondylosis*. This type of syndrome or disease process is very

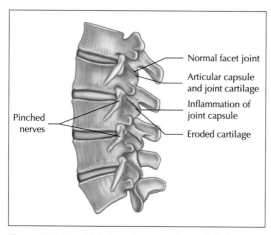

Figure 10.6. Facet joint syndrome and spondylosis.

Normal facet joint
Articular capsule and joint cartilage
Inflammation of joint capsule
Eroded cartilage
Pinched nerves

common in many patients presenting with ongoing chronic back pain.

Lumbar Spine as a Cause of Pelvis Dysfunctions

I have mentioned on numerous occasions the concept of the pelvis and possibly the hip joint being the key areas that are responsible for the presentation of pain in the lumbar spine and pelvic girdle regions. However, there have to be certain times (and, of course, there are) that some other structures (apart from those already mentioned) might need to be incorporated into the bigger picture in order to solve the problem; the structures that I am going to talk about might actually play an even greater role. Once you understand the next concept, I hope it will help you to place the jigsaw puzzle pieces in the correct sequence, so that a clearer picture will begin to appear.

It could be that the underlying issue is hidden and dormant and not showing itself as a dysfunction: the musculoskeletal problem is lying quietly in the grass and minding its own business. Let's consider for a moment the possibility that the problem is actually within the lumbar spine, and this structure could be the key to solving the mystery, as well as being the main reason for maintaining the pelvic dysfunctions.

For example, a patient has ongoing recurrent pelvic dysfunctions that you have been correcting time and time again to no avail; you constantly feel as if you are banging your head against the wall, because what you are doing (in terms of treatment) does not seem to be the key to solving the problem, whereas it might have been with other patients you have treated in the past. The problem potentially lies within the lumbar spine, and it is this skeletal structure that is the underlying causative factor maintaining and controlling the ongoing dysfunctional pelvic pattern. If there is a rotational component at the lumbosacral junction (L5/S1), this has been recognized as one of the causes of recurrent pelvic malalignment.

Let's look at an example where the lumbar spine is the root cause. If we have a clockwise rotation (i.e. to the right) of L5, the right-sided TP will rotate backward (posteriorly). There are soft tissue attachments onto the L4 and L5 TPs for the iliolumbar ligament, and this ligamentous tissue attaches directly to the iliac crest. The induced rotation increases the tension within the iliolumbar ligament, and also the L5 rotation to the right will force the right innominate to rotate posteriorly; the left TP of L5 is rotating anteriorly and this creates an anterior position (anterior rotation) of the left innominate (Figure 10.7). Farfan (1973) reasoned that the shorter the TP, the longer the iliolumbar ligament and the greater the torsional force.

The L5 *right* inferior facet will be in a relatively open position on the superior facet of S1; the *left* inferior facet, however, will be in a closed position on the superior facet of S1. If the left facet joint is compressed, and the position is maintained and continued, it can now become a pivot point (fulcrum). This fixation (left) of the L5/S1 facet joint will now start to encourage the sacrum to rotate to the right axis (R-on-R), which will eventually force the whole pelvis unit into a right rotated position (Figure 10.7).

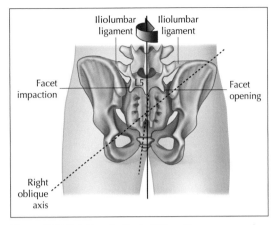

Figure 10.7. Rotational effect of L5 on the sacrum and on the innominate (via the attachment to the iliolumbar ligament).

So how do we go about correcting a dysfunction of the lumbar spine? Well, the assessment of the pelvis in Chapter 12 contains snippets of valuable information that will help you ascertain if a lumbar dysfunction exists. Once you have read and understood how to determine a lumbar dysfunction in your patient, you will then need to read the appropriate text in Chapter 13, which explains in detail how to correct any possible dysfunctions that may be found within the lumbar spine complex.

> **Note:** I would still recommend that you first treat any pelvic dysfunctions, before embarking on realigning specific dysfunctions that you find within the lumbar spine complex.

Sacroiliac Joint Screening

Before I set about guiding you through a comprehensive assessment protocol for the pelvis, I believe that it makes sense to look first at the standard testing procedures for screening the SIJ. In this way we might be able to determine if the actual SIJ is responsible (or partly responsible) for a patient's presenting symptoms; the screening process, on the other hand, may lead us to conclude that the SIJ is not involved.

Let me give you an example of why I might do the screening tests for the SIJ first. When patients present to my clinic with pain in the area of, let's say, the lower lumbar spine and/or pelvis, I will naturally always screen the hip joints for any underlying pathology (as I demonstrated in Chapter 7 on the hip joint), because I personally consider this area of the body (hip joint) to potentially be responsible in part for their presenting symptoms of back or pelvic pain. In this case I can at least then decide if I need to investigate the hip pathology/dysfunction a little further. These clinical findings would probably make me reconsider and alter my treatment strategy to now focus on the area of the hip joint complex rather than specifically on the area of the lumbar spine or pelvis, especially if I wanted

my treatment to have a longer-lasting effect of reducing my patient's ongoing painful symptoms in their lower back and pelvis.

Schamberger (2013) talks about the concept of malalignment syndrome and considers that 80–90% of all adults present with their pelvis out of alignment. Rotational malalignment is by far the most frequently seen, with an anterior rotation to the right innominate bone and a compensatory posterior rotation to the left innominate bone by far the most common (in approximately 80% of patients). This type of rotational malalignment can occur either on its own or in combination with other presentations (upslip/out-flare/in-flare; see "Pelvic Girdle Dysfunctions" section in Chapter 12). An upslip presents on its own in around 10% of patients, and in combination with the other types (rotational/out-flare/in-flare) in another 5–10% of patients. Out-flares and/or in-flares are present in approximately 40–45%, either in isolation or in combination with one or both of the other types.

Klein (1973) also shows that malalignment of the pelvis is present in 80–90% of high-school graduates. Of these, around one-third are asymptomatic and two-thirds are symptomatic, where they present with, for example, lower back or groin pain. Klein talks about three common presentations that account for 90–95% of those subjects found to be out of alignment:

1. Rotational malalignment—either an anterior or a posterior innominate rotation, or a combination of both (approximately 80–85%).
2. Out-flare/in-flare (40–50%).
3. Upslip (15–20%).

Remember, the history taking for your patient is one of the most important components when trying to decide on what you consider to be the actual condition/dysfunction that the patient is presenting with. It is very common for an examiner during a consultation to ask a patient where their pain is. Suppose, in the particular case of assessing the pelvis, the patient points to the area inferior and medial to the PSIS (Figure 11.1(a)), and is able to do this consistently twice and also within a radius of 0.4" (1cm) each time; according to Fortin and Falco (1997), this is a positive sign of SIJ dysfunction.

The above is an example of what is commonly called the *Fortin finger test*; I consider this test to be of value, but only in combination with the

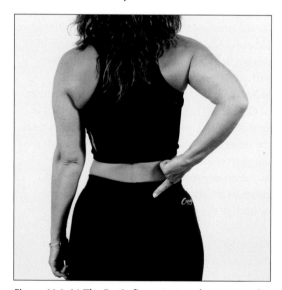

Figure 11.1. (a) The Fortin finger test, as demonstrated by the patient pointing to the area of pain.

provocation tests described below, especially the FABER (Patrick's) test.

Schamberger (2013) mentions that localized pain may arise from one or both SIJs: those with hypomobility or "locking" of one SIJ not infrequently complain of pain from the region of the other, supposedly "normal," SIJ. One explanation for this pain is the increased stress placed on this "normal" joint and its capsule and ligaments as it tries to compensate for the lack of mobility of the impaired SIJ.

In the 1997 study, the Fortin finger test was used as a means of identifying patients with lower back pain and SIJ dysfunction. Provocation-positive SIJ injections were used to confirm or discount the applicability of this clinical sign for the identification of patients with SIJ dysfunction. A total of 16 subjects were chosen from 54 consecutive patients by using the Fortin finger test. All 16 patients subsequently had provocation-positive joint injections, validating SIJ abnormalities. These results indicate that a positive finding of the Fortin finger test, a simple diagnostic measure, successfully identifies patients with SIJ dysfunction.

Fortin et al. (1994) carried out an earlier study on pain pattern mapping for the SIJ and injected the contrast material Xylocaine into the actual SIJ in 10 volunteers. These authors reported that their sensory examination immediately after the injection revealed an area of buttock hypoesthesia extending approximately 4" (10cm) caudally (inferiorly) and 1.2" (3cm) laterally to the PSIS (Figure 11.1(b)). This area of hypoesthesia corresponded to the area of maximal pain noted upon administration of the injection.

In terms of SIJ referral patterns, however, there has been a lot of debate about the exact location to which the SIJ refers: Fortin said 4" (10cm) caudally by 1.2" (3cm) laterally to the PSIS. In contrast, a study conducted by Slipman et al. (2000) called "Sacroiliac joint pain referral zones" recorded significant differences from Fortin's

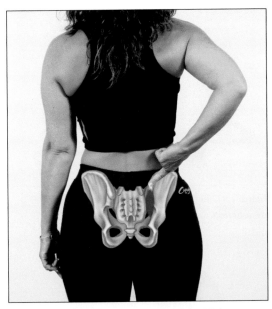

Figure 11.1. (b) The referral pattern of the SIJ from Fortin et al.'s 1994 study.

findings. Using fifty consecutive patients who satisfied clinical criteria and demonstrated a positive diagnostic response to a fluoroscopically guided SIJ injection, Slipman's study yielded the following results. Forty-seven patients (94.0%) described buttock pain, and thirty-six (72.0%) described lower lumbar pain. Twenty-five patients (50.0%) described associated lower-extremity pain. Fourteen patients (28.0%) described leg pain distal to the knee, groin pain was described in seven patients (14.0%), and six patients (12.0%) reported foot pain. Eighteen patterns of pain referral were observed. A statistically significant relationship was identified between pain location and age, with younger patients more likely to describe pain distal to the knee. It was concluded that pain referral from the SIJ does not appear to be limited to the lumbar region and buttock.

SIJ Provocative/Screening Tests

Based on very rigorously reviewed research, there are numerous ways of screening the SIJ.

I, however, currently utilize only five of these provocation tests—those which I consider to be of real value to the clinician and which are used on a day-to-day basis throughout the UK (and the rest of the world) to commonly diagnose SIJ disorders. These SIJ provocation tests, when used in combination rather than in isolation, can be very accurate, as the feedback response from the SIJ can be very sensitive and specific, especially when giving information about the potential effectiveness of an SIJ dysfunction. These tests are not all specific in their application to the SIJ, because they also stress the hip joint and the lumbosacral region. Compressive types of testing motion are more likely to ascertain pain directly from within the joint, whereas distraction types of testing will provoke pain from the corresponding ligaments and joint capsule.

The presence of an SIJ dysfunction can be assumed if one achieves three out of five positive results with the following tests:

1. FABER
2. Compression
3. Thigh thrust
4. Distraction
5. Gaenslen

1. FABER Test

You may recall that I discussed the FABER (flexion, abduction, external rotation) test in Chapter 7, as it is commonly used to screen for any underlying hip pathology; however, it is also a very effective test for ascertaining SIJ dysfunction. The main reason why this test can help the therapist identify the presence of an SIJ dysfunction is the fact that the test induces a motion of the innominate bone in a posterior and external direction relative to the sacrum; this innominate motion encourages sacral nutation and subsequently stresses the associated ligaments (sacrotuberous, sacrospinous, and

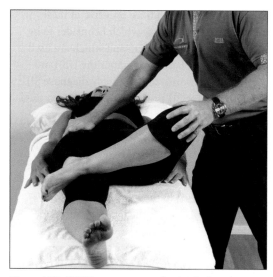

Figure 11.2. FABER test to screen for SIJ dysfunction.

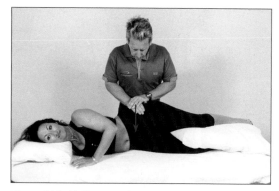

Figure 11.3. (a) Compression test to screen for SIJ dysfunction.

interosseous). The posteriorly rotated innominate position also becomes a lever that can be used to compress the SIJ posteriorly and open the joint anteriorly, which will then stretch the anterior capsule and associated ligaments.

The therapist places the patient's hip into a position of flexion, abduction, and external rotation. The opposite side of the pelvis (at the ASIS) is stabilized, and a gentle, steadily increasing pressure is applied to the same-side knee of the patient, exaggerating the motion of hip flexion, abduction, and external rotation (Figure 11.2). If there is a restriction (in the hip joint mainly) or pain posteriorly in the area of the SIJ, a pathological change/dysfunction within the SIJ might be indicated.

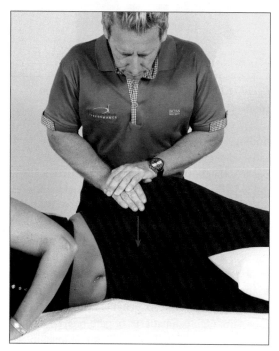

Figure 11.3. (b) Close-up view of the compression test.

2. Compression Test

The patient is placed in a side-lying position, facing away from the therapist, with a pillow between the knees for comfort. The therapist applies a gradual downward pressure through the anterior aspect of the innominate, between the greater trochanter of the femur and the iliac crest, to check if pain in the corresponding SIJ is present (Figure 11.3(a–b)).

3. Thigh Thrust Test

The patient lies in a supine position with one hip flexed to 90 degrees. The therapist stands on the same side as the flexed leg and stabilizes the patient's pelvis by applying pressure to the opposite ASIS. Gradually increasing pressure is then applied through the axis of the femur, to determine if pain is present within the SIJ (Figure 11.4(a–b)).

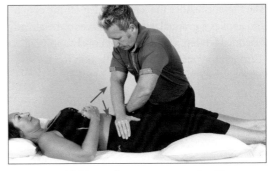

Figure 11.4. (a) Thigh thrust test to screen for SIJ
dysfunction.

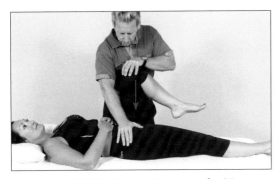

Figure 11.5. (a) Distraction test to screen for SIJ
dysfunction.

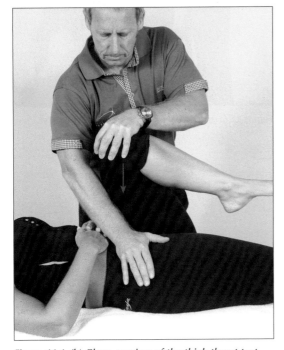

Figure 11.4. (b) Close-up view of the thigh thrust test.

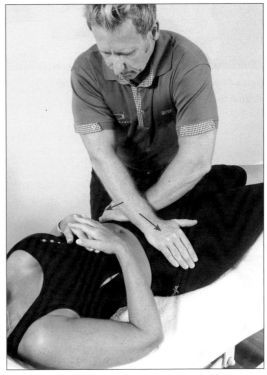

Figure 11.5. (b) Close-up view of the distraction test.

4. Distraction Test

The patient lies in a supine position with a
pillow under their knees for support. With
arms crossed and elbows relatively straight,
the therapist places their hands on the anterior
aspects of the patient's left and right ASISs of the
innominate bones. A gradual pressure is then
applied laterally, to encourage a distraction of the
SIJ (Figure 11.5(a–b)). The presence of any pain
is noted.

5. Gaenslen Test

The patient lies in a supine position near the left
edge of the couch. They are asked to flex the right
hip by pulling their right knee to their chest, a
movement which rotates the right innominate
posteriorly, while allowing the left innominate
to rotate anteriorly; this particular action has
the effect of locking the SIJ at the same time.

The therapist slides the left lower leg off the couch and applies a gradual extension force to the already extended left leg, while simultaneously applying (through the patient's hands) a flexion force through the right leg (Figure 11.6(a–b)).

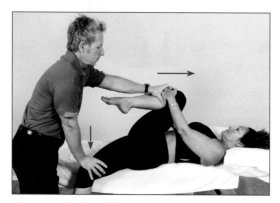

Figure 11.6. (a) Gaenslen test to screen for SIJ dysfunction.

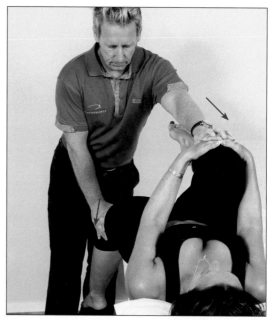

Figure 11.6. (b) Close-up view of the Gaenslen test.

Assessment of the Pelvis

Once you have screened the SIJ by following the five provocation tests as recommended in Chapter 11, you will at least be able to confirm or discount the presence of pain and possible dysfunction directly located within the SIJ. The next step will be to carry out an assessment of the pelvis.

The assessment procedure I will present in this chapter is very similar to the examination protocol that I personally follow with my own patients at my clinic in Oxford; however, you are not expected to initially follow every single process, especially during the first consultation. It could take a lot of time for you to gather all the information from the individual tests; moreover, once that has been done, you would need to assimilate all that necessary information in order to come up with a plan of action.

I am sure that there are numerous therapists out there who can help patients with only one session, and I believe that is the same for me. That said, I think it still takes a few physical therapy sessions to truly have a good understanding of the patient's individual musculoskeletal biomechanical framework. That is why I might not include all the tests I demonstrate in this chapter during my initial consultation, as some of the specific testing criteria might be more relevant in the second, or even third or fourth, follow-on session.

I hope that you will use this text, and specifically this chapter, time and time again as a reference point, especially when you are faced with a patient for the first time who presents with pelvis and lumbar spine pathology. I would love to think that this book will assist you greatly in trying to understand this fascinating area as well as in correcting any presenting pelvic malalignments.

Assessment Procedure: Part 1

The following assessment tests will be covered in this section:

- Pelvic balance
- Mens active straight leg raise
- Standing forward flexion
- Backward bending
- Seated forward flexion
- Stork
- Hip extension

- Lumbar side bending
- Pelvic rotation

Table A1.3 in Appendix 1 will be useful for noting down the relevant positional landmarks for your patient in the standing position. Similarly, Table A1.4 can be used to record the clinical findings for any type of pelvic dysfunction that exists.

Pelvic Balance Test

With the patient standing, the comparative levels of the following are noted:

- Pelvic crest (posterior view)
- Posterior superior iliac spine (PSIS)
- Greater trochanter
- Lumbar spine
- Gluteal folds
- Popliteal folds
- Leg, foot, and ankle position (anterior/posterior view)
- Pelvic crest (anterior view)
- Anterior superior iliac spine (ASIS)
- Pubic tubercle

Posterior View

The patient is asked to stand with their weight equally distributed on both legs. The therapist sits or kneels behind the patient, and places their hands on the top of the iliac crest to ascertain the level (Figure 12.1(a–b)).

It is very common to find the right innominate slightly higher if there is a presentation of a right-sided anterior rotation (the most common finding) or an iliosacral upslip. Be careful, however—the right-side innominate could actually appear lower, even though it is still in an anterior rotation: this could be because of an anatomically longer left leg (true LLD). In the sitting and the lying prone positions, on the other hand, the iliac crest might actually be higher on the right side that is fixed in

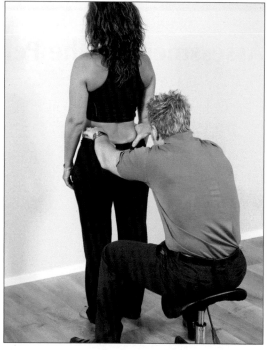

Figure 12.1. Pelvic balance test: (a) Posterior view of the pelvic crest—hand position for ascertaining the level.

an anteriorly rotated position, because the effect of the LLD has now been removed from the equation.

The therapist then places the pads of their thumbs under the PSIS and compares the levels (Figure 12.1(c)).

Next, the therapist places their hands (fingertips) on top of the greater trochanters, again to

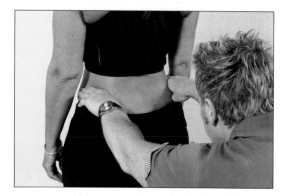

Figure 12.1. (b) Close-up view of the hand position.

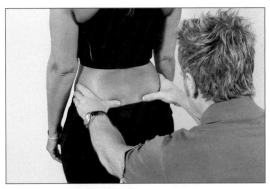

Figure 12.1. (c) Hand position for comparing the height of the PSIS on the left and right sides.

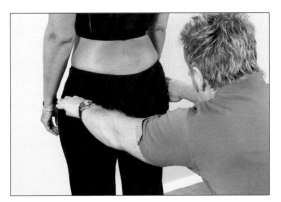

Figure 12.1. (d) Hand position for ascertaining the height of the greater trochanter.

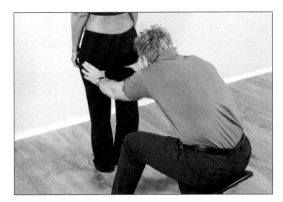

Figure 12.1. (e) Hand position for ascertaining the level of the gluteal fold and the position of the ischial tuberosity.

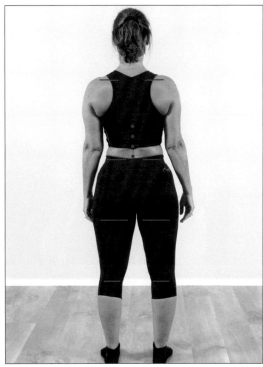

Figure 12.1. (f) Observation of the lumbar spine, gluteal fold, and popliteal fold, as well as the relative position of the leg, foot, and ankle.

determine the height (Figure 12.1(d)). The therapist then palpates the gluteal folds and the ischial tuberosities (Figure 12.1(e)).

The therapist observes the position of the lumbar spine, gluteal folds, and popliteal (knee) folds for asymmetry, then observes the relative position of the leg, foot, and ankle (Figure 12.1(f)), looking in particular for an external rotation of the lower leg and for over-pronation (pes planus), supination (pes cavus), or a neutral position (pes rectus). (Think back to Chapter 5 on LLD.)

Anterior View

The patient is asked to stand with their weight equally distributed on both legs. The therapist sits or kneels in front of the patient, and places their

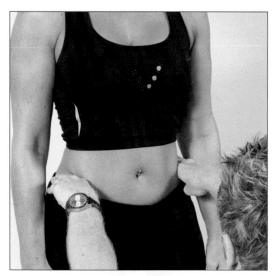

Figure 12.1. (g) Anterior view of the pelvic crest—hand position for ascertaining the level.

hands on the top of the iliac crest to ascertain the level (Figure 12.1(g)).

The therapist then places the pads of their thumbs under the ASIS and compares the levels (Figure 12.1(h)).

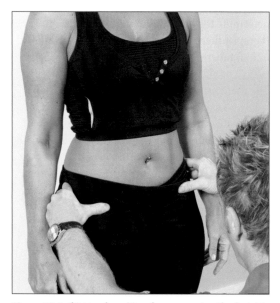

Figure 12.1. (h) Hand position for comparing the height of the ASIS on the left and right sides.

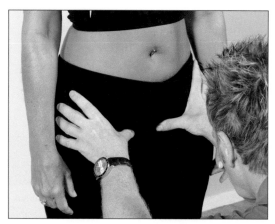

Figure 12.1. (i) Hand position for ascertaining the height of the pubic tubercle.

The therapist can also palpate the height/level of the pubic tubercles to ascertain their position (Figure 12.1(i)).

> **Note:** The most common finding in terms of initial observation is the right leg in a slight position of external rotation and the right foot in a relative position of pronation, compared with the left side (relative supination). If these observations are made, it is possible that a rotational malalignment dysfunction of a right anterior innominate rotation, with a compensatory left posterior innominate rotation is present. If you obtain similar findings on the opposite (left) side, a left anterior innominate rotation with a right posterior innominate rotation dysfunction possibly exists (less common).

If either the iliac crest or the greater trochanter is lower on one side, this means an anatomically shorter leg; if the greater trochanters are level but the iliac crest is asymmetric, this can equate to a pelvic dysfunction.

Mens Active Straight Leg Raise Test

Mens et al. (1999, 2001, 2002) have developed a diagnostic test for SIJ dysfunction. They studied the relationship between the active straight leg raise (ASLR) test and mobility of the pelvic joints with and without the application of a pelvic belt. The sensitivity and specificity of the test proved to be high for patients with pelvic girdle pain (PGP). They also found that the test was suitable for discriminating between patients with PGP and healthy individuals.

Test Procedure

The patient is asked to adopt a supine position; when they are relaxed, they are asked to lift one of their legs an inch (2.5cm) or so off the couch. This is repeated on the contralateral side (opposite side) and then back on the ipsilateral side (same side) approximately three or four times (Figure 12.2). The patient is then requested to say whether or not the movement of the individual leg lift increases their SIJ symptoms. The patient is also asked which leg feels *heavier* or simply *harder* to lift off the couch.

The starting movement of the leg lift is performed by the contraction of the iliacus and rectus femoris muscles, which initially induces an anterior rotation of the innominate; this movement reduces the tension in the corresponding sacrotuberous ligament and hence decreases form closure. The anterior rotation could also indicate decreased activation of the dynamic stabilizers (force closure).

Mens et al. (1997) described how a decreased ability to actively perform a straight leg raise while lying supine seemed to correlate with an abnormally increased mobility of the pelvic girdle.

To continue with the assessment process, I will add six components to assist in the form and force closure. However, before I demonstrate these, I need to go through an example to help you understand the following process. Imagine that when you initially observed the patient lifting their leg, the *left* leg was deemed to be the *heavier* leg; that simply means the contralateral side will now be the right leg (lighter leg) and the ipsilateral side will obviously be the left leg (heavier leg) in this particular case.

Snijders et al. (1993a) made the following observation. Provided the local and global systems (inner and outer cores) are functioning normally, the overall effect of carrying out a right-sided ASLR is a stabilization of both the lumbosacral junction and the right SIJ, which in turn allows a more effective load transfer from the spine to the leg on that side.

The six additional components are:

Contralateral (opposite side) con-traction of the right latissimus dorsi of the posterior oblique sling increases force closure (see Figure 12.3). With simultaneous contraction of the right latissimus muscle, the left leg should now feel *lighter* when lifted.

Contralateral (opposite side) con-traction of the right anterior oblique sling increases force closure

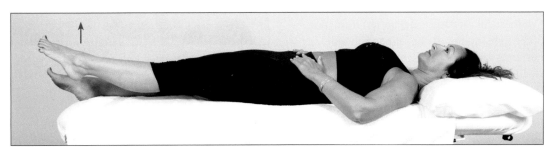

Figure 12.2. Mens ASLR: the patient alternately lifts each leg and indicates which feels heavier.

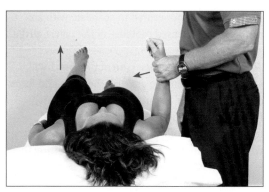

Figure 12.3. Posterior oblique sling activation while lifting the left leg.

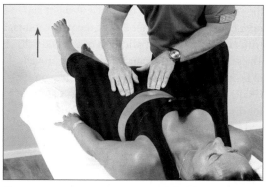

Figure 12.5. Inner core activation while lifting the left leg.

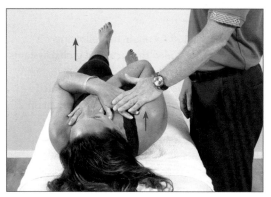

Figure 12.4. Anterior oblique sling activation while lifting the left leg.

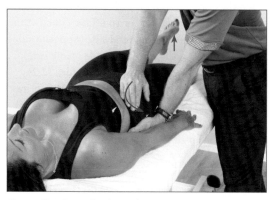

Figure 12.6. Posterior innominate rotation (opposite side) while lifting the left leg.

(Figure 12.4). With simultaneous contraction of the right oblique muscles, the left leg should now feel *lighter* when lifted.

Activation of the inner core muscles, TVA, increases force closure (Figure 12.5). With simultaneous contraction of the TVA, the left leg should now feel *lighter* when lifted.

Contralateral (opposite side) posterior rotation of the right innominate bone (opposite side) decreases force closure (Figure 12.6). The left leg should now feel *heavier* to lift.

Ipsilateral (same side) posterior rotation of the left innominate bone (same side) increases force closure (Figure 12.7). The left leg should now feel *lighter* when lifted.

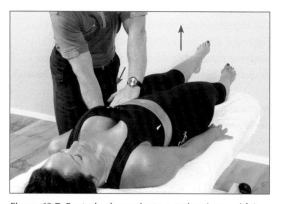

Figure 12.7. Posterior innominate rotation (same side) while lifting the left leg.

Bilateral compression of the innominate bones will increase form closure (Figure 12.8). The left leg should now feel *lighter* when lifted.

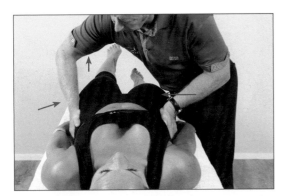

Figure 12.8. Bilateral compression of the innominate while lifting the left leg.

Without appropriate bracing of the deep abdominal muscles, the hip flexor muscles (such as the iliacus) can pull the ilium anteriorly, creating a counter-nutated position of the SIJ. Counter-nutation is typical for unloaded situations such as when lying supine, as demonstrated by Mens et al. (1999).

Shadmehr (2012) suggested there is reduced tonicity in the erector spinae, Gmax, biceps femoris, and external oblique muscles during ASLR testing of patients with SIJ pain.

Standing Forward Flexion Test (Iliosacral Dysfunction)

During forward bending of the trunk, the left and right innominate bones and the pelvic girdle rotate as a whole in an anterior direction on the femur, as I explained in Chapter 2. Initially, the innominate bones rotate anteriorly to roughly 60 degrees as the sacrum goes through nutation. This ROM is normal and occurs because the posterior structures (posterior oblique muscles, sacrotuberous ligament, thoracolumbar fascia, and hamstrings) become taut and will naturally limit sacral nutation. The sacrum is now held in what is known as *relative counter-nutation*, which causes an unstable

position of the SIJ. The common reason for excessive counter-nutation, and the subsequent instability of the SIJ, is generally shortened and tight hamstrings.

Test Procedure

The patient is asked to stand with equal weight on both legs. The therapist places their hands onto the patient's innominate bones, with the pads of the thumbs lightly placed just inferior to the level of the PSIS (Figure 12.9).

The patient is then asked to fully flex the trunk slowly toward the floor, as far as they can without bending the knees, while the therapist's contact to the PSIS is maintained. The therapist observes the motion of the innominate bones, but pays extra attention to the motion of each PSIS (see Figure 12.10).

Flexion of the spine carries the base of the sacrum anteriorly, and motion is then introduced to the SIJs. There is a natural pause before the sacrum takes the innominate into anterior rotation; this is why you should feel the left and right PSISs rise equally in a cephalic (superior) direction (see Figure 12.11).

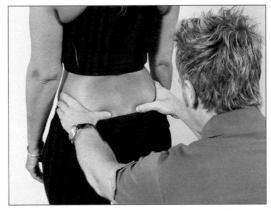

Figure 12.9. Standing forward flexion test: the therapist places their thumbs inferior to the PSIS.

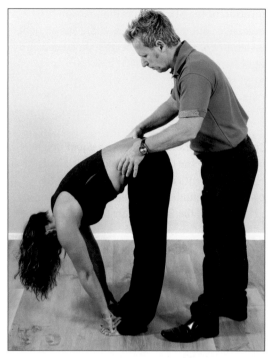

Figure 12.10. The therapist observes their thumbs as the patient forward bends.

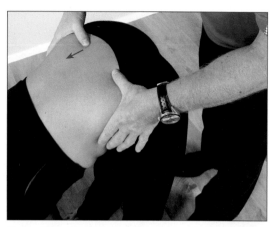

Figure 12.12. The right thumb is seen to be in a higher (cephalic) position, compared with the opposite side, indicating an iliosacral dysfunction on the right side.

has been described is that the iliosacral joint has locked too early on that side, causing the PSIS to rise sooner than normal, compared with the other side.

False-Positive Result

A false-positive result might be noted if the contralateral (opposite side) hamstring is held in a shortened and subsequently tight position, thus limiting the motion of the opposite innominate bone. For example, the right-side PSIS traveling further than that on the left during the standing forward flexion test could be caused by the left hamstrings being held in a shortened and tight position; in other words, the left innominate bone is being held back (fixed) by the short hamstring muscles.

Moreover, if the ipsilateral (same side) QL muscle is held in a shortened and tight position, this too will also give a false-positive result, but on the same side. For example, if the right-side PSIS was seen to travel further, the QL on the right side might be held in a shortened position; as a result, this muscle will be pulling the innominate bone forward sooner rather than later (Figure 12.13).

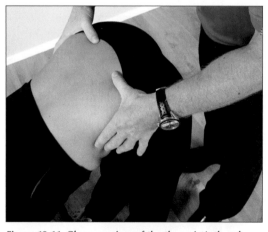

Figure 12.11. Close-up view of the therapist's thumbs as the patient adopts a forward-bent position.

If one thumb is seen to move more superiorly (cephalically) during flexion, this could be an indication that the innominate bone is fixed to the sacrum on that side (Figure 12.12); this is known as an *iliosacral dysfunction*. Another way that this

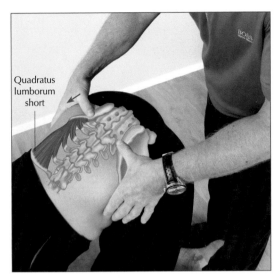

Figure 12.13. The position of the right thumb is higher than that on the opposite side, possibly indicating a tightness of the right QL muscle.

Note: The standing forward flexion test does not tell you the actual nature of the dysfunction, i.e. whether it is a rotation, flare, or slip; it only guides the examiner as to the side on which the innominate bone is fixed in relation to the sacrum. We will decide later on in this chapter, through further testing and palpation, what type of iliosacral dysfunction exists. Chapter 13 will then show you how to correct all these iliosacral dysfunctions that are commonly found in patients. For now, I would simply get used to practicing the standing forward flexion test, as I consider this to be one of the main tests to use in your own clinic setting.

Backward Bending Test

The patient is asked to stand with equal weight on both legs. The therapist places their hands on the patient's innominate bones, with the pads of the left and right thumbs lightly placed just inferior to the level of the PSIS. The patient is then asked to fully extend their trunk backward, while the

therapist's contact to the PSIS is maintained. The therapist observes the motion of the innominate bones, but pays extra attention to the motion of each PSIS. Normally, the PSIS is seen to move very slightly caudally (inferiorly), as shown in Figure 12.14(a–b).

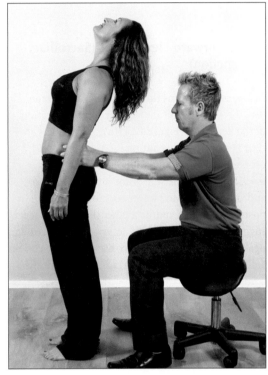

Figure 12.14. Backward bending test: (a) The therapist places their thumbs inferior to the PSIS and asks the patient to backward bend.

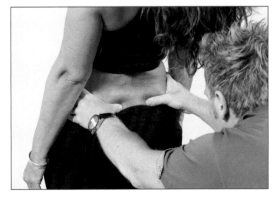

Figure 12.14. (b) Close-up view of the therapist's thumbs as the patient backward bends.

During backward bending, the innominate bones and sacrum remain in the same position, and so there should be no relative change felt in the position of the thumbs; however, the sacrum should be seen and felt to nutate slightly in order to maintain stability of the SIJ during the backward bending motion.

Seated Forward Flexion Test (Sacroiliac Dysfunction)

Before one performs the seated forward flexion test, it is very important to ascertain the position of the iliac crest (Figure 12.15(a)). Schamberger (2013) mentions that sitting is likely to present problems, as the ischial tuberosities are at different levels, raised on the side of the anterior rotation and/or an upslip, and lower on the side of the posterior rotation and/or a downslip. It has been suggested that, with a right anterior rotation or an upslip, the right ischial tuberosity can easily end up 0.4" (1cm) off the seating surface, the weight now being borne primarily by the left tuberosity.

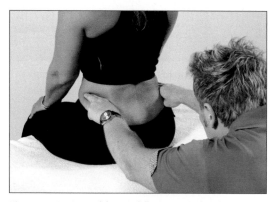

Figure 12.15. Seated forward flexion test: (a) The therapist places their fingers on top of the iliac crest to ascertain the position.

Position 1

The patient is asked to sit on the edge of a couch, with their feet flat on the floor, or in a comfortable

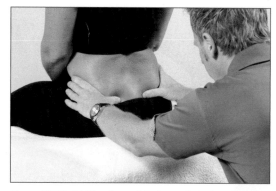

Figure 12.15. (b) The therapist places their thumbs inferior to the left and right PSIS.

position on the couch. The therapist places their hands on the patient's innominate bones, with the pads of the thumbs lightly placed just below the level of the left and right PSIS (Figure 12.15(b)).

The patient is then asked to slowly fully flex their trunk, by rolling their chin to their chest, and continue as far as they can, with their hands on their knees for support (Figure 12.15(c)).

The therapist observes the motion of the innominate bones, as well as focusing on the specific motion of the PSIS. If one of the thumbs, which is located inferior to the PSIS, is seen to move more superiorly (cephalically) during flexion, this could mean that the sacrum is fixed to the innominate bone on that side

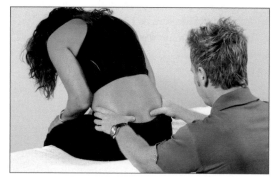

Figure 12.15. (c) The therapist observes their thumbs as the patient forward bends in the seated position.

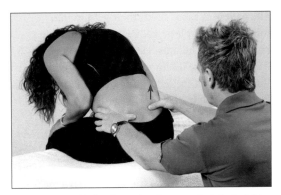

Figure 12.15. (d) The therapist observes that their right thumb travels more cephalically than their left thumb, indicating an SIJ dysfunction on the right side.

(Figure 12.15(d)); this is known as a *unilateral sacroiliac dysfunction*.

Position 2

With the patient in the neutral position, the therapist moves the pads of their thumbs from the original position (inferior to the PSIS) to the posterior aspect of the sacral apex, and in particular to the ILA, in order to ascertain the level/position (Figure 12.16(a)).

Note if one side of the ILA is asymmetric compared with the opposite ILA; this information will be used as part of the process of assessing for

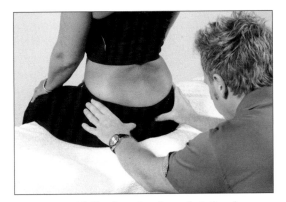

Figure 12.16. (a) The therapist places their thumbs on the sacral apex and observes the relative position of the ILA.

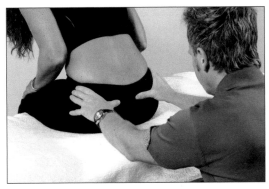

Figure 12.16. (b) The therapist observes the relative position of the ILA as the patient forward bends.

sacroiliac dysfunction. The patient is then asked to forward bend and the motion/position of the ILA is observed (Figure 12.16(b)).

> **Note:** The seated forward flexion test does not tell you what type of SIJ dysfunction is present: it only guides you as to which side the sacrum is fixed (in relation to the innominate bone). The test removes the influence of the legs and pelvis on the sacrum (because of the sitting position), and allows you to decide if an actual SIJ fixation is present. (Please be aware that the QL muscle, if held in a shortened position, is still capable of giving a false-positive result for the same side.)

Iliosacral or Sacroiliac

Suppose your right thumb, which is located inferior to the PSIS, travels further (cephalically) than the left thumb in both the standing forward flexion test and the seated forward flexion test; in other words, the left thumb remains lower than the right thumb. This means you have found both an iliosacral and a sacroiliac dysfunction on the right side at the same time. If the right thumb is seen to move only during the standing forward flexion test, however, this indicates the presence of an *iliosacral* dysfunction on the right side. On the other hand, if the right thumb is seen to move only during the seated forward flexion test, then a *sacroiliac* dysfunction on the right side is present.

Stork Test (One-Legged)

The stork test (also known as the *Gillet test*) consists of two elements: the upper pole and the lower pole.

Test 1: Upper Pole

With the patient standing, the therapist sits or kneels behind the patient. The therapist places their left hand on top of the patient's left innominate bone, and the pad of their left thumb under the inferior part of the PSIS. The therapist's right hand is positioned on the right innominate bone, while the pad of the right thumb is in contact with the level of S2 (this is in line with the corresponding PSIS), as shown in Figure 12.17.

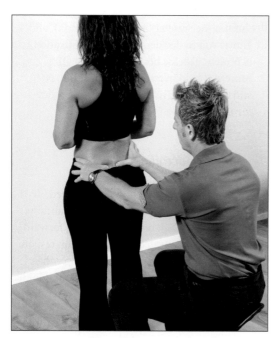

Figure 12.17. Stork test—upper pole: the therapist places their left thumb inferior to the PSIS, and their right thumb on S2.

The patient is asked to lift their left hip into full flexion, to at least above the level of the hip joint. The therapist's left hand remains in contact with the left innominate and monitors the movement: the left thumb on the PSIS should be seen to rotate posteriorly, medially, and inferiorly (caudally), with respect to the right thumb, which still maintains contact with S2 (Figure 12.18(a–b)).

Note: I consider that the specific movement of the stork test indicates the ability of the innominate bone to posteriorly rotate on

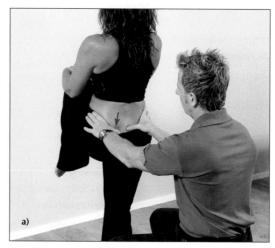

Figure 12.18. (a) The therapist observes for normal inferior motion of the innominate bone while the patient flexes their hip.

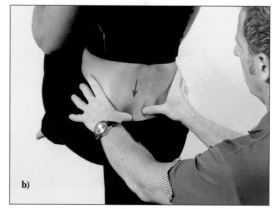

Figure 12.18. (b) Close-up view of the therapist's hand and thumb in contact with the PSIS and S2.

the sacrum, even though research does not actually confirm this hypothesis. Most therapists I have talked to in the past say that when they perform the stork test, they simply look for the movement described earlier (inferior motion of the thumb), and if the movement is restricted in any way, then an iliosacral dysfunction is present. Again, this test does not tell you the type of the iliosacral dysfunction; it only signals that one is present and that it is located on the side that tests positive in the stork test.

If the standing forward flexion test and also the stork test are positive on the same side, you know that there is an iliosacral dysfunction present; the following tests in this chapter will help you determine the type of this dysfunction. The contralateral (opposite) side is then tested for comparison.

A test is positive when the thumb located on the PSIS is not seen to move medially and inferiorly, or is seen to move in a cephalic direction (Figure 12.19(a–b)).

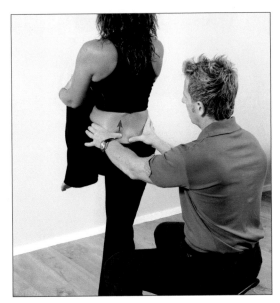

Figure 12.19. (a) The altered motion of the innominate bone shows a dysfunction is present.

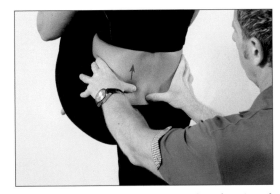

Figure 12.19. (b) Close-up view of the altered motion of the left innominate bone.

Test 2: Lower Pole

With the patient standing, the therapist sits or kneels behind the patient. The therapist places their left hand on top of the patient's left innominate bone, while placing the pad of their left thumb under the inferior part of the posterior inferior iliac spine (PIIS). The therapist's right hand is positioned on the right innominate bone, while the pad of the right thumb is in contact with the level of the S4 (near to the sacral hiatus), as shown in Figure 12.20.

The patient is asked to lift the left hip into full flexion, to at least above the level of the hip joint. The therapist's left hand remains in contact with

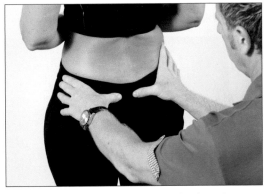

Figure 12.20. Stork test—lower pole: the therapist places their left thumb inferior to the PIIS, and their right thumb on S4.

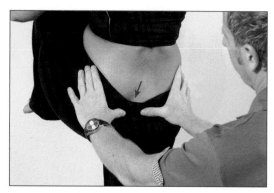

Figure 12.21. The therapist observes for normal anterior and lateral motion of the innominate bone while the patient flexes their hip.

the left innominate and monitors the movement: the left thumb on the PIIS should be seen to rotate anteriorly and laterally, with respect to the right thumb, which is palpating the level of the S4 (Figure 12.21).

A test is positive when the thumb located on the PIIS is not seen to move, or is seen to move in a cephalic direction (Figure 12.22).

> **Note:** These specific tests for the upper and lower poles are sensitive to the motion of the SIJ as well as to the motion of the iliosacral joint (as mentioned earlier). Other authors consider that if the upper pole tests positive, a posterior (backward) torsion of the SIJ dysfunction is present, and if the lower pole tests positive, an anterior (forward)

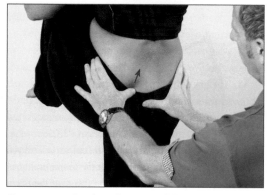

Figure 12.22. The altered motion of the innominate bone shows a dysfunction is present.

torsion of the sacroiliac dysfunction exists. However, it is very difficult to prove with these tests that an SIJ dysfunction is actually present, as the research regarding their validity is currently limited. Even so, I think that these tests will give the therapist some important palpatory feedback that might be useful in making an overall diagnosis and developing a subsequent treatment plan.

Hip Extension Test

With the patient standing, the therapist sits or kneels behind the patient. The therapist places their right hand on top of the patient's right innominate, while placing the pad of their right thumb under the inferior part of the right PSIS. The therapist's left hand is positioned on the left innominate, while the pad of the left thumb is in

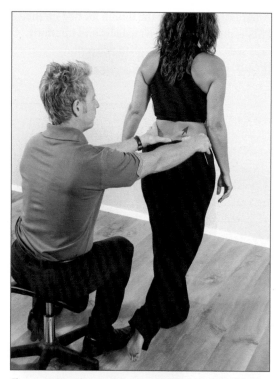

Figure 12.23. Hip extension test: with their right thumb inferior to the PSIS, the therapist observes for normal superior and lateral motion of the innominate bone while the patient extends their hip.

contact with the level of S2 (this is in line with the corresponding PSIS), as shown earlier in Figure 12.17.

The patient is asked to lift their right hip into full extension, as far as comfortable. The therapist's hand remains in contact with the right innominate bone and monitors the movement: the right thumb on the PSIS should be seen to rotate superiorly and laterally (cephalically), with respect to the left thumb, which is palpating the level of S2 (Figure 12.23). This indicates the ability of the innominate bone to anteriorly rotate with respect to the sacrum. The contralateral (opposite) side is then tested for comparison.

A test is positive when the thumb located on the PSIS is not seen to move superiorly and laterally, or is seen to move in a caudal direction (Figure 12.24).

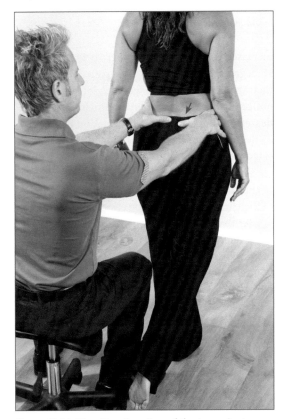

Figure 12.24. The altered motion of the innominate bone shows a dysfunction is present.

Lumbar Side Bending Test

The patient is asked to stand with their feet shoulder-width apart. The therapist sits or kneels behind the patient, and places their hands on top of the patient's iliac crests, with the pads of the thumbs on the posterior part of the PSIS.

The patient is asked to side bend to the left (without forward flexing their spine) as far as comfortable. The therapist observes the lumbar spine and looks for a smooth "C" curve with a fullness of the erector spinae on the side of the convexity (right side in this case); this fullness is seen on the side opposite to the induced side bending, because of Type I, or neutral, spinal mechanics (Figure 12.25(a)).

A positive finding during the observation is either fullness on the side of the concavity (same side as the side bending), see Figure 12.25(b), or a possible straightening of the lumbar curve. These positive findings tend to indicate a non-neutral spinal mechanics type of dysfunction (Type II).

> **Note:** When looking at the lumbar curvature, the therapist should also be aware of the palpatory findings for the PSIS. The normal motion of trunk side bending to the right will induce a lumbar rotation to the left, and this in turn will induce (through the normal

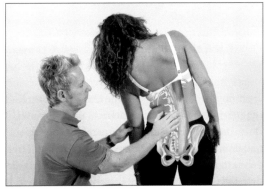

Figure 12.25. Lumbar side bending test: (a) A normal motion is seen by a fullness of the erector spinae on the right side as the patient side bends to the left.

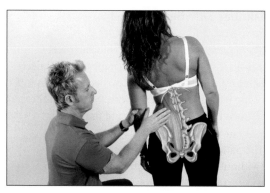

Figure 12.25. (b) An altered motion is seen by a fullness of the erector spinae on the left side (same side) as the patient side bends to the left.

Type I neutral spinal mechanics) a rotation of the sacrum to the opposite (right) side.

In simple terms, if the patient has normal lumbosacral motion, when they side bend their lumbar spine to the right side, a coupled rotation to the left side (Type I mechanics/neutral) is induced. As a result of the lumbar spine side bending right and rotating left, the sacrum should also be felt to go through the opposite motion, i.e. a side bending to the left, which will induce a rotation this time to the right. This movement of the sacrum can be palpated through the light contact of your right thumb, which is positioned on the right-side PSIS. This is all because of the fact that the lumbar spine will have rotated to the left (opposite side to the bending, because of Type I mechanics).

Pelvic Rotation Test

When you assess the patient in the standing-erect position, it is very common to consider the pelvis to be in an asymmetrical position. If the patient presents with a typical rotational malalignment syndrome, you may notice the pelvis to have rotated in an anticlockwise (left) direction, especially if they present with the most common finding of a right anteriorly rotated innominate and a left posteriorly rotated innominate (Figure 12.26(a)); it is usual for this

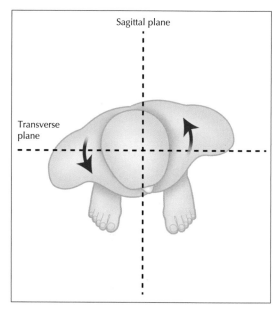

Figure 12.26. Pelvic rotation test: (a) The most common malalignment type of syndrome—right anterior innominate rotation with a compensatory left posterior innominate rotation.

increased rotation to be anywhere between 5 and 10 degrees. If you now ask your patient to rotate their trunk to the right (Figure 12.26(b)), you will notice further right rotation (approximately 45 degrees), compared with a left rotation of around 35 degrees when the trunk is rotated to the left (Figure 12.26(c)).

In the above example, the reason why rotation of the trunk to the right side (clockwise) is greater than to the left (even though the pelvis has rotated slightly to the left side because of the presenting dysfunction) is that the left innominate bone already starts out in a posteriorly rotated position (because of the dysfunctional pattern). This basically means that the left-side innominate is capable of rotating further in an anterior direction, to its available end ROM, than it would if it actually started out in a normal position. The same is true for the right-side innominate, which has already anteriorly rotated; the right side is now capable of traveling through a greater ROM in a posterior direction, giving the appearance of further rotation to the right side (clockwise).

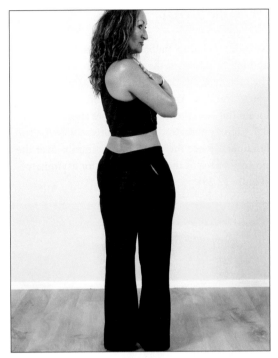

Figure 12.26. (b) The patient is asked to rotate to the right side (clockwise) and approximately 45 degrees is seen.

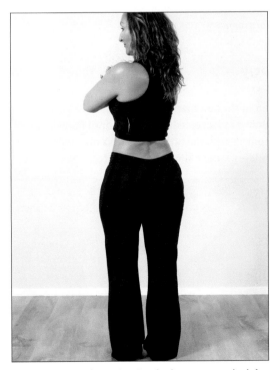

Figure 12.26. (c) The patient is asked to rotate to the left side (anticlockwise) and approximately 35 degrees is seen.

Schamberger (2013) also says that on account of the wedging of the sacrum, the left innominate already flares slightly inward, and the right slightly outward. Overall, this translates into more degrees of clockwise rotation.

> **Note:** If the pelvis position appeared to be neutral, with no obvious asymmetry/ rotation present (contrary to the example above), one would expect pelvic rotation of the trunk to the left side (anticlockwise) to equal the available rotation of the trunk to the right side (clockwise).

Assessment Procedure: Part 2

Palpatory Assessment—Patient Prone

In this part of the assessment criteria we will be looking for asymmetry of the anatomical landmarks, as outlined below. The patient is asked to adopt a prone position on the couch. The therapist stands next to the patient and observes for the levels of the following areas using their dominant eye:

- Gluteal fold
- Ischial tuberosity
- Sacrotuberous ligament
- Inferior lateral angle (ILA) of the sacrum
- Posterior superior iliac spine (PSIS)
- Sacral sulcus
- Lumbar spine (L5)
- Iliac crest
- Greater trochanter

Table A1.5 in Appendix 1 can be of value to the therapist for noting down any asymmetries found during the prone palpatory assessment.

Gluteal Fold and Ischial Tuberosity

First observe the level of the gluteal fold and then lightly palpate this area to ascertain the position. From the gluteal fold, move your

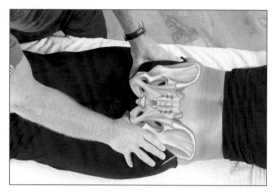

Figure 12.27. Palpation of the gluteal fold and ischial tuberosity for symmetry.

thumbs in a cephalic direction until contact with the ischial tuberosity is made. Place your thumbs in a horizontal plane against the inferior aspect of the ischial tuberosity, and note the level (Figure 12.27).

Sacrotuberous Ligament

After the ischial tuberosity has been palpated, the thumbs are now directed medially and cephalically until the sacrotuberous ligament is found (Figure 12.28). Gently palpate the ligament, feeling for increased tension or laxity as well as increased tenderness, as these can be associated with sacroiliac or iliosacral dysfunction.

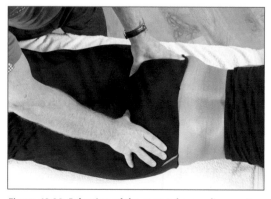

Figure 12.28. Palpation of the sacrotuberous ligament.

ILA of the Sacrum

Next, if you lightly palpate the ischial tuberosity and follow it toward the proximal component of the sacrotuberous ligament, it will naturally take you to the ILA. Another way of finding it is to locate the sacral hiatus and palpate approximately 0.8" (2cm) lateral to this area—this will be the ILA landmark. Place the pads of your thumbs over the posterior area of the ILA to check for asymmetry (Figure 12.29).

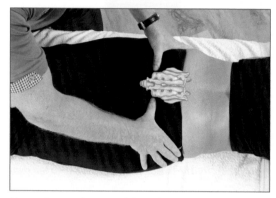

Figure 12.29. Palpation of the inferior lateral angle (ILA) for symmetry.

PSIS

From the landmark of the ILA, now place your thumbs in a cephalic direction until they make contact with the bony landmarks on either side—i.e. the PSIS (Figure 12.30(a)). From this

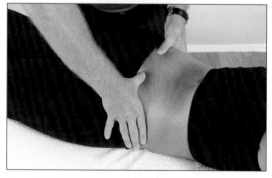

Figure 12.30. (a) Palpation of the PSIS for symmetry.

position, look at each of the contact thumbs on the PSIS and note down any asymmetry that is found.

Iliac Crest

From the PSIS, it is advisable to ascertain the position of the iliac crest to check the level by lightly placing the fingers on top of the crest (Figure 12.30(b)).

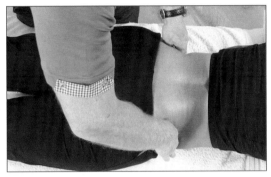

Figure 12.30. (b) Palpation of the iliac crest for symmetry.

Sacral Sulcus

The sacral sulcus is the area that is naturally formed by the junction of the sacral base with the corresponding ilium on either side. You might notice an overlying dimple that will correspond to the sacral sulcus: these left and right dimples are known as the *dimples of Venus*. From the position of the PSIS, the thumbs are now directed (gently) at an angle of 45 degrees medially toward the junction of L5/S1, until the sacral base is contacted. It is best to wait a moment for the tissues to settle down before deciding on the appropriate position. You are trying to determine what is termed the *depth* of the sacral sulcus (located between the sacral base and the PSIS); the normal depth is approximately 0.4–0.6" (1.0–1.5cm), but it is usually less, because of the soft tissues overlying the sulcus. Normal findings are that the thumbs palpate as equal, or level, within the sacral sulcus/base (Figure 12.31).

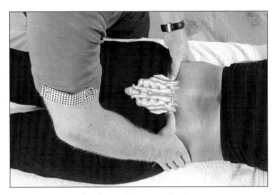

Figure 12.31. Palpation of the sacral sulcus for symmetry/depth.

Sacral Rotation

Imagine for a moment that when you palpate the sacral sulcus you convince yourself that your thumbs look asymmetric: for example, the right thumb seems to sink (palpate) deeper and the left thumb palpates shallow within the sacral base. This finding might possibly indicate either an *anterior* (or forward) sacral base (nutated) on the deeper *right* side, or a *posterior* (or backward) sacral base (counter-nutated) on the shallower *left* side. Either way, the sacrum in this case would still be "rotated" to the *left* (Figure 12.32).

In the article "Sacroiliac joint mechanics revisited" by Jordan (2006), I was very interested

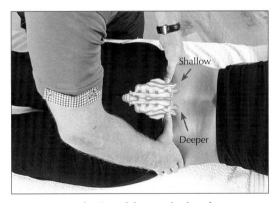

Figure 12.32. Palpation of the sacral sulcus for symmetry—the right thumb (in this case) appears deeper and the left thumb appears shallower.

to read in particular about the area of palpation for identifying the depth of the sacral sulcus. The clinician mentioned that when one palpates into the sacral sulci and checks for the relative sacral sulcus depth, the relative depth does not reflect the sacral position, but rather the multifidus muscle thickness, even in petite patients. In addition, overlying the multifidus is the lumbosacral fascia, a very thick layer of collagenous connective tissue, which can feel quite solid and be mistaken for bone. If one side of the multifidus muscle is more contracted than the other, a greater cross-sectional area is produced, and consequently the sacral sulcus will naturally appear *shallower*.

True though this may be, please remember that palpation of the sacral sulcus is only one component of the assessment process. You can think of the assessment process as a jigsaw puzzle, and palpation of this sulcus will only be one piece of the puzzle. As I have said before, there are lots of other pieces in the puzzle, so try not to rely on just one piece.

While I am on the subject of the relative depth of the sacral sulci, one also has to consider the position of the innominate bone. For example, if the right sacral sulcus palpated as *shallow,* this could indicate an *anteriorly* rotated innominate on the right (iliosacral dysfunction, and a common finding). A different type of rotational malalignment can also relate to the opposite finding: if the sacral sulcus palpated as *deeper* on the right side, this could correspond to a *posteriorly* rotated innominate bone on the right (a less common finding).

Remember from earlier that the most common malalignment condition found is *rotational*, and typically this will be a right anterior rotation, along with a compensatory left posterior innominate rotation. In terms of palpation for the depth of the sacral sulci with this common finding, the right thumb would palpate shallow and the left thumb would palpate deep, even though the sacrum is in a relatively neutral position by comparison.

In this case it is the innominate bone that is the dysfunctional (iliosacral) structure, but the impression of a right rotated sacrum is given (even though it is not right rotated), mainly because the left side of the sacral sulcus palpates as deeper as a result of the posteriorly rotated left innominate bone.

I have already discussed in Chapters 2 and 4 that we know the sacrum is capable of side bending with a coupled motion of rotation, since this is what your sacrum undergoes during the walking cycle, as you shift your weight from one leg to the other. The sacral motion follows Type I motion, and side bending and rotation are coupled to the opposite side: we call this type of movement *torsion.* So, for example, if the left sacral base is posterior, the sacrum will be left rotated, or left torsioned, and side bent to the right. If, when we palpate the sacral base as well as the position of the ILA in a neutral position (patient prone), we find asymmetry of the sacral base and also of the ILA, then we can safely say a dysfunction occurs and there is some SIJ fixation.

The question I ask you is this: how do you determine which is the fixed side? Well, you have already partly answered this question without actually realizing it. Why? Because you have already performed the seated forward flexion test, and this particular SIJ test will indicate the side of the body on which the dysfunction is located. Suppose, for example, the *left* side tests positive (left thumb travels cephalically, compared with the right thumb) during the seated forward flexion test; in addition, when you palpate the left sacral sulcus, the left thumb sinks further into the sulcus than the right thumb (i.e. it palpates *deeper* on the left side). You then know that the sacrum has to be in a position of anterior/forward nutation on the left side, because it has rotated to the right and side bent to the left, as in what we call a *R-on-R sacral torsion* (Figure 12.33).

Let's look at another scenario: the seated forward flexion test still gives a positive result on the left side, but this time the left sacral sulcus now

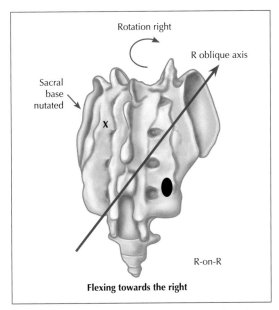

Figure 12.33. Anterior/forward (nutated) sacral torsion R-on-R. X = Anterior or deep. ● = Posterior or shallow.

palpates as *shallow* instead of deep. Hopefully, you now know that the left side of the sacrum is in a position of counter-nutation: the sacrum has rotated to the left and side bent to the right, as in a *L-on-R sacral torsion* (posterior/backward sacral torsion on the left), as shown in Figure 12.34.

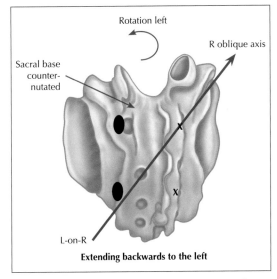

Figure 12.34. Posterior/backward (counter-nutated) sacral torsion L-on-R. X = Anterior or deep.

● = Posterior or shallow.

Posterior/Backward (Counter-Nutated) Fixed Sacral Torsion

Let's move on to the next part of the assessment, which will continue on the theme of sacral torsion. We will now be looking at confirming or discounting the actual presence of a sacral dysfunction/torsion by asking the patient to simply backward and forward bend their trunk, to ascertain what happens to the depth of the sacral sulci.

Let's continue with the concept of the above example, where the left sacral base is posterior in neutral. From this position, you now ask your patient to forward bend their trunk, and the sacral dysfunction appears to disappear (your thumbs become level). When you ask your patient to perform a backward-bending motion (sphinx test—explained later) the rotation seems to increase: the position of the sacral base becomes worse—i.e. the left thumb appears shallower on the left side (or the sacral sulcus palpates as deeper on the right side). This will confirm that the left sacral base is fixed posteriorly, which is what we call a L-on-R sacral torsion. Why? Think about it for a minute. As you ask the patient to extend their lumbar spine, the sacrum should bilaterally anteriorly nutate (think "opposite motion to that of the lumbar spine"). If the left side is fixed in a backward/posterior position, this means that the left side will be unable to anteriorly nutate (to go forward), so it must be fixed in a counter-nutated position (posterior or backward sacral torsion). Another way of looking at it is that in backward bending, the left sacral base stays where it is—in a posterior fixed position; however, the right sacral base moves further into an anterior position as the patient backward bends, thereby making the rotation appear to worsen (increase).

When you ask the patient to perform a forward bending motion, the left sacral base will stay fixed posteriorly (counter-nutated on the left), as the right side of the sacrum is able to continue its motion and rotate back posteriorly (counter-nutate on the right); the sacral sulcus will now appear to become level, so that the rotation seems to disappear.

Sphinx Test/Trunk Extension

One maneuver I particularly like to ask my patients to perform, as a guide to ascertaining the presence of a posterior torsion of the sacrum, is the sphinx test. The patient is asked to adopt a prone position on the couch. Standing next to the patient, place the pads of your thumbs or index fingers directly over the left and right sacral bases, with your dominant eye facing the pelvis.

The test is rather simple: ask the patient to raise themselves onto their elbows (i.e. a sphinx position), as in reading a book. If a posterior sacral torsion exists, the sacral sulcus will be asymmetrical (posterior sacrum on the shallow side). The sacral torsion will be a L-on-R if the sacral sulcus is shallow on the left side (or the right sacral sulcus is deeper), as shown in Figure 12.35; likewise, the sacral torsion will be a R-on-L if the sacral sulcus is shallow on the right side (or the left sacral sulcus is deeper).

> **Note:** If the sacral sulcus diminishes or normalizes (becomes level) during the sphinx test, an anterior sacral torsion is present. This forward torsion will either be a R-on-R or a L-on-L (this will be explained in the section "Anterior/Forward (Nutated) Fixed Sacral Dysfunction").

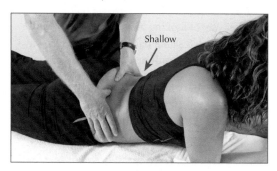

Figure 12.35. Sphinx test: a L-on-R (posterior/backward) sacral torsion is indicated (the left thumb becomes shallower in this case).

Lumbar Flexion Test

Let's continue with the case of a L-on-R sacral torsion (left side of the sulcus is fixed in counter-nutation). After the patient has adopted the sphinx position and the level of the sacral sulcus has been noted, you ask the patient to perform a forward bending motion of the trunk (lumbar flexion). Because the left sacral base in this example is fixed posteriorly, the right side of the sacrum is able to rotate back normally in a posterior direction (counter-nutation); this will make the sulci appear to become level, so that the rotation seems to disappear (Figure 12.36(a)).

If you prefer the patient to flex their lumbar spine from a prone position rather than a sitting

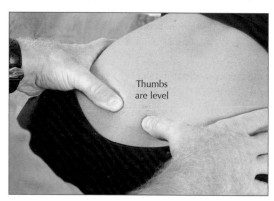

Figure 12.36. (a) Forward flexion test for the lumbar spine: a L-on-R (posterior/backward) sacral torsion is indicated (both thumbs now become level).

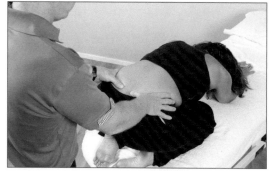

Figure 12.36. (b) Alternative lumbar flexion test: a L-on-R (posterior/backward) sacral torsion is indicated (both thumbs now become level).

position, you can ask them to sit back onto their heels with their arms stretched forward (Figure 12.36(b)).

Anterior/Forward (Nutated) Fixed Sacral Dysfunction

Let's look at another example of a forward sacral torsion. This time, when we palpate the left sacral sulcus in a neutral position (patient prone), the thumb appears to sink deeper on that side; in addition, the seated forward flexion test is positive on the left side. Because of these two findings, we can almost conclude that a R-on-R forward sacral torsion is present. We will now confirm this by asking the patient to forward bend, with your thumbs in light contact with the patient's sacral sulci. The left sacral base appears to get worse (deeper) in this position (Figure 12.37), and becomes level in a backward-bent (sphinx) position (Figure 12.38).

This means that the opposite of what I said at the beginning is present: we have an anteriorly nutated fixation on the left side (R-on-R). Why? When your patient forward bends, their left sacral base stays fixed in an anteriorly nutated position, but their right sacral base moves further into posterior nutation (counter-nutation), which will thus make the rotation appear to

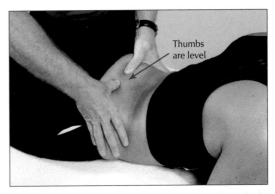

Figure 12.38. Sphinx test, indicating a R-on-R (anterior/forward) sacral torsion (both thumbs become level).

worsen (left thumb appears to sink even deeper). When the patient is asked to backward bend, the left sacral base is still fixed in an anteriorly nutated position; however, the right sacral base is able to move into its normal anteriorly nutated position. This now shows that the dysfunctional rotation of the sacrum seems to disappear, and palpation of the sacral sulcus on each side now indicates they are level.

Lumbar Spine (L5)

Spring Test

The patient is asked to adopt a prone position on the couch, and the therapist stands facing the patient. The therapist observes the lumbar spine for the following positions: flat back (flexed), increased lordosis (extended), or neutral. If the patient has a relatively flat back, this indicates the lumbar spine is in a position of flexion, and the sacrum will be in a position of relative counter-nutation. If the patient has a lordotic posture, this means the lumbar spine is now in a position of extension, and the sacrum will be in a position of relative nutation. After observing the positions of the lumbar and sacral spines, the therapist places the heel of their dominant hand directly over the spinous process of L5 and exerts a gentle but firm pressure toward the couch (see Figure 12.39).

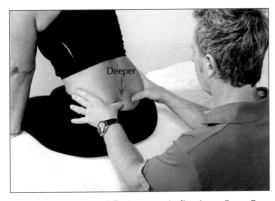

Figure 12.37. Forward flexion test, indicating a R-on-R (anterior/forward) sacral torsion (left thumb becomes deeper).

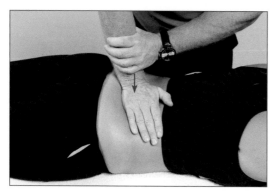

Figure 12.39. Lumbar (L5) spring test: either a posterior or an anterior sacral torsion is indicated.

A positive test is where there is firm resistance to the applied pressure to L5, with no obvious movement in the underlying tissues; a firm resistance indicates a locking of the L5 facets into a flexed position. This finding demonstrates that either the sacrum has bilaterally (on both sides) counter-nutated, or a unilateral (one-sided) posterior/backward sacral torsion (L-on-R or R-on-L) is present.

If the spring test is negative (there is some available motion, i.e. spring) and the lumbar spine appears to have an increased lordosis (curvature increased), then either the sacrum has bilaterally nutated, or a unilateral anterior/forward sacral torsion (L-on-L or R-on-R) is present.

> **Note:** The spring test will also be negative if the patient is in a neutral position, as there is some natural lordosis of the lumbar spine in this case.

L5 Position—Neutral

Once you have decided on the relevant position of the sacral base for ascertaining any underlying sacral torsions, position your thumbs and direct them to the level of the L5 spinous process. From the spinous process of L5, direct the pads of the thumbs and place them equally and lateral (approximately 1–1.4", or 2.5–3cm) to the L5 spinous process; this placement should be in

line with the corresponding left and right TPs, so that the relevant position of L5 is identified. If a shallow side is palpated, let's say on the right side, then in this particular case we know that L5 has rotated to that side (right), as shown in Figure 12.40(a–b).

However, think back to Chapter 6: just because L5 has rotated to the right, we don't know whether the right-side facet joint of L5/S1 is fixed in a closed position, or whether the left-side facet joint of L5/S1 is fixed in an open position. As I have already explained in Chapter 6, we would need to ascertain the position of the L5/S1 facet joint by the use of specific motions, whereby the patient is asked to perform extension and flexion movements of the trunk.

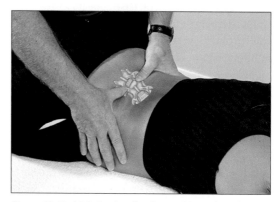

Figure 12.40. (a) Palpation for the position of L5: the shallow side is seen on the right, indicating a right rotation of L5.

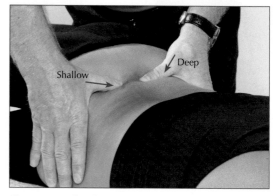

Figure 12.40. (b) Close-up view of the position of L5, with the shallow side on the right.

Note: Generally speaking, the position of L5 is particularly dependent on the position of the sacral base. L5 will be in a different position for each of the four sacral torsion positions discussed in earlier chapters.

Remember from earlier that L-on-L and R-on-R sacral motions are classified as *normal* physiological motions of the sacrum, which will elicit typical Type I spinal mechanics (side bending and rotation are coupled to the opposite side) of the lumbar spine during the gait cycle. However, my own thought process tells me that if the sacrum is fixed in a forward/nutated (Examples 1–2 below) or backward/counter-nutated (Examples 3–4 below) torsional position for a significant period of time, then through the natural compensatory processes the lumbar spine in some way has to alter its position and possibly adopt Type II spinal mechanics; in this case the side bending and rotation are now coupled to the same side (either in flexion or in extension), as explained by the following examples.

Example 1

A *L-on-L* sacral torsion typically causes L5 to adopt neutral Type I spinal mechanics of right rotation with left side bending. If the sacral dysfunction has become chronic, however, the altered position of the sacrum can potentially change the position of L5: this is known as an *ERS(R)*—the L5/S1 facet joint is closed on the right side.

Why? The motion of L5 will be opposite (right) to the nutated motion of the sacrum (left), which means L5 will be in a position of extension, side bending, and rotation to the right side, i.e. an ERS(R). Put simply, the sacrum is rotating in an anterior (nutated) direction to the left, so L5 will rotate in a posterior direction to the right. This right rotation of the lumbar spine is in part classified as normal Type I mechanics because of the induced left rotation of the sacrum; however, if the lumbar spine increases

its lordotic curvature as a result of the forward (nutated) sacral torsion, L5 will be forced into Type II mechanics and subsequently develop the position of an ERS(R).

Example 2

A *R-on-R* sacral torsion potentially causes L5 to adopt a position known as an *ERS(L)*—the L5/S1 facet joint is closed on the left side.

The motion of L5 will be opposite to that of the sacrum, so the vertebra will be in an ERS(L) position. Why? Put simply, the sacrum is rotating in an anterior direction to the right side, which means L5 will rotate in a posterior direction to the left side.

Example 3

A *L-on-R* sacral torsion sacral torsion potentially causes L5 to adopt a position known as an *FRS(R)*—the L5/S1 facet joint is open on the left side (remember, it is the side opposite to the side of rotation).

The motion of L5 will be opposite to that of the sacrum, so the vertebra will be in an FRS(R) position. Why? Put simply, the sacrum is rotating in a posterior (counter-nutated) direction to the left side, which means L5 will rotate in an anterior direction to the right side.

Example 4

A *R-on-L* sacral torsion sacral torsion potentially causes L5 to adopt a position known as an *FRS(L)*—the L5/S1 facet joint is open on the right side (remember, it is side opposite to the side of rotation).

The motion of L5 will be opposite to that of the sacrum, so the vertebra will be in an

FRS(L) position. Why? Put simply, the sacrum is rotating in a posterior (counter-nutated) direction to the right side, which means L5 will rotate in an anterior direction to the left side.

Exceptions to the Above Rule

Please bear in mind, from the discussion of spinal mechanics in Chapter 6, that in exceptional circumstances the motion of L5 can also be to the same side as the sacral torsion. For instance, it is common with very chronic lumbar spine/pelvic dysfunctions to find the sacrum rotated to the right side and L5 rotated to the same side; likewise, it is possible for a left rotation of the sacrum to cause L5 to rotate to the same side. An example (explained in Chapter 10) of the above is where you have a primary lumbar spine dysfunction that causes the sacrum to rotate to the same side as the vertebral rotation; in this case the lumbar spine dysfunction will need to be treated first.

Iliac Crest—Posterior View

Place your hands on top of each of the patient's iliac crests and note the relevant positions. A higher side might indicate a shortness of the QL, a pelvic rotation, or even an iliosacral upslip (Figure 12.41).

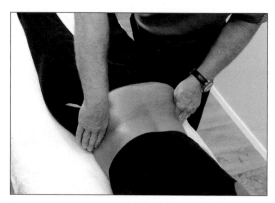

Figure 12.41. Palpation for the position of the iliac crest: a higher side is indicated on the right.

Greater Trochanter

From palpating the iliac crests, next direct your hands to the greater trochanter, to check for relevant levels (Figure 12.42).

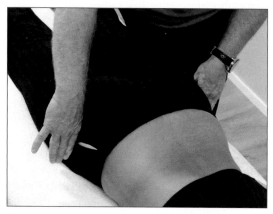

Figure 12.42. Palpation for the position of the greater trochanter.

Palpatory Assessment—Patient Supine

The patient is asked to adopt a supine position on the couch, and the therapist stands next to the patient and observes, using their dominant eye, for the levels in the following areas:

- Anterior superior iliac spine (ASIS)
- Iliac crest
- Pubic tubercle
- Inguinal ligament
- Medial malleolus

Table A1.6 in Appendix 1 can be used to note down any asymmetries found during the supine palpatory assessment.

ASIS

After initially observing the level of the ASIS, palpate the inferior aspect of the ASIS to ascertain the position (Figure 12.43).

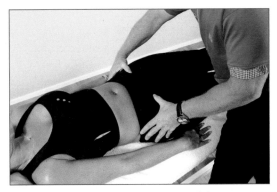

Figure 12.43. Palpation for the position of the ASIS.

Iliac Crest—Anterior View

From the ASIS, place your hands on top of the iliac crests to check for the position (Figure 12.44).

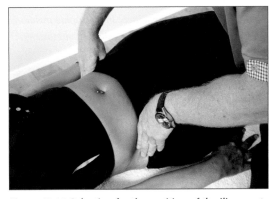

Figure 12.44. Palpation for the position of the iliac crest.

Pubic Tubercle and Inguinal Ligament

Ask the patient to relax and inform them (also requesting their consent) about what is about to happen in this procedure. Using the heel of your hand, and starting with light contact from the abdominal area, gently move caudally down until the pubic tubercle is felt beneath the hand. Place the pads of the thumbs or index fingers on top of each of the pubic tubercles (symphysis pubis joint) and check for the position (Figure 12.45(a)). A positive finding

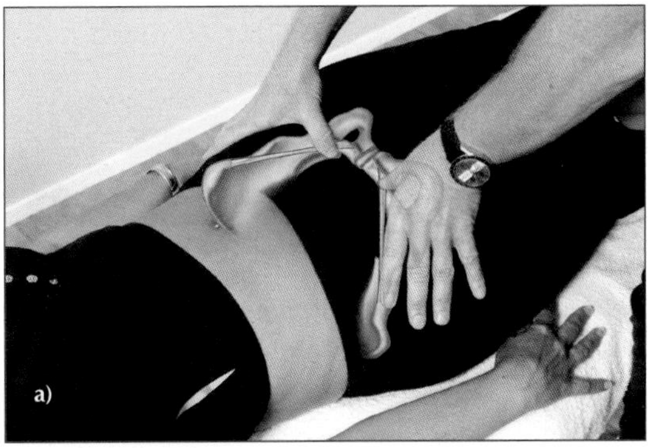

![Figure 12.45 a]

Figure 12.45. Palpation for the position of (a) the pubic tubercle.

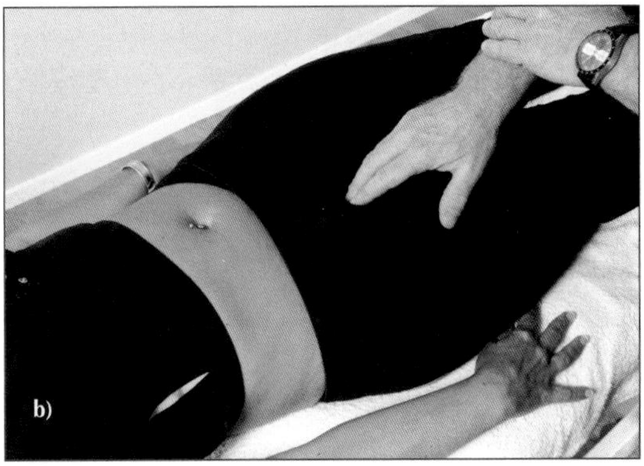

![Figure 12.45 b]

Figure 12.45. Palpation for the position of (a) the pubic tubercle, and (b) the inguinal ligament.

is if one of the pubic tubercles appears in either a superior or an inferior position, when comparing them with each other.

Once you have palpated the left and right pubic tubercles, let your thumbs drift laterally and superiorly, to contact the inguinal ligament, which attaches from the pubic tubercle to the ASIS. Another positive finding for a dysfunction is if the soft tissue structure of the inguinal ligament is tender on palpation (Figure 12.45(b)).

Medial Malleolus (Leg Length)

Before the position of the medial malleoli (leg length) is ascertained, grasp the patient's legs

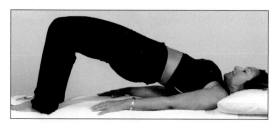

Figure 12.46. (a) Patient lifts their pelvis off the couch two or three times, to encourage leveling of the pelvis.

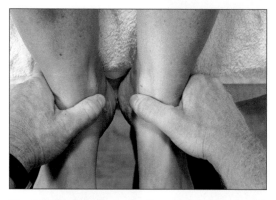

Figure 12.46. (b) Palpation for the position of the medial malleoli (leg length).

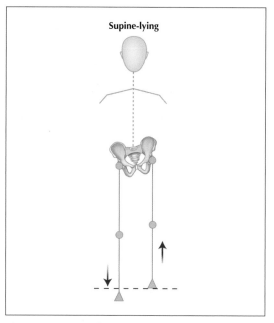

Supine-lying

Figure 12.46. (c) With the patient in the supine position the left medial malleolus appears shorter and the right medial malleolus appears longer.

above the ankles and ask the patient to bend both knees to 90 degrees. Next ask them to lift their pelvis off the couch two or three times (Figure 12.46(a)), and then to straighten their legs (this has the effect of encouraging the pelvis to become level). After this, take hold of the patient's ankles and place your thumbs under their medial malleoli, to identify which leg appears longer, shorter, or level (Figure 12.46(b)).

Supine to Long Sitting Test (Back to Supine)

The aim of this test is to determine the relevance of the SIJ to an apparent or true LLD. The patient lies in a supine position and the therapist compares the two medial malleoli, to see if there is any difference in position. Let's say, for instance, when the patient is in a supine lying position you notice that the left medial malleolus appears to be shorter and that

the right medial malleolus appears to be longer (Figure 12.46(c)).

Ask the patient to sit up, while keeping their legs extended. Compare the position of the medial malleoli again, to see if there is any change (Figure 12.46(d)). If there is a *posterior* innominate present on the left side, the leg that appeared shorter will now *lengthen* as the patient sits up. If there is an *anterior* innominate present on the right, the leg that appeared longer will now *shorten* during the sitting-up motion.

From the long sitting position, it would make sense to ask the patient to lie back down, so that they adopt the starting supine position, and to observe what happens to the medial malleoli during this maneuver. If you notice that the right leg in the *long sitting position* appears to be *shorter* than the left, and that the right leg appears to be *longer* than the left in the *supine lying position*, then you have probably confirmed a right anterior innominate rotation with a left posterior innominate rotation.

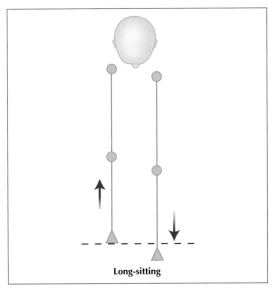

Figure 12.46. (d) Observation of the positions of the medial malleoli (leg length) after the supine to long sitting test. The right leg appears shorter and the left leg appears longer, confirming right anterior and left posterior innominate rotations.

Schamberger (2013) has a general rule for remembering this process—the rule of the five Ls, which relates to the side of the anteriorly rotated innominate:

"**Leg Lengthens Lying, Landmarks Lower**"

So let's recap on that thought process just for a moment. Schamberger (2013) calls the test the *sitting–lying test* rather than what I call it, the *supine to long sitting test*. What Schamberger says is basically the same, but in reverse. He looks at the patient's medial malleoli in a long sitting position to start with, noting the position, and observes if one malleolus appears to get "longer" when the patient lies back to adopt a supine position. If, for instance, it is found that the right-side malleolus appears to get longer (compared with the left side), as shown in Figure 12.46(e), then the right side is more than likely to be locked in an anteriorly rotated position (think back to the rule of the five Ls), with a compensatory left posteriorly rotated innominate.

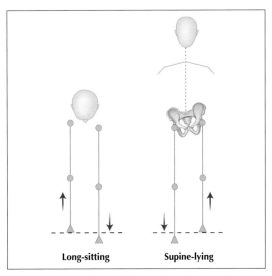

Figure 12.46. (e) Observation of the positions of the medial malleoli. The right leg appears shorter in long sitting, and appears longer in supine lying, indicating a right anterior rotation.

True LLD

If a true LLD exists, the right leg will appear longer both in the supine position and in the long sitting position (Figure 12.46(f)). Remember that all the pelvic landmarks are higher on the side of the

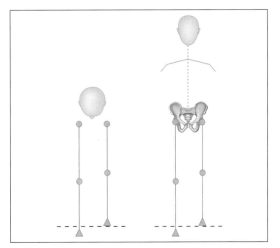

Figure 12.46. (f) Observation of the positions of the medial malleoli. The right leg appears longer both in long sitting and in supine lying, indicating a true LLD of the right leg.

longer leg, but only in a standing posture; the bony pelvic landmarks will be level when sitting and lying, as shown in the figure.

Upslip

An upslip on the right side, for example, means that the right leg will appear shorter in the supine lying position, and subsequently shorter in the long sitting position (Figure 12.46(g)). You will notice that the pelvic landmarks are all cephalic on the right side compared with the left side, indicating a possible right iliosacral upslip.

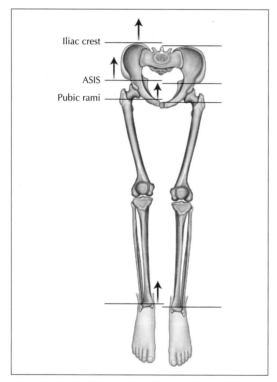

Figure 12.46. (g) Observation of the position of the medial malleolus for a right upslip. The right leg appears shorter in both the supine and long sitting position.

Out-Flare/In-Flare

When a patient presents with an out-flare or an in-flare iliosacral dysfunction, there will be no difference between the medial malleoli in the supine or long sitting positions.

The tests demonstrated above can help in differentiating between a true LLD and a sacroiliac/iliosacral dysfunction. The reason why the supine to long sitting and back to supine test is of value is that in a supine position the acetabulum lies in an anterior position relative to the ischial tuberosity, and that on moving from the supine to the long sitting position, the pelvis tilts forward and eventually pivots over the ischial tuberosity. As a result of this motion, the legs appear to lengthen equally if there is no dysfunction present. If a rotational dysfunction is present, however, the pelvis moves independently on each side rather than as a single unit, and hence the leg length appears to either shorten or lengthen.

Schamberger (2013) mentions that a shift in leg length demonstrated in the long sitting to supine lying test serves as a probable indicator of the presence of a "rotational malalignment" and is useful for differentiating it from an anatomical (true) LLD and an upslip; nevertheless, a coexisting anatomical LLD, an upslip, or both cannot be ruled out. The test also provides the person doing the assessment with an easy way of determining which side has rotated anteriorly or posteriorly.

Just to confuse the picture a little, as in reality it is never as straightforward as it seems (and I apologize for that), Schamberger (2013) also says: "A knowledge of which iliac crest is higher when standing is not helpful for predicting which leg will be longer in long sitting or supine lying. Nor does it help us to determine the side of an 'anterior rotation' or 'upslip.'"

The fact of the matter is that differences as much as 0.8–1.6" (2–4cm) may be observed to reverse completely when changing from the long sitting position to the supine position; yet, with realignment, most of the people affected will turn out to have legs of equal length!

Remember that only 6–12% of us actually have evidence of an anatomical (true) LLD of 0.2" (5mm) or more, once in alignment, as demonstrated by Armour and Scott (1981) and by Schamberger (2002).

Pelvic Girdle Dysfunctions

According to some authors (myself included), at least 14 potential different dysfunctions can occur within the pelvic girdle complex. It is also common to find musculoskeletal dysfunctions coexisting between all of the three areas—iliosacral, sacroiliac, and symphysis pubis joints—and possibly all occurring at the same time.

Iliosacral Dysfunction (Fixation)

The following six iliosacral dysfunctions or fixations are possible:

- Anteriorly rotated innominate
- Posteriorly rotated innominate
- Superior shear (cephalic)—upslip
- Inferior shear (caudal)—downslip
- Innominate out-flare
- Innominate in-flare

Tables 12.1 and 12.2 overleaf summarize all of the specific testing and palpatory findings for each of the six types of iliosacral dysfunction.

Anteriorly/Posteriorly Rotated Innominate

Whenever I am giving lectures for my courses around the world, the terminology of anterior and posterior rotational components of the pelvis always crops up; we can therefore almost take it for granted that these rotations are a common dysfunctional pattern scenario for the innominate bone to follow. Hopefully, by now you will know that the rotation is classified as an *iliosacral* (and not sacroiliac) dysfunction, as it is the innominate bone that has rotated with respect to the sacrum.

If you look at Tables 12.1 and 12.2, you will notice that the indicated anterior and posterior rotations

Table 12.1. Iliosacral dysfunctions—left side.

Dysfunction	Left side	Standing flexion test	Medial malleolus	ASIS	PSIS	Sacral sulcus	Ischial tuberosity	Sacrotuberous ligament
Anterior rotation	Left	Left	Long left	Inferior	Superior	Shallow left	Superior	Lax left
Posterior rotation	Left	Left	Short left	Superior	Inferior	Deep left	Inferior	Taut left
Out-flare	Left	Left	No change	Lateral left	Medial left	Narrow left	No change	No change
In-flare	Left	Left	No change	Medial left	Lateral left	Wide left	No change	No change
Upslip	Left	Left	Short left	Superior left	Superior left	No change	Superior	Lax left
Downslip	Left	Left	Long left	Inferior left	Inferior left	No change	Inferior	Taut left

Table 12.2. Iliosacral dysfunctions—right side.

Dysfunction	Right side	Standing flexion test	Medial malleolus	ASIS	PSIS	Sacral sulcus	Ischial tuberosity	Sacrotuberous ligament
Anterior rotation	Right	Right	Long right	Inferior	Superior	Shallow right	Superior	Lax right
Posterior rotation	Right	Right	Short right	Superior	Inferior	Deep right	Inferior	Taut right
Out-flare	Right	Right	No change	Lateral right	Medial right	Narrow right	No change	No change
In-flare	Right	Right	No change	Medial right	Lateral right	Wide right	No change	No change
Upslip	Right	Right	Short right	Superior right	Superior right	No change	Superior	Lax right
Downslip	Right	Right	Long right	Inferior right	Inferior right	No change	Inferior	Taut right

alter the positions of the ASIS, PSIS, and medial malleoli (leg length). These types of iliosacral dysfunction are initially found (as well as by observation and other testing procedures) by the key test known as the *standing forward flexion test*. For example, if the standing forward flexion test is positive on the left side, and on palpation, when compared with the opposite side, the left ASIS is superior, the left PSIS is inferior, and the left medial malleolus (leg length) is shorter, then you have now found a left posterior rotation of the innominate. This dysfunction would be classified as a *left iliosacral posterior rotation* (Figure 12.47). On the other hand, if the standing forward flexion test is positive on the right side, but this time the right ASIS is inferior, the right PSIS is superior, and the right medial malleolus (leg length) appears longer, then one can assume a *right iliosacral anterior rotation* (the most common) is present (Figure 12.48).

Let's go through a thought process for just a moment and assume that the patient has the most common presentation: a right anterior innominate rotation and a left compensatory

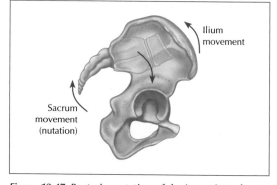

Figure 12.47. Posterior rotation of the innominate bone.

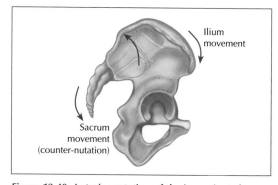

Figure 12.48. Anterior rotation of the innominate bone.

posterior innominate rotation, so that the right SIJ is considered to be *locked* (Figure 12.49(a)). In this Figure you can see three things: (1) the right pubic bone has displaced inferiorly (caudally) compared with the right side; (2) the sacrum has compensated for the rotational malalignment by rotating left on the left oblique axis (L-on-L); and (3) the lumbar spine has also compensated by rotating into the convexity to the left side.

With the most common presentation of a right anterior innominate rotation and a compensatory left posterior rotation, you will see in Figure 12.49(b) that a patient demonstrating a reaching motion toward their toes on the right side is able to do this with no restriction; however, on the left side (Figure 12.49(c)), the patient is clearly prevented from touching their toes.

Figure 12.49(d) demonstrates an improvement after a realignment technique has been performed (Chapter 13). The reason why the patient had a restriction to the left side is that the left innominate is locked into a posterior rotation, and that the reaching forward type of motion (as shown in the figures) demands an anterior motion of the innominate bone. The treatment

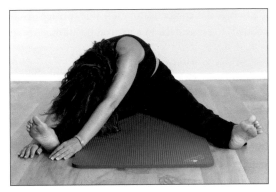

Figure 12.49. (b) The patient's reach to the right is normal.

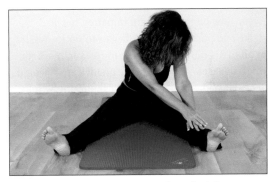

Figure 12.49. (c) The patient's reach to the left is impaired.

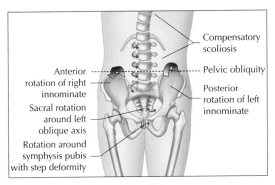

Compensatory scoliosis

Pelvic obliquity

Anterior rotation of right innominate

Posterior rotation of left innominate

Sacral rotation around left oblique axis

Rotation around symphysis pubis with step deformity

Figure 12.49. (a) Presentation of the most common rotational malalignment syndrome—right anterior and left posterior rotation. The compensations are shown by both the symphysis pubis joint and the sacrum having rotated left on the left oblique axis (L-on-L), and by the lumbar spine also having rotated left into the spinal convexity.

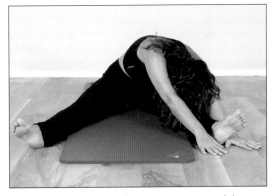

Figure 12.49. (d) After realignment treatment of the rotation of the right innominate bone, the patient can now reach to the left.

technique (see Chapter 13) is to correct the right anterior innominate rotation and not the left posterior innominate rotation; this will then encourage the compensatory left side (posteriorly rotated) to come back to a neutral position.

Case Study

On looking at the excellent book by Schamberger (2013) on malalignment syndrome, I was interested to read that the author was a very fit marathon runner, but he himself had suffered from right heel pain that had lasted many years. His ankle and foot were in a position of over-pronation, especially the right foot; he had tried orthoses but they failed to correct the position. Every time he ran, the pain impaired his heel-strike and push-off, and he began to notice wasting in all of his right leg muscles; moreover, his right thigh muscles—especially the quadriceps—would ache. He had an injection of local anesthetic into the area of the heel pain, but this did not even give him any short-term relief.

As time passed, the heel pain persisted. At some point he went to a medical conference, where one of the speakers talked about the sacrotuberous and sacrospinous ligaments referring pain to

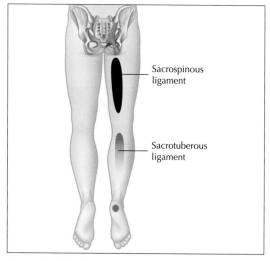

Figure 12.49 (e). Referral pattern for the sacrotuberous and sacrospinous ligaments, specific in particular to the area of the heel bone.

the leg, and especially to the heel (Figure 12.49(e)). That same afternoon, Schamberger was checked out by an osteopath, who noticed that he was out of alignment and said that his right innominate was rotated anteriorly; the osteopath proceeded to perform a corrective MET technique (Chapter 13) to correct the right anterior rotation. The applied technique was very simple and miraculously made the heel pain disappear completely, because of the fact that Schamberger was now realigned. The best part was to come, as later that day he ran for 12 miles (20km) and, for the first time in years, finished the run without an ache in his right thigh muscles or any pain in his heel.

Superior/Inferior Shear—Upslip/Downslip

An iliosacral *upslip* (superior shear, also known as *hipbone shear*) dysfunction normally relates to some type of trauma or accident: perhaps the person in question has had a motor accident, tumbled down some stairs from a height and landed on one side of their ischial tuberosity, fallen from a height (such as from a horse), or even simply missed a step when running or walking. It has even been considered that a strain of the QL muscle sustained while picking up a heavy load from the floor could be responsible for an upslip.

Williams and Warwick (1980) found that the degrees of freedom of the SIJ normally permit approximately 2 degrees of upward (cephalic) and downward (caudal) translation of the innominate relative to the sacrum. These dysfunctions tend to be less common (approximately 10–20%, compared with around 80% for innominate rotations) in patients who present with chronic back and pelvic pain. This type of dysfunction needs to be corrected by treatment, as it is very difficult for the patient to self-correct it (a very effective treatment protocol for this will be demonstrated in Chapter 13).

The initial diagnosis is indicated by the standing forward flexion test. In addition, on the side that tested positive in this test, the anatomical landmarks of the ASIS, PSIS, iliac crest, and pubic bone (potentially a 0.08–0.12", or 2–3mm, step deformity could be palpated at the symphysis pubis joint), as well as the ischial tuberosity, will all appear to be *cephalic* or *superior* (compared with the opposite side), as shown in Figure 12.50(a). On the higher (dysfunctional) side, the sacrotuberous ligament will be lax and the medial malleolus (leg length) will appear to be shorter.

An upslip can coexist with a rotation (anterior) and/or an out-flare/in-flare of the innominate bone, which means that some of the palpatory landmarks can be "hidden"; it will therefore be less obvious that an upslip is present (Figure 12.50(b)). This type of dysfunction is possible, especially if the corresponding knee joint is straight but the hip is not in a neutral position when the trauma is sustained, as this might cause a rotational force to the innominate, as well as producing an upslip.

Through his experiences, Schamberger (2013) discovered that the high side of the pelvis in standing or sitting does not always correspond

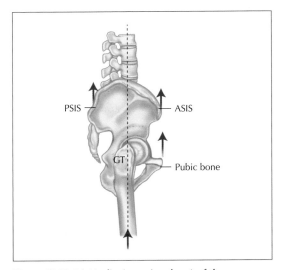

Figure 12.50. (a) Upslip (superior shear) of the innominate bone.

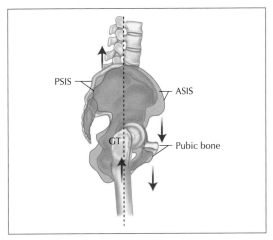

Figure 12.50. (b) Upslip is "hidden" as a result of the anterior rotation of the innominate bone.

with the side of the upslip. For example, the iliac crest is high on the right side in standing, sitting, and lying prone; in those with a left upslip present, with the left iliac crest high in lying, it is usually the right iliac crest that is high in standing and sitting. These findings suggest that the upslip may be associated with some rotation of the pelvis. In other words, if someone presents in this case with a right upslip, in combination with a right anterior and left posterior rotation, then some of the landmarks may alter: the step deformity of the symphysis pubis joint disappears, the ASIS becomes level compared with the opposite side, and the PSIS on the right becomes accentuated compared with the left side. Schamberger says that a correction of the rotational malalignment will reveal the underlying right upslip, with all the landmarks on the right side of the pelvis now in a superior position relative to those on the left.

If you suspect that your patient has an iliosacral *downslip* (inferior shear), the initial diagnosis is carried out through a standing forward flexion test: on the side that tests positive, the anatomical landmarks of the ASIS, PSIS, iliac crest, and ischial tuberosity will all appear to be *caudal* or *inferior* (compared with the opposite side). On the low (dysfunctional) side, the sacrotuberous ligament

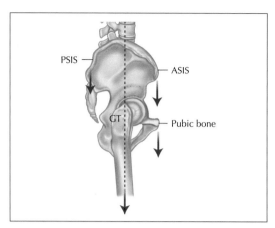

Figure 12.51. Downslip (inferior shear) of the innominate bone.

will be taut and the medial malleolus (leg length) will appear to be longer (Figure 12.51).

Dysfunctions of this type tend to be self-correcting when you walk. If you think about it logically, if a downslip is suspected on the right side, when the weight is placed onto the right leg, the right-side back of the pelvis is naturally pushed to a neutral position; in general, therefore, no treatment is actually required.

Innominate Out-Flare/In-Flare

Out-flare and in-flare refer to the movement of the innominate bones in outward and inward directions respectively. An out-flare motion is considered to be combined with the anterior rotation of the innominate bone, while an in-flare motion is considered to be combined with a posterior rotation of the innominate bone; this is because the innominates need to perform this specific type of rotary motion during the gait cycle, as well as during forward bending of the trunk.

DonTigny (2007) stated that SIJ dysfunction is essentially caused by an anterior rotation of the innominate bones and an out-flare relative to the sacrum. In-flare occurs with a posterior rotation of the innominate bone relative to the sacrum

and with sacral nutation. According to Kapandji (1974), during the initial 50–60 degrees forward flexion of the trunk when standing up, the sacrum nutates and the ilia rotate anteriorly and flare outward.

Think back to earlier when you were palpating the ASIS: I mentioned that it is important to look at your thumbs for equal symmetry of the two bony landmarks of the innominate bones, and to note down if you found any asymmetry. If you notice a difference between the two sides, you now need to imagine a straight line down the center of the body, which typically passes through the area of the umbilical (belly button). Now compare how far each thumb is from the centerline of the umbilicus. If you observe that your left thumb on the patient's right ASIS seems further away from the umbilicus than the opposite side, you have probably discovered an in-flare or an out-flare (Figure 12.52(a)).

How do you decide what type of dysfunction is present? Yes, you have guessed correctly—the good old standing forward flexion test and also the stork test. If these two tests are positive, for example on the patient's right side, you have now found an *iliosacral out-flare* (Figure 12.52(b)). Conversely, if the standing forward flexion test and the stork test were positive on the left side, you would conclude that an *iliosacral in-flare* is present (Figure 12.52(c)).

DeStefano (2011) is a particularly interesting read, and includes the following abstract:

"The two dysfunctions out-flare and in-flare are quite rare and they are only found in those SIJs

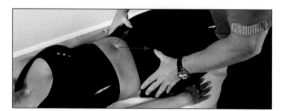

Figure 12.52. (a) Palpation assessment from the ASIS to the umbilicus, looking for an out-flare/in-flare.

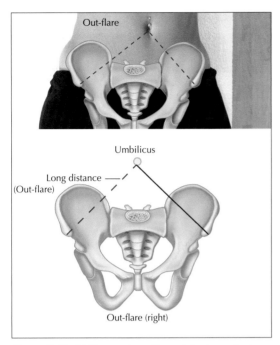

Figure 12.52. (b) Iliosacral out-flare of the innominate bone.

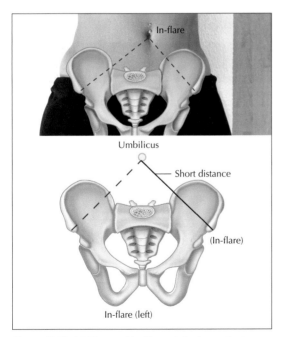

Figure 12.52. (c) Iliosacral in-flare of the innominate bone.

that have altered convex-to-concave relationships to S2 with convexity on the sacral side and concavity on the ilia side. They can only be diagnosed after the correction of any hipbone rotational dysfunction that is present."

Sacroiliac Dysfunction

The following sacroiliac dysfunctions are possible:

- L-on-L anterior sacral torsion
- R-on-R anterior sacral torsion
- L-on-R posterior sacral torsion
- R-on-L posterior sacral torsion
- Bilaterally nutated sacrum
- Bilaterally counter-nutated sacrum

Tables 12.3, 12.4 and 12.5 summarize all of the specific testing and palpatory findings for all of the sacral torsions and sacral dysfunctions.

I would like to recap just for a moment. By the time you have got to this stage of the book you should know that a dysfunction of the SIJ can result from how the pelvis (innominates) impacts on the sacrum, and, vice versa, from how the sacrum impacts on the pelvis (innominates). If the pelvis is fixed on the SIJ, then (as explained in previous chapters) we call it an *iliosacral dysfunction*; if the sacrum is fixed on the pelvis, then we call it a *sacroiliac joint dysfunction*.

Let's look at trying to find sacral torsions in a way that is different from (but hopefully simpler than) the one I have already explained. Your patient is lying in a prone position, and hopefully in a position of neutral; your thumbs are sitting nicely within the left and right sacral sulci. In this position, you feel that your right thumb is *shallow* and your left thumb is *deeper*. What does this mean? Think about it before reading on—yes, either the right side of the sacral base is posterior and also right rotated, or the left side is anterior but again right rotated. If the

Table 12.3. Anterior/forward sacral torsions (normal physiological motion).

	L-on-L sacral torsion (forward/nutation)	**R-on-R sacral torsion (forward/nutation)**
Deep sacral sulcus	Right	Left
Shallow sacral sulcus	Left	Right
ILA posterior	Left	Right
L5 rotation	Right—ERS(R)	Left—ERS(L)
Seated flexion test	Right	Left
Lumbar spring	Negative	Negative
Sphinx (extension) test	Sulci level	Sulci level
Lumbar flexion test	Right sacral sulcus deep	Left sacral sulcus deep
Lumbar lordosis	Increased	Increased
Medial malleolus (leg length)	Short left	Short right

sacral base is rotated in neutral, it therefore has to be dysfunctional: either the right side is fixed posteriorly (counter-nutation) or the left (deeper) side is fixed anteriorly (nutation).

How to Decide on the Fixation?

With the patient still prone and our thumbs sitting on the left and right sacral sulci, we can

Table 12.4. Posterior/backward sacral torsion (non-physiological motion).

	L-on-R sacral torsion (backward/counter-nutation)	**R-on-L sacral torsion (backward/counter-nutation)**
Deep sacral sulcus	Right	Left
Shallow sacral sulcus	Left	Right
ILA posterior	Left	Right
L5 rotation	Right—FRS(R)	Left—FRS(L)
Seated flexion test	Left	Right
Lumbar spring	Positive	Positive
Sphinx (extension) test	Left sacral sulcus shallow (right sacral sulcus deeper)	Right sacral sulcus shallow (left sacral sulcus deeper)
Lumbar flexion test	Sulci level	Sulci level
Lumbar lordosis	Decreased	Decreased
Medial malleolus (leg length)	Short left	Short right

Table 12.5. Bilaterally nutated and counter-nutated sacrum.

	Bilaterally nutated sacrum (forward)	Bilaterally counter-nutated sacrum (backward)
Standing flexion test	Negative	Negative
Seated flexion test	Positive bilateral	Positive bilateral
Stork (Gillet) test	Positive on both sides	Positive on both sides
Sacral base	Left and right anterior	Left and right posterior
ILA	Left and right posterior	Left and right anterior
Lumbar spring test	Negative	Positive
Lumbar lordosis	Increased	Decreased
Medial malleolus (leg length)	Equal	Equal

ask the patient to backward bend (come up onto the elbows, as in reading a book), and forward bend (ask the patient to tilt their pelvis posteriorly or to perform the lumbar flexion test, as shown previously) from the position they are in. If the rotation increases (gets worse) in a backward-bent position (right thumb becomes shallower and left thumb becomes deeper), and then the rotation is seen to disappear in a forward-bent position, you know that the right side has to be fixed in a posterior position and rotated to the right, as in a R-on-L sacral torsion. This is because when you ask your patient to backward bend, the sacrum has to be able to go in an anterior direction, which it cannot do. The right fixed sacrum therefore now becomes a fixed pivot point, and so is unable to perform this forward motion because of the fact that the right sacral base is fixed posteriorly; hence the rotation looks worse.

With these types of posterior fixation you will notice a reduction in lumbar lordosis (back flattens), and the L5 spring test will feel firm to palpation when pressure is applied (positive test).

Let's look at the other scenario whereby the left sacral base is fixed in an anterior position (nutation). We again ask the patient to perform

backward bending and forward bending motions. This time, however, the forward-bent position gives the appearance of the rotation increasing, and the backward-bent position seems to make the sacral base become level. This is because during the forward bending motion, the left sacral base stays fixed anteriorly, so it cannot move in a posterior direction; it therefore becomes a pivot point, but the patient's right sacral base moves further in a posterior direction and subsequently makes the rotation appear to become worse. This type of dysfunction is called a *R-on-R sacral torsion*.

With these types of anterior fixation, you will notice an increase in lumbar lordosis, and the L5 spring test will indicate some spring when pressure is applied (negative test).

Tip: A simple rule of thumb for determining which side is fixed is as follows. If the sacral rotation increases when the patient backward bends, then the side that the sacrum has rotated to (the shallow side) will be the side that is fixed posteriorly. This dysfunction is a counter-nutated sacral torsion as in a L-on-R sacral torsion or a R-on-L sacral torsion.

If, however, with your patient still in the backward-bent position, the sacral rotation becomes level (it seems to disappear), then the side opposite to the side of rotation (think back to the neutral test of sacral sulcus) is the side that is fixed anteriorly. This is a nutated sacral torsion as in a *R-on-R sacral torsion* or a *L-on-L sacral torsion*.

I like the way this is interpreted in DeStefano (2011), which contains the following statement (overleaf) regarding sacral torsions:

"Forward torsions become asymmetric in forward bending and become symmetric in backward bending. The posterior torsions are the reverse, they get more asymmetric in backward bending and symmetric in forward bending."

Bilaterally Nutated/Counter-Nutated Sacrum

I have left bilateral sacral nutation (forward) and bilateral sacral counter-nutation (backward) till the end of the discussion, since they only occur very rarely and are also often missed by an examiner. Most of the initial tests (such as the standing forward flexion test) will turn out to be negative, and also the levels of the sacral base and the ILA will be level; however, the stork test will demonstrate a bilateral restriction and is of value to the overall diagnosis. These sacral dysfunctions are generally related to L5; for instance, if the sacrum is bilaterally nutated, it will cause an extension position of L5, whereas if the sacrum is bilaterally counter-nutated, L5 will be held in a flexed position. The consequences will be the change in lordosis curvature and the positive or negative result from the lumbar spring test.

Symphysis Pubis Dysfunction

The pubic bone tends to be either superior or inferior, although some authors discuss other types of potential symphysis pubis dysfunction (SPD). Here we will focus on:

- Superior pubis
- Inferior pubis

Tables 12.6 and 12.7 summarize all of the specific testing and palpatory findings for SPDs.

To be honest, I feel that this area of the pelvic girdle (the symphysis pubis) is probably the least assessed and consequently the least treated, and this also applies to me, especially when I am with my own patients. I would say that some therapists more than likely tend to focus on the area of the pain, without realizing that part of the problem potentially lies in a different area. Recall the wise words of Dr. Ida Rolf: "Where the pain is, the problem is not." This could not be any truer than when looking for dysfunction within the SPJ.

Table 12.6. Symphysis pubis dysfunctions—left side.

	Superior pubis	**Inferior pubis**
Standing forward flexion test	Left	Left
Pubic tubercle	Superior	Inferior
Inguinal ligament	Tender on palpation	Tender on palpation

Table 12.7. Symphysis pubis dysfunctions—right side.

	Superior pubis	**Inferior pubis**
Standing forward flexion test	Right	Right
Pubic tubercle	Superior	Inferior
Inguinal ligament	Tender on palpation	Tender on palpation

Case Study

When an excellent physiotherapist and a personal friend of mine called Gordon Bosworth was mentoring me in my early osteopathy studies, I remember him assessing a young male who was part of the Olympic bobsleigh team; he had what had been diagnosed as a typical groin strain of the adductor longus muscle and the team doctor had recommended treatment through the use of a steroid injection.

The patient decided not to have the injection but to see the team's physiotherapist (Gordon) instead. I remember actually watching the patient being assessed (in a similar way to that mentioned in this chapter); Gordon came to the decision that this patient had an iliosacral dysfunction on the right side and corrected that dysfunction using the techniques I will be demonstrating in Chapter 13. I then watched Gordon assess the SPJ and once again he said a dysfunction was present and then proceeded to correct the underling issue by using a specific MET for the SPJ (also explained in Chapter 13). After performing the realignment techniques, he retested the area of the pain by doing a resisted adductor test; to my surprise, the pain had completely disappeared. From that moment on, I knew that this joint demanded a bit more love and attention, as it could just be the key to solving the overall problem.

When trying to decide on the side that is dysfunctional, the first thing that is relevant is the standing forward flexion test. So if, let's say, the standing forward flexion test is positive on the left side, you know that a dysfunction is present and that it is located specifically on the left side. The second thing to consider is palpation of the bony landmarks: if you palpate the area of the pubic tubercle and you determine the level to be cephalic/superior compared with the opposite side, you know that a superior pubis condition exists (only if the standing forward flexion test is positive on that side). The third thing that also confirms

the diagnosis is tenderness of the inguinal ligament on palpation.

How to Decide Which Dysfunction Exists

Out of all the tests I have shown you, I consider the key ones to be the standing and seated forward flexion. I say that because these tests specifically indicate the side of the body on which the dysfunction is present. If your patient bends forward in the standing position, and the left side of the PSIS travels further than the right side, the conclusion is that they have either an iliosacral dysfunction or a SPD on the left side. However, if the standing flexion test is negative (i.e. the thumbs move symmetrically when the patient forward bends), but you notice that your left thumb moves more cephalically than your right thumb during the seated forward flexion test, the indications are that a sacroiliac dysfunction is present on the left side.

The standing and seated forward flexion tests do not actually tell you what is wrong, in terms of the actual dysfunction that is present: they only give you some of the necessary information regarding the side on which the dysfunction exists. It therefore makes sense, especially as a starting point, to treat the side that tests positive in the standing/seated forward flexion tests. During the examination process, you may notice that what you consider to be the side of the fixation might not actually be the painful side for the patient's presenting symptoms. The side that is presenting with pain could be the side that is doing all the motion (hypermobile) and is compensating for the side that is fixed (hypomobile).

As a sort of recap (which I hope will help you to understand exactly what I am trying to put across), let's think about what I said in the previous paragraph. In general, if the standing flexion test is positive for the left side, then the dysfunction is present on that same side, possibly indicating an iliosacral or even an SPD. This test will be part of the process that will help you ascertain what the dysfunction is and formulate a treatment plan.

If, however, the seated flexion test is positive, this indicates a *sacroiliac dysfunction* on the tested side and not an iliosacral dysfunction or SPD. Just to complicate matters somewhat, you can have a standing forward flexion test indicating positive on the left side (iliosacral/pubic dysfunction), and a seated forward flexion test indicating positive on the right (SIJ dysfunction), both at the same time.

Unfortunately, it is never as easy as it might seem. Remember what Schamberger (2013) says: an iliosacral upslip (in isolation) and a true LLD have no correlation to the standing forward flexion test. With a right upslip, for example, the right PSIS remains higher than the left to an equal extent throughout the full range of flexion carried out in either a standing or a sitting position. Basically, it would appear to be a false positive because of the motion of the right PSIS; however, the left PSIS traveled an equal distance, making the test negative. Please bear these things in mind when you are reading other texts about the lumbopelvic complex, and try to be a little open-minded, especially when you are assessing your own patients and athletes.

recognizable picture. Perhaps the picture is not absolutely clear yet, but if you have understood what I am trying to say, then some image should at least have developed in your mind. Be honest with yourself: if you do not quite understand the content of each of the chapters, then I suggest you read them again, or at least certain parts, before continuing to Chapter 13 and beginning to actually treat common pelvic dysfunctions.

I say that because if you truly do not understand the concepts and the underlying biomechanics of the pelvic girdle, then how will you be able to treat patients effectively? That said, the techniques I demonstrate in the next chapter are very safe to perform, as the majority of them are soft tissue techniques, specifically METs. It would therefore be acceptable if you wanted to practice them on a colleague first, before actually using them on real patients with real symptoms. I would still recommend that you have a good understanding of all the potential dysfunctions that your patient could present with to your clinic, before you unreservedly say that you are an effective therapist and that what you plan to do in terms of treatment will be of value to your patient.

The Next Step

I hope that now you have reached this stage of the book, the jigsaw puzzle pieces are forming a

Treatment of the Pelvis

A s you will probably have guessed by now, this is the final chapter of the book and I hope you have enjoyed reading all of the other chapters leading up to it. I think it makes perfect sense to finish the book with a chapter that concentrates on one of the most important areas, namely the treatment of all the various types of pelvic girdle and lumbar spine dysfunctions that have been previously covered and discussed extensively throughout this text.

The focus of this particular chapter will therefore be on the application of specific realignment techniques for treating the three main areas of the pelvis: symphysis pubis, iliosacral, and sacroiliac types of dysfunction. These are the most common presentations typically found when assessing athletes and patients.

At the end of this chapter I will also include a treatment strategy for the area of the lumbar spine, because the lumbar spine is a naturally occurring connection to the pelvis. I always say the following to my students: if you have a primary pelvic girdle dysfunction, there must be some form of compensatory mechanism continuing on throughout the area of the lumbar spine, and even the thoracic spine and the cervical spine will

be involved in the compensation process; these areas could be a potential site of pain and a natural concern for your patients. Once you have applied some of the realignment techniques that I am about to demonstrate for the pelvic girdle, it would be sensible to make absolutely sure that the lumbar spine is also in a relatively level position through the appropriate treatment protocols discussed at the end of this chapter.

In previous chapters I discussed in great detail how to thoroughly assess the three areas of the pelvic girdle in order to confirm or discount the existence of any presenting malalignment syndromes. We now need to put everything that has been taught into practice by applying the following techniques to correct and normalize the various musculoskeletal dysfunctions that you might find during your initial assessment/screening process.

Treatment Strategy

Other experts in this complex field of manual medicine start the treatment strategy by initially correcting the position of the lumbar spine. They then move on to dysfunctions that are found within the iliosacral area, followed by the region of the sacroiliac, and finishing off with a treatment of the symphysis pubis joint.

In DeStefano (2011), Greenman's suggestion of the treatment sequence is: symphysis pubis, hipbone shear (upslip is considered a hipbone shear) dysfunction, sacroiliac dysfunction, and iliosacral dysfunction.

My personal preference is the following (and I like to think it is similar to Greenman's approach, as I was taught his manual medicine principles early on in my osteopathy training). I would recommend starting the corrective treatment with the symphysis pubis joint, followed by treatment of iliosacral dysfunctions (upslip first), and then moving on to sacroiliac dysfunctions. I would finish the treatment, if I felt it was necessary, with any compensatory dysfunctions that are present within the region of the lumbar spine.

Greenman in DeStefano (2011) recommends treating the symphysis pubis joint early on during the assessment process. The reason for this is that SIJ dysfunctions are typically found in a patient in the prone position; if a symphysis pubis dysfunction is present at the front of the body, the patient is not symmetric in the prone position, resting on the tripod formed by the two ASISs and the symphysis pubis.

Greenman also suggests treating superior shear (upslip) after the symphysis pubis, as he found that the presence of shear restricts all other motions within that SIJ: therefore, he says shear deserves attention early on in the treatment process. He mentions that you need to have two symmetric hipbones available in order to assess the position of the sacrum between these two bones.

In terms of assessing and treating patients, I consider my concept/approach to be similar to Greenman's. When I give lectures to my students about the pelvis and SIJ, I like to recommend

Greenman's Principles of Manual Medicine (DeStefano 2011), as I think it is a great book for assisting students in learning about this area. However, I also highly recommend other physical therapy books to my students (see Bibliography), such as those by the experts Lee, Vleeming, and Schamberger. I would like to think that in time, if students of physical therapy endeavor to read some, or indeed all of the books I have recommended (as well as this book), they will hopefully be able to competently assess, identify, and treat their own patients and athletes in their own clinical settings.

> **Note:** The realignment techniques demonstrated in this chapter mainly consist of soft tissue techniques, specifically METs, as explained in Chapter 7. However, since I am an osteopath and have trained in the skill of spinal manipulation, the word "thrust" or the words "high-velocity thrust" (or abbreviation HVT) will be mentioned from time to time. These advanced techniques should only be incorporated into the treatment plan if one has the necessary training and qualifications to perform them.

Most of the techniques I will show you are very safe to perform in your own clinic. If you are unsure of which technique (depending on your skill level and qualifications) is best applied to your patient, I would follow the soft tissue MET approach initially, as generally these techniques will cause no harm but are very effective at correcting any malalignment presentations, especially when used properly. However, there will come a time when you will feel a thrust technique (HVT) is needed, so you have a choice: either you can train in the appropriate field of manual therapy, e.g. osteopathy or chiropractic, or it might be easier (in my opinion) to simply refer your patient to a suitably qualified practitioner who is skilled in the art of spinal manipulation.

Part 1: Treatment Protocol for Symphysis Pubis Dysfunctions

Symphysis pubis dysfunctions (SPDs) are very common but are generally neglected in terms of treatment by the physical therapist; I feel that this is probably because of the lack of symptomatic pain within the SPJ. The pubic bone tends to be either superior or inferior (although other types of potential dysfunction are discussed by some authors). For this text, we will focus on:

- Superior/inferior SPD
- Left superior SPD
- Right inferior SPD

Diagnosis: Superior/Inferior SPD

Treatment: MET/Thrust technique (shotgun technique)
Position: Supine

The patient adopts a supine position with the knees and hips bent and the feet flat. The therapist stands at the side of the couch and places their hands on the outsides of the patient's knees.

The patient is asked to abduct their hips against a resistance for 10 seconds (Figure 13.1(a)), which causes an RI effect in the adductors; this isometric contraction is repeated approximately three times. The therapist then places a clenched fist between the patient's knees, and the patient is asked to squeeze the fist tightly (adduction), as shown in Figure 13.1(b). This motion of adduction is generally enough to cause a realignment of the symphysis pubis joint—it is very common for a noise (due to cavitation) to be heard from the joint, indicating a release. There is no direct thrust involved with this technique, so it is very safe to perform.

If there is no sign of cavitation using the above technique, and you still consider the joint to be dysfunctional, a thrust/HVT

technique is appropriate. After the patient has abducted the hip three times (Figure 13.1(a)), the therapist places their hands on the insides of the patient's knees (see Figure 13.2(a)), or even their forearms (if easier), see Figure 13.2(b). The patient is then asked to adduct quickly and strongly against the applied resistance. As the patient adducts, the therapist can apply a rapid abduction motion (see Figure 13.3). If a dysfunction is present, this specific technique will cause a cavitation of the symphysis pubis joint; hence this technique is known as the *shotgun*.

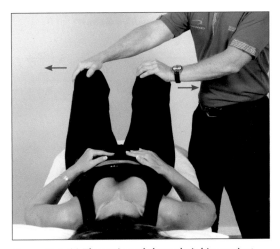

Figure 13.1. (a) The patient abducts their hips against a resistance applied by the therapist.

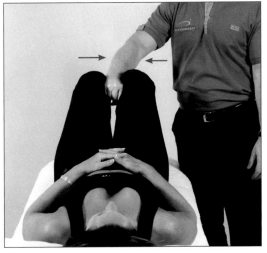

Figure 13.1. (b) The therapist places their clenched fist between the patient's knees as they adduct firmly.

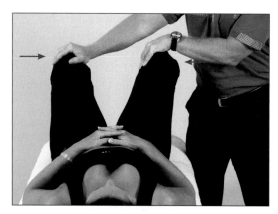

Figure 13.2. (a) The therapist places their hands between the patient's knees as they adduct firmly.

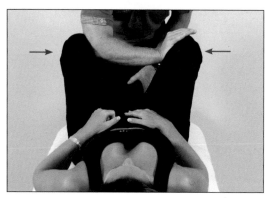

Figure 13.2. (b) The therapist places their forearms between the patient's knees as they adduct firmly.

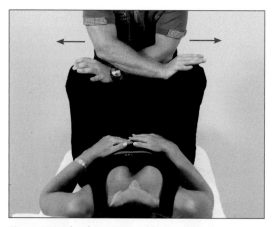

Figure 13.3. The therapist quickly separates the patient's knees while they are still adducting. A noise is sometimes heard as the symphysis pubis joint undergoes cavitation.

Diagnosis: Left Superior SPD

Treatment: MET
Position: Supine

The patient adopts a supine position and lies at the edge of the couch with their arms placed across their body for extra support. The therapist stands on the same side as the dysfunction and places the patient's left leg so that it hangs off the couch. The therapist stabilizes the right side of the patient's pelvis with their left hand, and places their right hand above the left patella, to stabilize the patient's left leg (Figure 13.4).

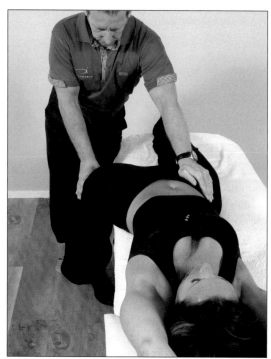

Figure 13.4. The therapist supports the patient, whose left leg hangs off the couch.

From this position, the patient is asked to flex their left hip against a resistance applied for 10 seconds by the therapist (Figure 13.5). On the relaxation phase, the therapist guides the patient's left leg into further extension, as this will encourage the left side of the symphysis pubis joint to move inferiorly (Figure 13.6).

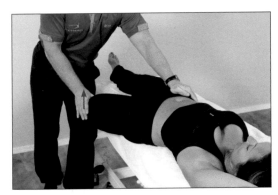

Figure 13.5. The patient lifts their left hip into flexion against a resistance applied by the therapist.

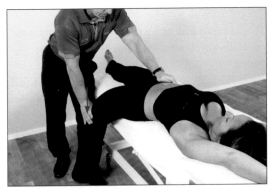

Figure 13.6. After the 10-second contraction, the therapist takes the leg into further extension, which encourages the left side of symphysis pubis to move inferiorly.

Diagnosis: Right Inferior SPD

Treatment: MET
Position: Supine

The patient adopts a supine position and lies at the edge of the couch with their arms placed across their body for extra support. The therapist stands on the side opposite to the dysfunction.

The therapist then flexes and adducts, with a slight internal rotation, the patient's right leg; this motion will encourage superior motion of the right side

of the symphysis pubis. Using the patient's leg as a lever, the therapist lifts the right side of the patient's pelvis off the couch, so that they can place their left hand and hook onto the patient's ischial tuberosity (Figure 13.7).

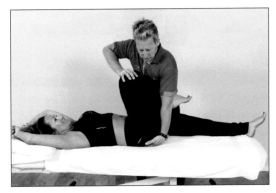

Figure 13.7. The patient's right hip is guided into flexion, adduction, and internal rotation.

The therapist lowers the pelvis down onto their hand; from this position the patient is asked to extend their right hip against a resistance applied for 10 seconds by the therapist (Figure 13.8). On the relaxation phase, the therapist encourages the patient's right leg into further flexion, while at the same time pressure is applied to the ischial tuberosity (see Figure 13.9); this will encourage the right side of the symphysis pubis joint to move superiorly.

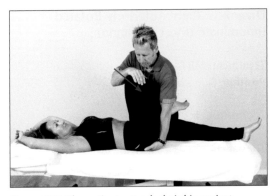

Figure 13.8. The patient extends their hip against a resistance applied by the therapist.

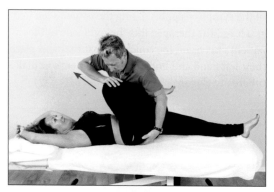

Figure 13.9. The therapist guides the patient's leg into further flexion while applying pressure to the ischial tuberosity.

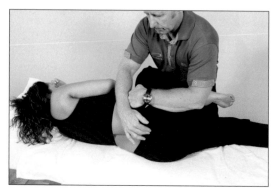

Figure 13.10. (a) The therapist cradles the patient's knee and hip at 90 degrees while controlling the innominate bone.

Part 2: Treatment Protocol for Iliosacral Dysfunctions

The following iliosacral dysfunctions are possible:

- Anteriorly rotated innominate
- Posteriorly rotated innominate
- Superior shear (cephalic)—upslip
- Inferior shear (caudal)—downslip
- Iliosacral out-flare (lateral rotation of innominate)
- Iliosacral in-flare (medial rotation of innominate)

Diagnosis: Right Anteriorly Rotated Innominate (Most Common)

Treatment: MET
Position: Side lying

Technique 1

The patient adopts a side-lying position and the therapist stands on the same side as the dysfunction. The patient's hip and knee are flexed to approximately 90 degrees and brought over the edge of the couch. The therapist stabilizes the patient's right innominate with their left hand and palpates the patient's PSIS with their right hand (Figure 13.10(a)).

The therapist fine-tunes this position by palpating the PSIS with their right hand as they flex the patient's hip until a barrier (point of bind) is felt at the level of the PSIS. From this position and using approximately 20% effort, the patient is asked to extend their hip (Gmax and hamstrings) against a resistance applied by the therapist for 10 seconds (Figure 13.10(b)).

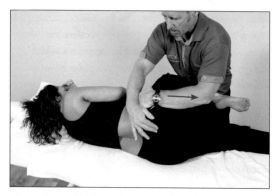

Figure 13.10. (b) The patient extends their hip against a resistance applied by the therapist.

After the contraction, and on complete relaxation, the right innominate bone is guided by the therapist's left hand into a posteriorly rotated position, while at the same time the hip and knee are being flexed (Figure 13.10(c)). This is repeated (normally three times) until a new barrier has been achieved.

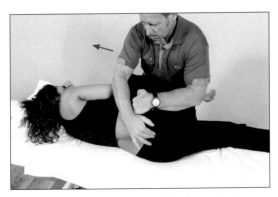

Figure 13.10. (c) The therapist guides the patient's innominate bone into a posteriorly rotated position as the knee and hip are being flexed.

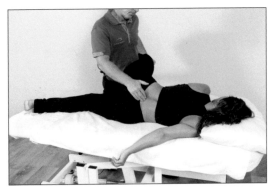

Figure 13.11. (a) The patient's torso is placed in a right rotation. The therapist cradles the patient's hip at 90 degrees while palpating the left PSIS.

Diagnosis: Left Anteriorly Rotated Innominate (Less Common)

Treatment: MET
Position: Side lying

Technique 2

(An alternative technique to correct a left anterior innominate rotation)

This is a similar technique to that explained above, with a few modifications: this time the dysfunction relates to a left anterior innominate rather than a right anterior innominate. The patient adopts a side-lying position and the therapist stands on the same side as the dysfunction. The patient's upper torso is placed in a right rotation, as this induces tension down to the lumbosacral junction and prevents unnecessary motion of the lumbar spine. Next, the therapist places the patient's left hip into flexion, and the patient's posterior thigh is rested against the therapist's hip (the patient hooks their left leg around the therapist), as shown in Figure 13.11(a). The patient's right lower leg is placed in an extended position.

The therapist palpates the PSIS and encourages flexion of the hip until a point of bind is felt. From this position and using approximately 20% effort, the patient is then asked to extend their hip (Gmax and hamstrings) against a resistance applied for 10 seconds by the therapist (Figure 13.11(b)).

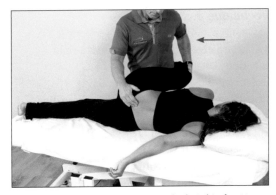

Figure 13.11. (b) The patient extends their hip for 10 seconds while the therapist palpates the left PSIS.

On complete relaxation, the left innominate bone is guided into a posteriorly rotated position by the therapist's right hand, while at the same time the hip and knee are being flexed (see Figure 13.11(c)). This is repeated (normally three times) until a new barrier has been achieved.

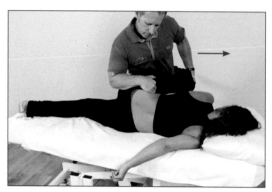

Figure 13.11. (c) The therapist guides the patient's innominate bone into a posteriorly rotated position as the knee and hip are being flexed.

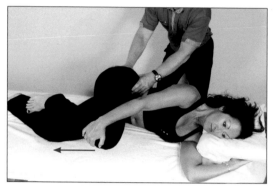

Figure 13.12. The therapist cradles the patient's innominate bone, and the patient holds their knees at 90 degrees. The patient then extends their hip against a resistance applied by their own hands.

Diagnosis: Right Anteriorly Rotated Innominate (More Common)

Treatment: MET
Position: Side lying

Technique 3

(An alternative technique to correct a right anteriorly rotated innominate)

The following technique is another alternative method for correcting anterior innominate rotation, in this case on the right side. This time the therapist stands behind the patient and cradles the right innominate with both hands, as the patient holds onto their knees at 90 degrees.

From this position, the therapist fines-tunes the innominate bone in a posterior rotation direction, in order to isolate the position of bind. The patient is then asked to resist hip extension against pressure applied by their own hands for 10 seconds (Figure 13.12).

After the 10-second contraction, and on complete relaxation, the patient is asked to slowly pull their right hip into full flexion at the same time as their right innominate is being guided by the therapist into a posteriorly rotated position (Figure 13.13).

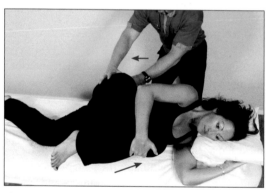

Figure 13.13. The therapist guides the patient's innominate into a posteriorly rotated position, as the patient flexes their hip.

Diagnosis: Left Posteriorly Rotated Innominate (Common)

Treatment: MET
Position: Prone

Technique 1

The patient adopts a prone position and the therapist stands on the same side as the dysfunction. The patient is asked to lift their left leg a few inches, so that the therapist can place their right arm under the patient's left thigh; the therapist interlocks their hands, so that their forearm rests on the patient's left PSIS.

The therapist fine-tunes this position by slowly extending and adducting the patient's hip joint until a barrier is felt. From this barrier, the patient is then asked to gently flex the hip of the affected side against a resistance for 10 seconds (Figure 13.14).

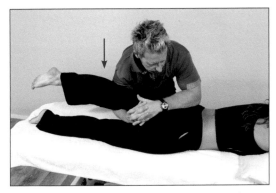

Figure 13.14. The therapist supports the patient's leg while controlling the innominate bone with their forearm. The patient then flexes their hip against a resistance applied by the therapist.

On complete relaxation, the therapist takes the extended leg further into hip extension and adduction, while gently encouraging anterior innominate rotation with their forearm. This combined movement of the hip joint and pelvis induces an anterior rotation of the innominate bone (Figure 13.15). This is repeated (normally three times) until a new barrier has been achieved.

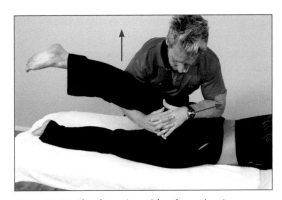

Figure 13.15. The therapist guides the patient's innominate bone in an anterior rotation direction, as the hip is extended and adducted at the same time.

Diagnosis: Right Posteriorly Rotated Innominate (Less Common)

Treatment: MET
Position: Prone

Technique 2

(An alternative technique, for a less common right posterior innominate rotation)

Some patients' legs can be extremely heavy; because of the increased weight of the leg in this case, I consider the following alternative technique a little easier to perform.

This time the therapist stands on the side (the left side) opposite to the dysfunction (the right side is fixed posteriorly). The patient is asked to lift their left leg a few inches, so that the therapist can place their right hand under the patient's right knee, while the left hand rests just at the level of the patient's right PSIS.

The therapist fine-tunes this position by slowly extending and adducting the right hip until a barrier is felt. From this barrier, the patient is asked to gently flex the right hip against a resistance applied by the therapist for 10 seconds (Figure 13.16).

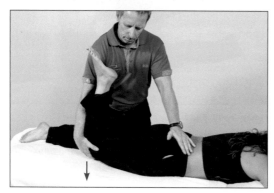

Figure 13.16. The therapist supports the patient's leg, while controlling the innominate bone with their hand. The patient then flexes their hip against a resistance applied by the therapist.

On complete relaxation, the therapist takes the right leg further into hip extension and adduction, while applying pressure with their left hand to the patient's right PSIS. This combined movement induces an anterior rotation of the right innominate bone (Figure 13.17). This is repeated (normally three times) until a new barrier has been achieved.

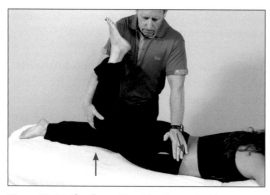

Figure 13.17. The therapist guides the patient's innominate in an anterior rotation direction, as the hip is extended and adducted at the same time.

Diagnosis: Right Superior Shear (Cephalic)—Upslip

Treatment: MET/Mobilization/Thrust technique
Position: Prone

The patient adopts a prone position and the therapist stands on the same side as the dysfunction. The patient is asked to slide down the couch until their knees are just off the edge. The patient is then asked to look to one side (any) and not to hold on to anything. The therapist straddles the patient's right leg and internally rotates the patient's thigh to cause a close-packed position of the hip joint (Figure 13.18).

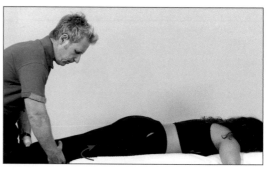

Figure 13.18. The therapist straddles the patient's right leg and internally rotates their hip in order to establish a close-packed position of the hip joint.

The therapist's right hand palpates the patient's right PSIS as their left hand stabilizes either the sacrum or the left thigh. With their thigh, the therapist slowly starts to grip the patient's right leg, while applying some traction to the leg by inducing a caudal pull to the right leg until the barrier is reached.

At the barrier, an MET is applied by asking the patient to hitch their pelvis up by activating their QL muscle for 10 seconds against a resistance applied by the straddling of the therapist's legs (Figure 13.19).

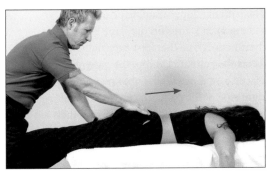

Figure 13.19. Using their QL muscle, the patient hitches the pelvis up in a cephalic/superior direction for 10 seconds.

After the contraction, and during the relaxation phase, a new barrier is found by gently applying a caudal/inferior traction to the leg (Figure 13.20). This technique is repeated three times. A mobilization or a manipulation (thrust) technique can also be performed from this position, to encourage a caudal/downward movement of the right innominate bone.

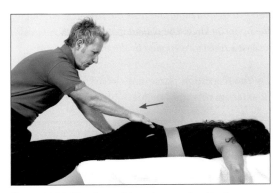

Figure 13.20. The therapist performs a traction/ mobilization or a manipulation (thrust) technique to the leg in a caudal direction after the initial MET contraction/treatment.

Diagnosis: Left Superior Shear (Cephalic)—Upslip

Treatment: MET/Mobilization/Thrust technique
Position: Supine

The patient adopts a supine position, with their right knee bent at 90 degrees (this prevents unnecessary motion of the right innominate bone). The therapist stands on the same side as the dysfunction and internally rotates the patient's thigh to introduce a close-packed position of the left hip joint.

The therapist gently grips the patient's lower leg with their hands and starts to apply light traction to the left leg by inducing a caudal pull to engage the barrier. At the barrier, a mobilizing technique, MET, or high-velocity thrust (HVT) is performed to encourage a caudal/downward movement of the innominate bone (Figure 13.21).

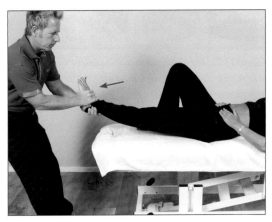

Figure 13.21. The therapist has the choice of performing an MET, a mobilization, or a manipulation technique from this specific position.

Diagnosis: Right Iliosacral Out-Flare (Lateral Rotation of Innominate)

Treatment: MET
Position: Supine

The patient adopts a supine position and the therapist stands on the same side as the dysfunction. The therapist flexes the patient's right hip and knee, then lifts the pelvis to the left using the leg as a lever, so that they can place their hand on the patient's right PSIS. The therapist lowers the patient's pelvis down until it rests on their hand, and then adducts the patient's hip with their right hand until a barrier is felt for the internal rotation of the innominate bone.

From this position of bind, the patient is asked to externally rotate and abduct their hip for 10 seconds (Figure 13.22).

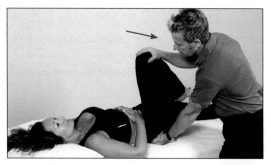

Figure 13.22. The therapist puts the patient's right hip into flexion and places their hand on the patient's PSIS. The patient then externally rotates against a resistance applied by the therapist.

On the relaxation phase, a new barrier of internal rotation is achieved, while at the same time the therapist is applying a traction technique to the patient's right PSIS (Figure 13.23).

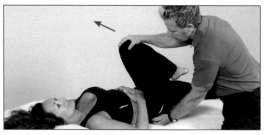

Figure 13.23. The therapist guides the patient's right hip into internal rotation while applying traction to the PSIS to encourage a neutral position of the innominate.

Diagnosis: Left Iliosacral In-Flare (Medial Rotation of Innominate)

Treatment: MET
Position: Supine

The patient adopts a supine position and the therapist stands on the same side as the dysfunction. The therapist externally rotates and flexes the patient's left hip; the patient's left foot is placed just above their right knee. Stabilizing the right side of the patient's pelvis with their right hand, and the patient's left knee with their left hand, the therapist encourages external rotation until a barrier is felt.

From this position of bind, the patient is asked to internally rotate their hip for 10 seconds (Figure 13.24).

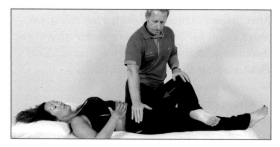

Figure 13.24. The therapist places the patient's left hip into external rotation, and rests the patient's left foot on the opposite knee. The patient then internally rotates against a resistance applied by the therapist.

On the relaxation phase, a new barrier of external rotation is achieved (Figure 13.25).

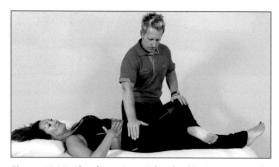

Figure 13.25. The therapist guides the hip into external rotation and encourages a neutral position of the innominate.

Part 3: Treatment Protocol for Sacroiliac Dysfunctions

The following sacroiliac dysfunctions are possible:

- L-on-L anterior (forward) sacral torsion
- R-on-R anterior (forward) sacral torsion
- L-on-R posterior (backward) sacral torsion
- R-on-L posterior (backward) sacral torsion
- Bilateral anterior sacrum (nutated)
- Bilateral posterior sacrum (counter-nutated)

Diagnosis: L-on-L Anterior (Forward) Sacral Torsion

Treatment: MET
Position: Sims

In this dysfunction the sacrum has rotated left (side bent right) on the left oblique axis, and the right sacral base has anteriorly nutated (Figure 13.26).

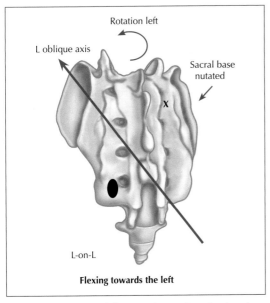

Figure 13.26. Left-on-left (L-on-L) sacral motion/torsion. X = Anterior or deep. ● = Posterior or shallow.

The patient adopts a prone position on the couch, while the therapist stands on the right side of the couch and flexes the patient's knees to 90 degrees. The therapist turns the patient onto their left hip to achieve what is known as the *Sims position* (Figure 13.27). Note that the patient's left arm is held back and the right arm is held forward.

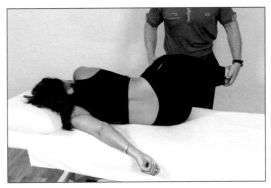

Figure 13.27. The therapist bends the patient's knees to 90 degrees and places the patient in the Sims position.

With the patient's knees placed on the therapist's left thigh, the lumbosacral junction is palpated using the left hand, while a left rotation of the patient's trunk is introduced until L5 is felt to rotate to the left (Figure 13.28).

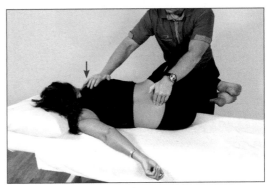

Figure 13.28. The therapist fine-tunes the position and introduces a rotation of L5 to the left.

From this position, the therapist palpates the lumbosacral junction and the right sacral base with their right hand, then, using the patient's legs as a lever, introduces a flexion motion to the trunk until a barrier is felt (Figure 13.29).

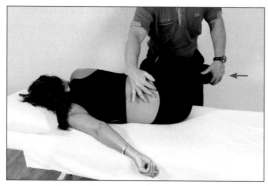

Figure 13.29. Using the patient's legs as a lever, the therapist flexes the patient's trunk until a barrier is felt at the lumbosacral junction.

The patient is asked to push their legs toward the ceiling against the therapist's resistance for 10 seconds (which activates the right piriformis muscle), as shown in Figure 13.30.

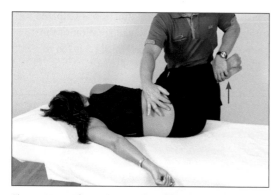

Figure 13.30. The patient pushes their legs toward the ceiling, as this motion activates the right piriformis muscle.

On the relaxation phase, the therapist takes the patient's legs toward the floor until they feel movement posterior to the right sacral base (Figure 13.31).

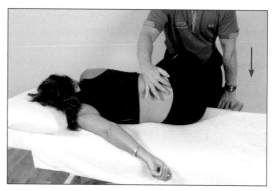

Figure 13.31. The therapist palpates the right sacral base and feels for posterior motion as the patient's legs are directed toward the floor.

Note: The Sims technique works well, as it challenges the sacral position to correct itself by using the motion of the lumbar spine as well as the motion from the lower limbs to facilitate the correction. For example, with a L-on-L type of dysfunction, we know that the right sacral base has migrated forward into a fixed position of nutation, so the restriction is due to the right sacral base being unable to counter-nutate. The first process in the technique is flexion of the lumbar spine, which encourages an extension of the sacrum. Second, left rotation is introduced to the lumbar spine, which encourages right rotation of the sacrum (a movement it cannot perform). The third phase is the combination of the motion and MET of the legs; this introduces the right piriformis muscle, to assist in restoring the sacral position.

Diagnosis: R-on-R Anterior (Forward) Sacral Torsion

Treatment: MET
Position: Sims

In this dysfunction the sacrum has rotated right (side bent left) on the right oblique axis, and the left sacral base has anteriorly nutated (Figure 13.32).

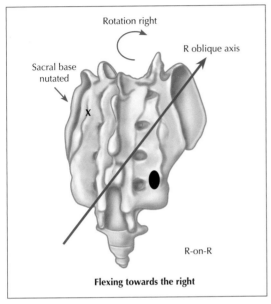

Figure 13.32. Right-on-right (R-on-R) sacral motion/ torsion. X = Anterior or deep. ◗ = Posterior or shallow.

The patient adopts a prone position on the couch, while the therapist stands on the left side of the couch and flexes the patient's knees to 90 degrees. The therapist turns the patient onto their right hip into the Sims position (left arm forward, right arm back), as shown in Figure 13.33.

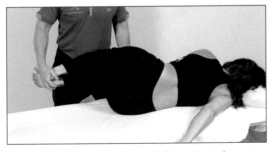

Figure 13.33. The therapist bends the patient's knees to 90 degrees and places the patient in the Sims position.

With the patient's knees placed on the therapist's right thigh, the lumbosacral junction is palpated using the right hand, while a right rotation of the patient's trunk is introduced until L5 is felt to rotate to the right (Figure 13.34).

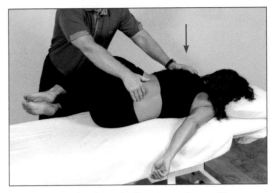

Figure 13.34. The therapist fine-tunes the position and introduces a rotation of L5 to the right.

From this position, the therapist palpates the lumbosacral junction and the left sacral base with their left hand, then, using the patient's legs as a lever, introduces a flexion motion to the trunk until a barrier is felt (Figure 13.35).

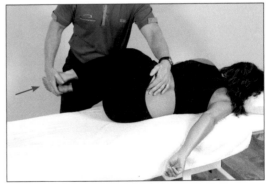

Figure 13.35. Using the patient's legs as a lever, the therapist flexes the patient's trunk until a barrier is felt at the lumbosacral junction.

The patient is asked to push their legs toward the ceiling against the therapist's resistance for 10 seconds (which activates the left piriformis muscle), see Figure 13.36.

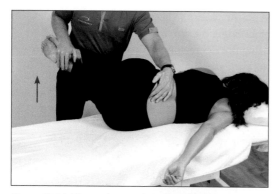

Figure 13.36. The patient pushes their legs toward the ceiling, as this activates the left piriformis muscle.

On the relaxation phase, the therapist takes the patient's legs toward the floor until they feel movement posterior to the left sacral base (Figure 13.37).

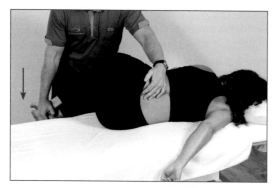

Figure 13.37. The therapist palpates the left sacral base and feels for posterior motion as the patient's legs are directed toward the floor.

Note: The R-on-R sacral torsion is the same concept as the L-on-L sacral torsion. The Sims technique again works well, as it challenges the sacral position to correct itself by using the motion of the lumbar spine as well as the motion from the lower limbs to facilitate the correction. For example, with a R-on-R type of dysfunction, we know that this time the left sacral base is fixed forward in a position of nutation, so the restriction is due to the sacral base being unable to counter-nutate on the

left side. The first process in the technique is to induce flexion of the lumbar spine, which encourages an extension of the sacrum. Second, right rotation is introduced to the lumbar spine, which encourages left rotation of the sacrum (remember, this is a movement it cannot perform). The third phase is the combined effect of the motion and the MET of the lower legs; this introduces the left piriformis muscle, to assist in restoring the sacral position.

Diagnosis: L-on-R Posterior (Backward) Sacral Torsion

Treatment: MET
Position: Side lying

In this dysfunction the sacrum has rotated left (side bent right) on the right oblique axis, and the left sacral base has posteriorly counter-nutated (Figure 13.38).

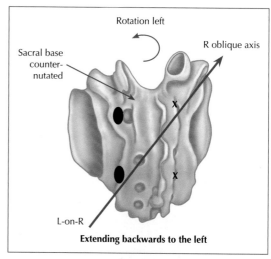

Figure 13.38. Left-on-right (L-on-R) sacral torsion. X = Anterior or deep. ● = Posterior or shallow.

The patient adopts a side-lying position on their right side, with their knees initially flexed to approximately 45 degrees, while the therapist stands facing the patient. Palpating the lumbosacral junction with their right hand, the therapist gently pulls the patient's right arm caudally (which introduces some extension to the lumbar spine, as well as right side bending and left rotation to the trunk) until L5 is felt to begin to rotate to the left (Figure 13.39).

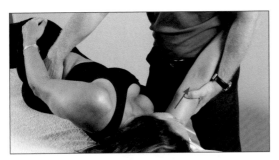

Figure 13.39. The therapist palpates L5 and feels for left rotation, as the patient is guided into position.

From this position, the therapist places the patient's right lower leg into extension with their right hand, while monitoring the left sacral base with their left hand until an anterior motion of the sacral base is felt (Figure 13.40).

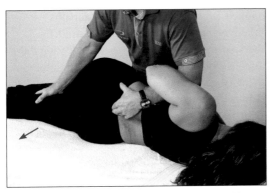

Figure 13.40. The therapist palpates the left sacral base for anterior (forward) motion, as the patient's lower leg is guided into the extension position.

Next, the therapist maintains contact with L5 as they lower the patient's left (top) leg off the side

of the couch, so that it faces toward the floor, and applies pressure to the distal femur (Figure 13.41).

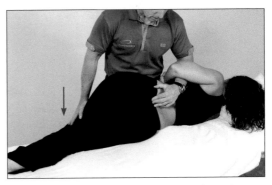

Figure 13.41. The therapist palpates L5 as the patient's left leg is guided toward the floor.

The patient is then asked to push their left (top) leg toward the ceiling for 10 seconds against the therapist's resistance (Figure 13.42). On the relaxation phase, two components are introduced: (1) the therapist continues to encourage the left leg toward the treatment couch/floor for a few seconds, and (2) while still monitoring the left sacral base, the therapist places the patient's right (bottom) leg into further extension (see Figure 13.43, overleaf). This resistance/relaxation procedure is repeated three to five times until an anterior motion of the left sacral base is felt.

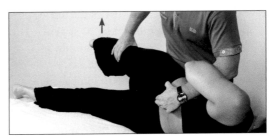

Figure 13.42. The patient lifts their left leg against the therapist's resistance, as this now introduces the left piriformis muscle, which will assist in restoring the sacral position. On the relaxation phase the therapist applies a downward pressure.

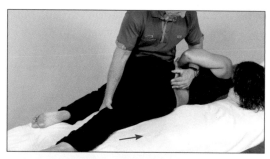

Figure 13.43. While monitoring the left sacral base, the therapist encourages further extension of the patient's right (bottom) leg.

Note: This technique works well, as it challenges the sacral position to correct itself by using the motion of the lumbar spine as well as the motion from the lower limbs to facilitate the correction. For example, with a L-on-R type of dysfunction, we know that the left sacral base has moved posteriorly, i.e. it has counter-nutated, so the restriction is due to the left sacral base being unable to nutate forward. The first process in the technique is to promote extension of the lumbar spine, which encourages a forward nutation motion of the sacrum. Second, left rotation is introduced to the lumbar spine, which encourages right rotation of the sacrum (the movement it cannot perform). In the third phase, we add the motion and the specific MET of the top leg being lowered (after the initial 10-second contraction), because this now introduces the left piriformis muscle as well as increasing side bending of the lumbar spine to the right, which will assist in restoring the sacral position. In addition, the extension of the lower leg promotes further nutation of the left sacral base and subsequent correction of the dysfunction.

Diagnosis: R-on-L Posterior (Backward) Sacral Torsion

Treatment: MET
Position: Side lying

In this dysfunction the sacrum has rotated right (side bent left) on the left oblique axis, and the right sacral base has posteriorly counter-nutated (Figure 13.44).

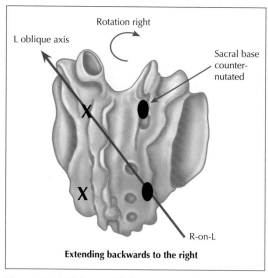

Figure 13.44. Right-on-left (R-on-L) sacral torsion. X = Anterior or deep. ● = Posterior or shallow.

The patient adopts a side-lying position on their left side, with their knees initially flexed to approximately 45 degrees, while the therapist stands facing the patient. Palpating the lumbosacral junction with their left hand, the therapist gently pulls the patient's left arm caudally (which introduces some extension to the lumbar spine, as well as left side bending and right rotation to the trunk) until L5 is felt to begin to rotate to the right (Figure 13.45).

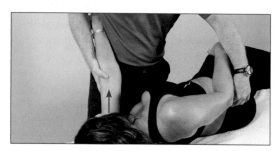

Figure 13.45. The therapist palpates L5 and feels for right rotation, as the patient is guided into position.

From this position, the therapist places the patient's left lower leg into extension with their left hand, while monitoring the right sacral base with their right hand until an anterior motion of the sacral base is felt (Figure 13.46).

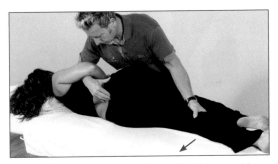

Figure 13.46. The therapist palpates the right sacral base for anterior (forward) motion, as the patient's lower leg is guided into the extension position.

Next, the therapist maintains contact with L5 as they lower the patient's right (top) leg off the side of the couch, so that it faces toward the floor, and applies pressure to the distal femur (Figure 13.47).

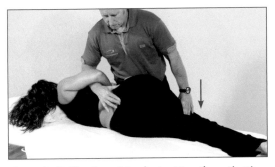

Figure 13.47. The therapist palpates L5 as the patient's right leg is guided toward the floor.

The patient is then asked to push their right (top) leg toward the ceiling for 10 seconds against the therapist's resistance (Figure 13.48). On the relaxation phase, two components are introduced: (1) the therapist continues to encourage the right leg toward the treatment couch/floor for a few seconds, and (2) while still monitoring the right sacral base, the therapist places the patient's left

(bottom) leg into further extension (Figure 13.49). This resistance/relaxation procedure is repeated three to five times until an anterior motion of the right sacral base is felt.

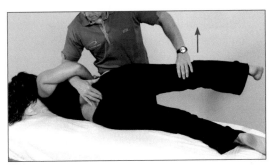

Figure 13.48. The patient lifts their right leg against the therapist's resistance, as this now introduces the piriformis muscle, which will assist in restoring the sacral position. On the relaxation phase the therapist applies a downward pressure.

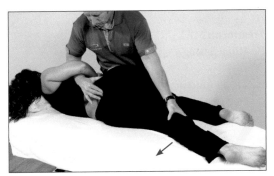

Figure 13.49. While monitoring the right sacral base, the therapist encourages further extension of the patient's left (bottom) leg.

Note: This technique works well, as it challenges the sacral position to correct itself by using the motion of the lumbar spine as well as the motion from the lower limbs to facilitate the correction. For example, with a R-on-L type of dysfunction, we know that the right sacral base has moved posteriorly, i.e. it has counter-nutated, so the restriction is due to the right sacral base being unable to nutate forward. The first process in the technique is to promote extension of the lumbar spine, which encourages a forward nutation motion of the sacrum. Second, right rotation is introduced to the lumbar spine, which encourages left rotation of the sacrum (the movement it cannot perform). In the third phase, we add the motion and the specific MET of the top leg being lowered (after the initial 10-second contraction), because this now introduces the right piriformis muscle as well as increasing side bending of the lumbar spine to the left, which will assist in restoring the sacral position. In addition, the extension of the lower leg promotes further nutation to the right sacral base and subsequent correction of the dysfunction.

Diagnosis: Bilateral Anterior Sacrum (Nutated)

Treatment: MET
Position: Sitting

In this dysfunction the sacrum has bilaterally nutated (Figure 13.50).

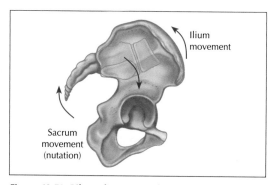

Figure 13.50. Bilateral nutation of the sacrum.

The patient adopts a sitting position on the couch, with their feet apart, while the therapist stands facing the patient's back. Palpating the sacral apex with their right hand, the therapist introduces flexion to the patient's trunk with their left hand until the sacrum is felt to begin to move (Figure 13.51).

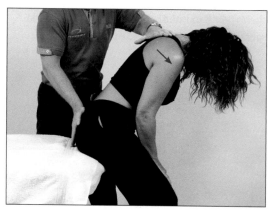

Figure 13.51. The therapist palpates the sacral apex and monitors motion, as the trunk of the patient is being flexed.

From this position, the patient is asked to lift their upper back toward the ceiling against a resistance applied by the therapist (Figure 13.52).

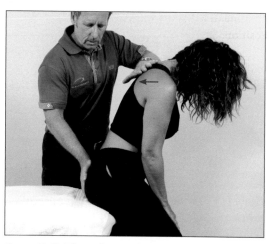

Figure 13.52. The patient performs trunk extension against a resistance applied by the therapist.

After 10 seconds, and during the relaxation phase, the therapist introduces further trunk flexion, while at the same time encouraging posterior sacral motion (counter-nutation) with their right hand (Figure 13.53).

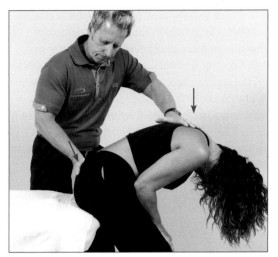

Figure 13.53. The therapist introduces further flexion and at the same time encourages the sacrum into counter-nutation.

Diagnosis: Bilateral Posterior Sacrum (Counter-Nutated)

Treatment: MET
Position: Sitting

In this dysfunction the sacrum has bilaterally counter-nutated (Figure 13.54).

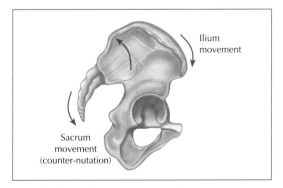

Figure 13.54. Bilateral counter-nutation of the sacrum.

The patient adopts a sitting position on the couch, with their feet apart, while the therapist stands facing the patient's back. Palpating the sacral base with their right hand, the therapist introduces

extension to the patient's trunk with their left hand until the sacrum is felt to begin to move (Figure 13.55).

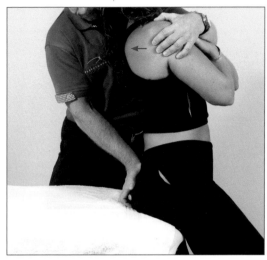

Figure 13.55. The therapist palpates the sacral base and monitors motion, as the trunk of the patient is being extended.

From this position, the patient is asked to flex their trunk against a resistance applied by the therapist (Figure 13.56).

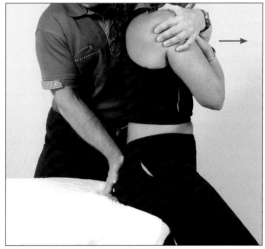

Figure 13.56. The patient performs trunk flexion against a resistance applied by the therapist.

After 10 seconds, and during the relaxation phase, the therapist introduces further trunk extension and at the same time encourages anterior sacral motion (nutation) with their right hand (Figure 13.57).

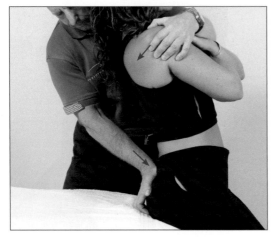

Figure 13.57. The therapist introduces further extension and at the same time encourages the sacrum into nutation.

Part 4: Treatment Protocol for Lumbar Spine Dysfunctions

I mentioned earlier that I consider lumbar spine dysfunctions to be caused by a compensatory mechanism associated with underlying malalignments of the pelvis. In my opinion, dysfunctions of the lumbar spine are a secondary type of dysfunction resulting from a primary dysfunction within the pelvic girdle complex; hence the main reason why I leave treating the lumbar spine till the end. There are exceptions to the rules, of course, where the lumbar spine is the primary cause rather than the compensatory secondary cause. Either way, the realignment techniques I will demonstrate shortly will be of value, as they will assist you in correcting the presentations that will commonly be found within the lumbar spine.

I would like to keep things simple to start with, even though this subject matter is by no means simple to understand. For the first example,

when I say that the facet joint is fixed in a closed position, this relates to the specific position of the inferior facet joint being closed in extension, side bending, and rotation (normally to one side) on the superior facet of the vertebra immediately below. Think back to the discussion of spinal mechanics in Chapter 6. I referred to this situation as an *ERS,* which is a Type II dysfunction (non-neutral mechanics), because the rotation and side bending are coupled to the same side but in an extended position, either to the left (ERS(L)) or to the right (ERS(R)).

The opposite motion, and the second example, therefore has to be where the facet joint is now fixed in an open position; in this case the motion is related to the specific position of the inferior facet joint being open in flexion, side bending, and rotation (normally to one side) on the superior facet of the vertebra immediately below. This type of spinal dysfunction is referred to as an *FRS,* which is also a Type II dysfunction (non-neutral mechanics), because the rotation and side bending are coupled to the same side but this time in a flexed position, either to the left (FRS(L)) or to the right (FRS(R)).

> **Note:** Regarding the position of a facet joint which is fixed in an open position, remember from earlier chapters that the joint will be open on the opposite side. For example, an FRS(L), i.e. flexion, rotation, and side bending left, indicates that the facet joint is fixed open on the right side.

The following lumbar spine dysfunctions are discussed:

- L5 ERS(L)
- L4 ERS(R)
- L5 FRS(L)

Diagnosis: L5 ERS(L)

Treatment: MET
Position: Side lying

This specific spinal dysfunction relates to the inferior facet joint of L5 being fixed in a position of extension, rotation, and side bending to the left side on the superior facet of S1. This basically means that the *left* facet joint of L5/S1 is fixed in a closed position (Figure 13.58). The subsequent motion restriction will affect movements on the side opposite the fixation, namely flexion, right rotation, and right side bending.

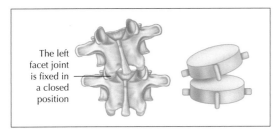

Figure 13.58. L5 ERS(L) on S1.

The patient adopts a side-lying position facing the therapist, with the posterior TP of the dysfunctional L5 toward the couch (i.e. dysfunction side down—in this case, left side down). While palpating the interspinous space of L4/5 with their left hand, the therapist cradles the patient's left arm and introduces flexion and right rotation of the patient's trunk down to the relevant lumbar level (Figure 13.59).

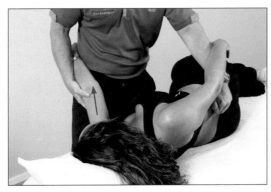

Figure 13.59. The therapist palpates the interspinous space of L4/L5 and introduces flexion and right rotation of the lumbar spine down to that level, to prevent over-locking of L5/S1.

The therapist cradles both of the patient's legs and introduces the hips into flexion, while at the same time palpating with the left hand the L5/S1 interspinous space for motion (Figure 13.60).

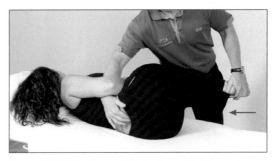

Figure 13.60. The therapist introduces hip flexion to both legs as they palpate the L5/S1 interspinous space for motion.

From this position, the patient is asked to push both their feet toward the floor (side bending left), as indicated by the arrow in Figure 13.61, for 10 seconds at a contraction of between 10 and 20% of maximum.

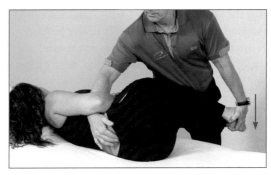

Figure 13.61. The patient pushes both feet toward the floor for 10 seconds.

After the contraction, and during the relaxation phase, the therapist encourages the patient's legs toward the ceiling, as this motion introduces right side bending of the lumbar spine (see Figure 13.62). This movement subsequently has the ability to open the left L5/S1 facet joint, which is fixed in a closed position.

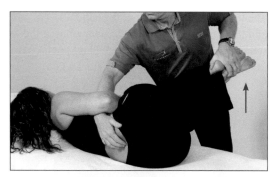

Figure 13.62. After the contraction the therapist introduces right side bending by using the motion from the legs toward the ceiling to open the left facet joint.

Diagnosis: L4 ERS(R)

Treatment: MET, Thrust technique (HVT)
Position: Side lying

This specific spinal dysfunction relates to the inferior facet joint of L4 being fixed in a position of extension, right rotation, and right side bending on the superior facet of L5. This basically means that the *right* facet joint of L4/5 is fixed in a closed position (Figure 13.63). The subsequent motion restriction will affect movements on the side opposite the fixation, namely flexion, left rotation, and left side bending.

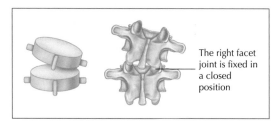

The right facet joint is fixed in a closed position

Figure 13.63. L4 ERS(R) on L5.

The patient adopts a side-lying position facing the therapist, with the posterior TP of L4 toward the ceiling (i.e. dysfunction side up—in this case, right side up). While palpating the interspinous space of L3/4 with their right hand, the therapist introduces

flexion and right rotation of the lumbar spine down to L4 with their left hand (Figure 13.64).

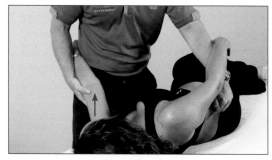

Figure 13.64. The therapist palpates the interspinous space of L3/4 and introduces flexion and right rotation of the lumbar spine down to L4.

Next, the patient's right hand is placed onto their right hip to stabilize the position. The therapist palpates the L4/5 interspinous space with their right hand and feels for specific motion as the patient's bottom leg is taken into flexion.

The patient's top leg is flexed and the foot is placed in the crease of the left knee. The therapist places their right hand through the natural gap formed by the patient's hand on their hip and palpates the L4/5 interspinous space. The patient's trunk is guided gently toward the floor by the therapist's left hand, which is placed on the patient's left knee and controls the motion (Figure 13.65).

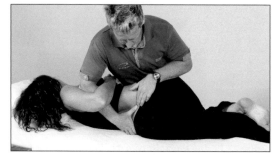

Figure 13.65. The therapist palpates L4 and fine-tunes the position by using the patient's top leg.

Once the position has been finely tuned, the patient is asked to abduct their right hip against a resistance applied by the therapist for 10 seconds (Figure 13.66).

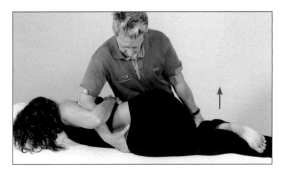

Figure 13.66. The patient abducts their right hip for 10 seconds.

After the contraction, and during the relaxation phase, the therapist encourages motion of the top leg toward the floor, as this type of movement introduces right side bending of the lumbar spine (Figure 13.67). This movement subsequently has the ability to open the right L4/5 facet joint, which is fixed in a closed position.

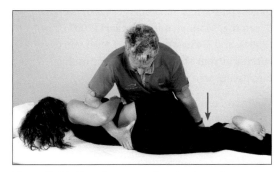

Figure 13.67. After the contraction the therapist introduces right side bending of the lumbar spine to open the right L4/5 facet joint.

If one is suitably qualified, then from the finely tuned position (as above) the therapist can apply a thrust technique (HVT) in the direction through the long lever of the femur toward the floor (Figure 13.68). This quick motion will cause a right side bending motion to L4/5, and a cavitation might be elicited from the joint.

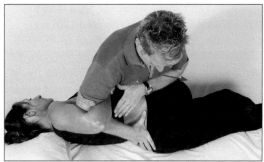

Figure 13.68. From the finely tuned position, the therapist applies a quick thrust technique to encourage right side bending of the lumbar spine, which may elicit a cavitation from the right L4/5 facet joint.

Diagnosis: L5 FRS(L)

Treatment: Soft tissue technique
Position: Prone

This specific spinal dysfunction relates to the inferior facet joint of L5 having become fixed in a position of flexion, left rotation, and left side bending on the superior facet of S1. This basically means that the *right* facet joint of L5/S1 is fixed in an open position (Figure 13.69). The subsequent motion restriction will affect movements on the side opposite the fixation, namely extension, right rotation, and right side bending.

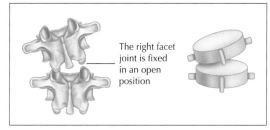

The right facet joint is fixed in an open position

Figure 13.69. L5 FRS(L) on S1.

With the patient lying prone, the therapist confirms by the position of the thumbs that the left TP of L5 is shallow and the right TP is deep, thus indicating a left rotation. When the patient backward bends, the left TP appearing shallower and the right TP becoming deeper confirms the presence of an FRS(L), where the right facet joint is fixed in an open position (Figure 13.70).

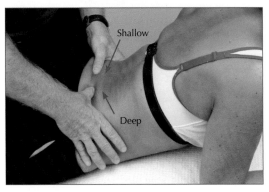

Figure 13.70. With the patient in a backward-bent position, the left thumb palpates shallow and the right thumb palpates deep, indicating an FRS(L).

The correction of this spinal dysfunction is very simple in some respects, as it can be treated from the backward-bent position. The therapist applies between 5 and 10lbs (2–4kg) of direct pressure directly onto the right L5 TP, either with a reinforced thumb (Figure 13.71), or with the elbow (Figure 13.72). The therapist then waits for the tissues to soften, before retesting the position to see if there has been any change.

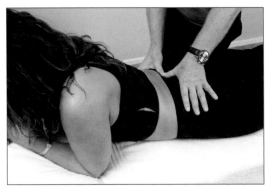

Figure 13.71. With the patient in a backward-bent position, the therapist applies pressure with a reinforced thumb directly onto the right L5 TP, to encourage a closure of the right facet joint.

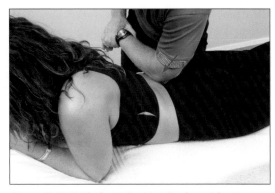

Figure 13.72. With the patient in a backward-bent position, the therapist applies pressure with their elbow directly onto the right L5 TP, to encourage a closure of the right facet joint.

In the case of an FRS(R), the opposite procedure would be performed.

If you have truly enjoyed reading this book and wish to continue on your journey toward understanding the pelvic girdle, along with all the complexities that naturally go with it, then I recommend in particular the following books to get you started: Schamberger (2002; 2013); Vleeming, Mooney, and Stoeckart (2007); Lee (2004); and DeStefano (2011). I wish you every success in your studies and practice in this fascinating area.

Tables for Dysfunction Testing

The following tables can be used in the therapist's own clinical setting (permission to reproduce is granted).

Hip Extension Firing Pattern

Table A1.1. Hip extension firing pattern—left side.

Left side	1st	2nd	3rd	4th
Gluteus maximus	○	○	○	○
Hamstrings	○	○	○	○
Contralateral erector spinae	○	○	○	○
Ipsilateral erector spinae	○	○	○	○

Table A1.2. Hip extension firing pattern—right side.

Right side	1st	2nd	3rd	4th
Gluteus maximus	○	○	○	○
Hamstrings	○	○	○	○
Contralateral erector spinae	○	○	○	○
Ipsilateral erector spinae	○	○	○	○

Initial Observation—Patient Standing

Table A1.3. Observation assessment—standing.

Observation	Left side	Right side
Pelvic crest (posterior)		
PSIS		
Greater trochanter		
Lumbar spine		
Gluteal folds		
Popliteal folds		
Foot/ankle position		
Pelvic crest (anterior)		
ASIS		
Pubic tubercle		

Evaluation of Pelvic Dysfunction

Table A1.4. Specific tests for the evaluation of pelvic dysfunction.

Test	Left side	Right side
Mens		
Standing forward flexion		
Backward bending		
Seated forward flexion		
Stork (Gillet)—upper pole		
Stork (Gillet)—lower pole		
Hip extension		
Side bending (trunk)		
Pelvic rotation		

Palpatory Assessment

Prone

Table A1.5. Palpation assessment—prone.

Palpation area	Left side	Right side
Gluteal fold		
Ischial tuberosity		
Sacrotuberous ligament		
ILA		
PSIS		
Sacral sulcus—neutral		
Sacral sulcus—extension (sphinx test)		
Sacral sulcus—flexion		
L5 spring test (neg. or pos.)		
L5 position		
Iliac crest		
Greater trochanter		

Supine

Table A1.6. Palpation assessment—supine.

Palpation area	Left side	Right side
ASIS		
Iliac crest		
Pubic tubercle		
Inguinal ligament		
Medial malleolus (leg length)		
Supine to long sitting test		
Long sitting to supine test		

Summary of Iliosacral Dysfunctions

Table A1.7. Iliosacral dysfunctions—left side.

Dysfunction	Left side	Standing flexion test	Medial malleolus	ASIS	PSIS	Sacral sulcus	Ischial tuberosity	Sacrotuberous ligament
Anterior rotation	Left	Left	Long left	Inferior	Superior	Shallow left	Superior	Lax left
Posterior rotation	Left	Left	Short left	Superior	Inferior	Deep left	Inferior	Taut left
Out-flare	Left	Left	No change	Lateral left	Medial left	Narrow left	No change	No change
In-flare	Left	Left	No change	Medial left	Lateral left	Wide left	No change	No change
Upslip	Left	Left	Short left	Superior left	Superior left	No change	Superior	Lax left
Downslip	Left	Left	Long left	Inferior left	Inferior left	No change	Inferior	Taut left

Table A1.8. Iliosacral dysfunctions—right side.

Dysfunction	Right side	Standing flexion test	Medial malleolus	ASIS	PSIS	Sacral sulcus	Ischial tuberosity	Sacrotuberous ligament
Anterior rotation	Right	Right	Long right	Inferior	Superior	Shallow right	Superior	Lax right
Posterior rotation	Right	Right	Short right	Superior	Inferior	Deep right	Inferior	Taut right
Out-flare	Right	Right	No change	Lateral right	Medial right	Narrow right	No change	No change
In-flare	Right	Right	No change	Medial right	Lateral right	Wide right	No change	No change
Upslip	Right	Right	Short right	Superior right	Superior right	No change	Superior	Lax right
Downslip	Right	Right	Long right	Inferior right	Inferior right	No change	Inferior	Taut right

Summary of Sacral Dysfunctions

Table A1.9. Anterior/forward sacral torsions (normal physiological motion).

	L-on-L sacral torsion (forward/nutation)	R-on-R sacral torsion (forward/nutation)
Deep sacral sulcus	Right	Left
Shallow sacral sulcus	Left	Right
ILA posterior	Left	Right
L5 rotation	Right—ERS(R)	Left—ERS(L)
Seated flexion test	Right	Left
Lumbar spring	Negative	Negative
Sphinx (extension) test	Sulci level	Sulci level
Lumbar flexion test	Right sacral sulcus deep	Left sacral sulcus deep
Lumbar lordosis	Increased	Increased
Medial malleolus (leg length)	Short left	Short right

Table A1.10. Posterior/backward sacral torsion (non-physiological motion).

	L-on-R sacral torsion (backward/counter-nutation)	R-on-L sacral torsion (backward/counter-nutation)
Deep sacral sulcus	Right	Left
Shallow sacral sulcus	Left	Right
ILA posterior	Left	Right
L5 rotation	Right—FRS(R)	Left—FRS(L)
Seated flexion test	Left	Right
Lumbar spring	Positive	Positive
Sphinx (extension) test	Left sacral sulcus shallow (right sacral sulcus deeper)	Right sacral sulcus shallow (left sacral sulcus deeper)
Lumbar flexion test	Sulci level	Sulci level
Lumbar lordosis	Decreased	Decreased
Medial malleolus (leg length)	Short left	Short right

Table A1.11. Bilaterally nutated and counter-nutated sacrum.

	Bilaterally nutated sacrum (forward)	Bilaterally counter-nutated sacrum (backward)
Standing flexion test	Negative	Negative
Seated flexion test	Positive bilateral	Positive bilateral
Stork (Gillet) test	Positive on both sides	Positive on both sides
Sacral base	Left and right anterior	Left and right posterior
ILA	Left and right posterior	Left and right anterior
Lumbar spring test	Negative	Positive
Lumbar lordosis	Increased	Decreased
Medial malleolus (leg length)	Equal	Equal

Summary of Symphysis Pubis Dysfunctions

Table A1.12. Symphysis pubis dysfunctions — left side.

	Superior pubis	Inferior pubis
Standing forward flexion test	Left	Left
Pubic tubercle	Superior	Inferior
Inguinal ligament	Tender on palpation	Tender on palpation

Table A1.13. Symphysis pubis dysfunctions — right side.

	Superior pubis	Inferior pubis
Standing forward flexion test	Right	Right
Pubic tubercle	Superior	Inferior
Inguinal ligament	Tender on palpation	Tender on palpation

Outer Core Stabilization Exercise Sheet

The following exercises can be used in the physical therapist's own clinical setting. For each exercise there is a blank space in which a patient's repetitions and sets can be recorded.

Exercise	SETS	REPS
1. Push		
2. Pull		
3. Squat—Bend to Extend		

Exercise	SETS	REPS
Progression 1: With Weight		
Progression 2: With Weight and Without a Core Ball		
4. Bend to Extend with Rotation		

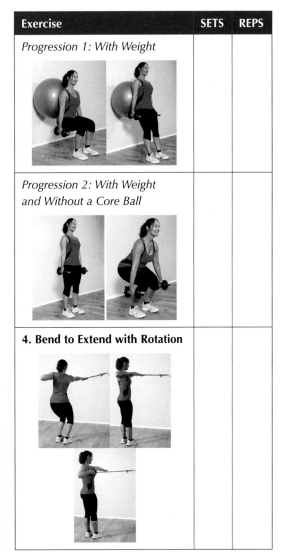

Exercise	SETS	REPS
5. Single-Leg Stance		
Lateral Sling and Posterior Oblique Sling		
6. Rotation		
Posterior Rotation		
Exercise Variations Combined Push–Pull		

Exercise	SETS	REPS
Combined Push–Pull on One Leg		
Push with Lunge		
Pull with Lunge		
Push on Unstable Base		
Pull on Unstable Base		

Exercise	SETS	REPS
Bend to Extend with Rotation on Unstable Base		
Bend High to Low (Wood Chop)		
Bend Low to High (Reverse Wood Chop)		
Bend Low to High (Single Arm)		

Exercise	SETS	REPS
Oblique Sling—Anterior Rotation on Unstable Base		
Oblique Sling—Anterior Rotation on One Leg		
Anterior Rotation While Kneeling		
Posterior Rotation While Kneeling		

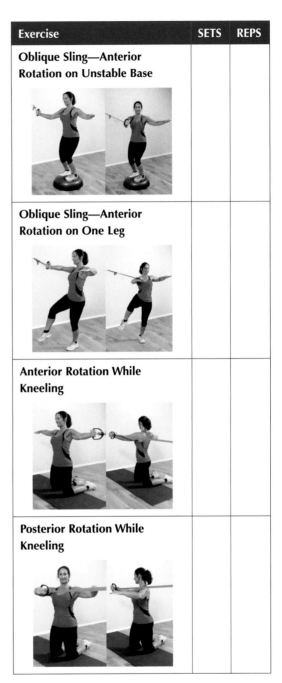

Bibliography

Abernethy, B., Hanrahan, S., Kippers, V., et al. 2004. *The Biophysical Foundations of Human Movement*, Champaign, IL: Human Kinetics.

Armour, P.C., and Scott, J.H. 1981. "Equalization of limb length," *J Bone Joint Surg* 63B, 587–592.

Basmajian, J.V., and De Luca, C.J. 1979. *Muscles Alive: Their Functions Revealed by Electromyography*, 5th edn, Baltimore, MD: Williams & Wilkins, 386–387.

Bullock-Saxton, J.E., Janda, V., and Bullock, M.I. 1994. "The influence of ankle sprain injury on muscle activation during hip extension," *Int J Sports Med* 15, 330–334.

Chaudhry, H., Schleip, R., Ji, Z., et al. 2008. "Three-dimensional mathematical model for deformation of human fasciae in manual therapy," *JAOA* 108(8), 379–390.

Chek, P. 1999. "The outer unit," C.H.E.K. Institute, Vista, CA.

Chek, P. 2009. *An Integrated Approach to Stretching*, Vista, CA: C.H.E.K. Institute.

Cohen, S.P. 2005. "Sacroiliac joint pain: A comprehensive review of anatomy, diagnosis, and treatment," *Anesth & Analg* 101, 1440–1453.

DonTigny, R.L. 2007. "A detailed and critical biomechanical analysis of the sacroiliac joints and relevant kinesiology: The implications for lumbopelvic function and dysfunction," in Vleeming et al. (2007), 265–278.

DeStefano, L. 2011. *Greenman's Principles of Manual Medicine*, 4th edn, Baltimore, MD: Lippincott Williams & Wilkins.

Egund, N., Olsson, T.H., Schmid, H., et al. 1978. "Movement of the sacroiliac joint demonstrated with roentgen stereophotogrammetry," *Acta Radiol Diagn* 19, 833–846.

Farfan, H.F. 1973. *Mechanical Disorders of the Back*, Philadelphia, PA: Lea and Febiger.

Fortin, J.D., and Falco, F.J.E. 1997. "The Fortin finger test: An indicator of sacroiliac pain," *Am J Orthop* 24(7), 477–480.

Fortin, J.D., Dwyer, A.P., West, S., and Pier, J. 1994. "Sacroiliac joint: Pain referral maps upon applying a new injection/arthrography technique. Part 1: Asymptomatic volunteers. Part 2: Clinical evaluation," *Spine* 19(13), 1475–1489.

Friel, K., McLean, N., Myers, C., and Caceras, M. 2006. "Ipsilateral hip abductor weakness after inversion ankle sprain," *J Athl Train* 41, 74–78.

Fryette, H.H. 1918. "Physiological movements of the spine," *J Am Osteopath Assoc* 18, 1–2.

Fryette, H. 1954. *Principles of Osteopathic Technic*, Indianapolis, IN: The Academy of Applied Osteopathy, 16.

Gibbons, J. 2011. *Muscle Energy Techniques: A Practical Guide for Physical Therapists*, Chichester, UK: Lotus Publishing.

Gibbons, J. 2014. *The Vital Glutes: Connecting the Gait Cycle to Pain and Dysfunction*, Chichester, UK/Berkeley, CA: Lotus Publishing/North Atlantic Books.

Gracovetsky, S. 1988. *The Spinal Engine*. New York: Springer-Verlag.

Grieve, G.P. 1983. "Treating backache—a topical comment," *Physiother* 69, 316.

Hall, T.E. 1955, in Wernham, S.G.J. (ed.), *Year Book 1956*. Maidstone, UK: The Osteopathic Institute of Applied Technique.

Hammer, W.I. 1999. *Functional Soft Tissue Examination and Treatment by Manual Methods: New Perspectives*, 2nd edn, Gaithersburg, MD: Aspen.

Inman, V.T., Ralston, H.J., and Todd, F. 1981. *Human Walking*, Baltimore, MD: Williams & Wilkins.

Janda, V. 1983. *Muscle Function Testing*, London: Butterworth-Heinemann.

Janda, V. 1987. "Muscles and motor control in low back pain: Assessment and management," in Twomey, L.T. (ed.), *Physical Therapy of the Low Back*, New York: Churchill Livingstone, 253–278.

Janda, V. 1992. "Treatment of chronic low back pain," *J Man Med* 6, 166–168.

Janda, V. 1996. "Evaluation of muscular imbalance," in Liebenson, C. (ed.), *Rehabilitation of the Spine: A Practitioner's Manual*, 1st edn, Baltimore, MD: Lippincott, Williams & Wilkins, 97–112.

Jordan, T.R. 2006. "Conceptual and treatment models in osteopathy. II. Sacroiliac mechanics revisited," *AAOJ*, 11–17.

Kampen, W.U., and Tillmann, B. 1998. "Age-related changes in the articular cartilage of human sacroiliac joint," *Anat Embryol* 198, 505–513.

Kapandji, I.A. 1974. *The Physiology of the Joints: III. The Trunk and Vertebral Column*, 2nd edn, Edinburgh: Churchill Livingstone/Elsevier.

Kendall, F.P., McCreary, E.K., Provance, P.G., et al. 2010. *Muscle Testing and Function with Posture and Pain*, 5th edn, Baltimore, MD: Lippincott, Williams & Wilkins.

Kiapour, A., Abdelgawad, A.A., Goel, V.K., et al. 2012. "Relationship between limb length discrepancy and load distribution across the sacroiliac joint—a finite element study," *J Orthop Res* 30, 1577–1580.

Klein, K.K. 1973. "Progression of pelvic tilt in adolescent boys from elementary through high school," *Arch Phys Med Rehabil* 54, 57–59.

Koushik physio 2011. "Fryette's Laws," *Truth about Fitness* (blog), November 19. http://koushikphysio. blogspot.co.uk/2011/11/fryettes-laws.html.

Lee, D.G. 2004. *The Pelvic Girdle: An Approach to the Examination and Treatment of the Lumbopelvic-Hip Region*, Edinburgh: Churchill Livingstone.

Lee, D.G., and Vleeming, A. 2007. "An integrated therapeutic approach to the treatment of the pelvic girdle," in Vleeming et al. (2007), pp. 621–638.

Lovett, R.W. 1903. "A contribution to the study of the mechanics of the spine," *Am J Anat* 2, 457–462.

Lovett, R.W. 1905. "The mechanism of the normal spine and its relation to scoliosis," *Boston Med Surg J* 13, 349–358.

Maitland, J. 2001. *Spinal Manipulation Made Simple: A Manual of Soft Tissue Techniques*, Berkeley, CA: North Atlantic Books.

Martin, C. 2002. *Functional Movement Development*, 2nd edn, London: W.B. Saunders Co.

Mens, J.M., Vleeming, A., Snijders, C.J., et al. 1997. "Active straight leg raising test: A clinical approach to the load transfer of the pelvic girdle," in Vleeming et al. (1997), 425–431.

Mens, J.M., Vleeming, A., Snijders, C.J., et al. 1999. "The active straight leg raising test and mobility of the pelvic joints," *Eur Spine J* 8, 468–473.

Mens, J.M., Vleeming, A, Snijders, C.J., et al. 2001. "Reliability and validity of the active straight leg raise test in posterior pelvic pain since pregnancy," *Spine (Phila Pa 1976)* 26, 1167–1171.

Mens, J.M., Vleeming, A, Snijders, C.J, et al. 2002. "Validity of the active straight leg raise test for measuring disease severity in patients with posterior pelvic pain after pregnancy," *Spine (Phila Pa 1976)* 27, 196–200.

Mitchell, B., McCrory, P., Brukner, P., et al. 2003. "Hip joint pathology: Clinical presentation and correlation between magnetic resonance arthrography, ultrasound, and arthroscopic findings in 25 consecutive cases," *Clin J Sport Med* 13, 152–156.

Mitchell, F.L., Sr. 1948. "The balanced pelvis and its relationship to reflexes," *Academy of Applied Osteopathy Year Book 1948*, 146–151.

Nelson, C.R. 1948, Calvin R. Nelson Papers, MS15, University Archives, UTHSC Libraries, The University of Texas Health Science Center at San Antonio.

Ober, F.R. 1935a. "Back strain and sciatica," *JAMA* 104(18), 1580–1581.

Ober, F.R. 1935b. "The role of the iliotibial band and fascia lata as a factor in the causation of low-back disabilities and sciatica," *J Bone Joint Surg Am* 18(1), 105–110.

Osar, E. 2012. *Corrective Exercise Solutions to Common Hip and Shoulder Dysfunction*, Chichester, UK: Lotus Publishing.

Richardson, C., Jull, G., Hodges, P., and Hides, J. 1999. *Therapeutic Exercise for Spinal Segmental Stabilization in Low Back Pain: Scientific Basis and Clinical Approach*, Edinburgh: Churchill Livingstone.

Richardson, C.A., Snijders, C.J., Hides, J.A., et al. 2002. "The relationship between the transversely oriented abdominal muscles, sacroiliac joint mechanics and low back pain," *Spine* 27(4), 399–405.

Sahrman, S. 2002. *Diagnosis and Treatment of Movement Impairment Syndromes*, 1st edn, St. Louis, MO: Mosby Inc.

Schamberger, W. 2002. *The Malalignment Syndrome: Implications for Medicine and Sport*, Edinburgh: Churchill Livingstone, 127–128.

Schamberger, W. 2013. *The Malalignment Syndrome: Diagnosing and Treating a Common Cause of Acute and Chronic Pelvic, Leg and Back Pain*, Edinburgh: Churchill Livingstone, Elsevier.

Schmitz, R.J., Riemann, B.L., and Thompson, T. 2002. "Gluteus medius activity during isometric closed-chain hip rotation," *J Sport Rehabil* 11, 179–188.

Shadmehr, A., Jafarian, Z., Talebian, S., et al. 2012. "Changes in recruitment of pelvic stabilizer muscles in people with and without sacroiliac joint pain during the active straight-leg-raise test," *J Back Musculoskelet Rehabil* 25, 27–32.

Sherrington, C.S. 1907. "On reciprocal innervation of antagonistic muscles," *Proc R Soc Lond [Biol]* 79B, 337.

Slipman, C.W., Jackson, H.B., Lipetz, J.S., et al. 2000. "Sacroiliac joint pain referral zones," *Arch Phys Med Rehab* 81(3), 334–338.

Snijders, C.J., Vleeming, A., and Stoeckart, R. 1993a. "Transfer of lumbosacral load to the iliac bones and legs. Part 1. Biomechanics of self-bracing of the sacroiliac joints and its significance for treatment and exercise," *Clin Biomech* 8(6), 285–295.

Snijders, C.J., Vleeming, A., and Stoeckart, R. 1993b. "Transfer of lumbosacral load to the iliac bones and legs. Part 2. The loading of the sacroiliac joints when lifting in a stooped posture," *Clin Biomech* 8(6), 295–301.

Stoddard, A. 1962. *Manual of Osteopathic Technique*, 2nd edn, London: Hutchinson.

Sturesson, B., Selvik, G., and Uden, A. 1989. "Movements of the sacroiliac joints: A roentgen stereophotogrammetric analysis," *Spine* 14(2), 162–165.

Sturesson, B., Uden, A., and Vleeming, A. 2000a. "A radiostereometric analysis of the movements of the sacroiliac joint in the reciprocal straddle position," *Spine* 25(2), 214–217.

Sturesson, B., Uden, A., and Vleeming, A. 2000b. "A radiostereometric analysis of the movements of the sacroiliac during the standing hip flexion test," *Spine* 25(3), 364–368.

Thomas, C.L. 1997. *Taber's Cyclopaedic Medical Dictionary*, 18th edn, Philadelphia, PA: F.A. Davis.

Tenney, H.R., Boyle, K.L., and DeBord, A. 2013. "Influence of hamstring and abdominal muscle activation on a positive Ober's test in people with lumbopelvic pain," *Physiother Can* 65(1), 4–11.

Umphred, D.A., Byl, N., Lazaro, R.T., and Roller, M. 2001. "Interventions for neurological disabilities," in Umphred, D.A. (ed.), *Neurological Rehabilitation*, 4th edn, St. Louis, MO: Mosby Inc., 56–134.

Vleeming, A., Stoeckart, R., and Snijders, D.J. 1989a. "The sacrotuberous ligament: A conceptual approach to its dynamic role in stabilizing the sacroiliac joint," *Clin Biomech* 4, 200–203.

Vleeming, A., Van Wingerden, J.P., Snijders, C.J., et al. 1989b. "Load application to the sacrotuberous ligament: Influences on sacroiliac joint mechanics," *Clin Biomech* 4, 204–209.

Vleeming, A., Stoeckart, R., Volkers, A.C.W., et al. 1990a. "Relation between form and function in the sacroiliac joint. Part 1: Clinical anatomical aspects," *Spine* 15(2), 130–132.

Vleeming, A., Volkers, A.C.W., Snijders, C.J., and Stoeckart, R. 1990b. "Relation between form and function in the sacroiliac joint. Part 2: Biomechanical aspects," *Spine* 15(2), 133–136.

Vleeming, A., Snijders, C.J., Stoeckart, R., et al. 1995. "A new light on low back pain," *Proc 2nd Interdisc World Congr Low Back Pain*, San Diego, CA.

Vleeming, A., Mooney, V., Dorman, T., et al. (eds) 1997. *Movement, Stability and Lower Back Pain: The Essential Role of the Pelvis*, Edinburgh: Churchill Livingstone, 425–431.

Vleeming, A., and Stoeckart, R. 2007. "The role of the pelvic girdle in coupling the spine and the legs: A clinical-anatomical perspective on pelvic stability," in Vleeming et al. (2007), 113–137.

Vleeming, A., Mooney, V., and Stoeckart, R. (eds) 2007. *Movement, Stability and Lumbopelvic Pain: Integration of Research and Therapy*, Edinburgh: Churchill Livingstone.

Vrahas, M., Hern, T.C., Diangelo, D., et al. 1995. "Ligamentous contributions to pelvic stability," *Orthoped* 18, 271–274.

Willard, F.H., Vleeming, A., Schuenke, M.D., et al. 2012. "The thoracolumbar fascia: Anatomy, function and clinical considerations," *J Anat* 221(6), 507–36.

Williams, P.L., and Warwick, R. (eds) 1980. *Gray's Anatomy*, 36th British edn, Edinburgh: Churchill Livingstone, 473–477.

Index